HAND KU-780-313

Veterinary Anesthesia

FOURTH EDITION

William W. Muir III, DVM, PhD, Dipl ACVA, Dipl ACVECC

Professor

John A. E. Hubbell, DVM, MS, Dipl ACVA

Professor

Richard M. Bednarski, DVM, MS Dipl ACVA

Associate Professor

Roman T. Skarda, Dr. Med Vet, PhD, Dipl ACVA

Professor (deceased)

All of the Department of Veterinary Clinical Sciences
The Ohio State University College of
Veterinary Medicine
Columbus, Ohio

Illustrations by Tim Vojt

with 138 illustrations

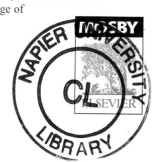

Can
636.089796 MUI

11830 Westline Industrial Drive
St. Louis, Missouri 63146

HANDBOOK OF VETERINARY ANESTHESIA

ISBN-13: 978-0-323-04678-7
ISBN-10: 0-323-04678-9

Notice

Knowledge and best practice in this field are constantly changing. As new research and experience broaden our knowledge, changes in practice, treatment and drug therapy may become necessary or appropriate. Readers are advised to check the most current information provided (i) on procedures featured or (ii) by the manufacturer of each product to be administered, to verify the recommended dose or formula, the method and duration of administration, and contraindications. It is the responsibility of the practitioner, relying on their own experience and knowledge of the patient, to make diagnoses, to determine dosages and the best treatment for each individual patient, and to take all appropriate safety precautions. To the fullest extent of the law, neither the Publisher nor the Authors assume any liability for any injury and/or damage to persons or property arising out or related to any use of the material contained in this book.

The Publisher

ISBN-13: 978-0-323-04678-7
ISBN-10: 0-323-04678-9

Acquisitions Editor: Anthony Winkel
Developmental Editor: Maureen Slaten
Publishing Services Manager: Deborah L. Vogel
Senior Project Manager: Steve Ramay
Designer: Teresa McBryan

HANDBOOK OF
Veterinary Anesthesia

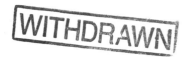

WITHDRAWN

The authors wish to dedicate the fourth edition
of *Handbook of Veterinary Anesthesia*
to
Dr. Roman Skarda
(1944-2005).

Romi was an inspiration
to everyone who had the opportunity
to meet and work with him.
He will be missed.

Preface
to the Fourth Edition

This edition of the *Handbook of Veterinary Anesthesia* was thoroughly reviewed and largely revised in order to provide the most up-to-date information available to veterinary anesthetists. As with previous editions, we have tried to provide a readily available and clinically useful source of information for producing anesthesia and reducing pain and suffering in animals. Emphasis has remained on those animals that are commonly treated by veterinarians, although specific chapters have been dedicated to anesthesia of exotic species and birds. We have reorganized several chapters and retained and updated chapters that encompass the full spectrum of the anesthetic experience, including anesthetic monitoring equipment, ventilators and ventilation, pain management, local anesthetic techniques and cardiopulmonary resuscitation.

This fourth edition is the result of the advice and labors of the Section of Anesthesiology of the Department of Veterinary Clinical Sciences at The Ohio State University. Recent critiques were provided by Dr. Phillip Lerche, Dr. Tokiko Kushiro, Dr. Elise Craft, Ashley Wiese, Gladys Karpa, Amanda English, Carl O'Brien, Theresa Weber, Heather Williams, Nicole Staten, Christina Duffey, and Barbara Lang. The authors would also like to thank Drs. John Dodam and Sheilah Robertson for their critical comments to the third edition.

William W. Muir III
John A. E. Hubbell

Contents

CHAPTER ONE

Introduction to Anesthesia

"There are no safe anesthetic agents; there are no safe anesthetic procedures; there are only safe anesthetists."

ROBERT SMITH

OVERVIEW

The art and practice of anesthesia are based on a general understanding of (1) the terms that describe the effects of anesthetic drugs in animals, (2) the pharmacology of anesthetic drugs and their antagonists, (3) the correct methods of anesthetic drug administration, and (4) appropriate therapy for anesthetic-related complications or emergencies. This chapter outlines commonly used terms, the general uses for anesthetics and the routes of administration of anesthetic drugs or drug combinations used to produce chemical restraint and anesthesia in animals.

GENERAL CONSIDERATIONS

I. Anesthesia and/or chemical restraint is a reversible process; the purpose of anesthesia is to produce a convenient, safe, effective, yet inexpensive means of chemical restraint so that medical or surgical procedures may be expedited with minimal stress, pain, discomfort, and toxic side effects to the patient or to the anesthetist

II. Criteria for selection of drugs and techniques
   A. Species, breed, age, and relative size of the patient
   B. Physical status and specific disease processes of the patient
   C. Concurrent medications
   D. Demeanor of the patient and the severity of pain
   E. Personal knowledge and experience (Fig. 1-1)

1

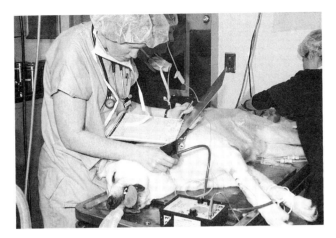

Fig. 1-1
Nothing is more necessary and important than an attentive, dedicated, and vigilant anesthetist.

    F. Availability and training of assistants
    G. Familiarity with available equipment
    H. Length and type of operation or procedure to be performed
  III. Patient responses can vary because doses and techniques are for the "average, normal, healthy" animal; thus it is essential that the practitioner knows how to modify anesthetic techniques
  IV. Definitions
    A. Medical terms used in the practice of anesthesia:
        Acupuncture: The stimulation of specific trigger points based on traditional Chinese medicine
        Agonist: A drug that produces an effect by interacting with a specific receptor site (e.g., opioid agonist morphine)
        Akinesia: Loss of motor response (movement) usually caused by blockade of motor nerves
        Allodynia: Pain evoked by a stimulus that does not normally cause pain
        Analgesia: Loss of sensitivity to pain

Anesthesia: Total loss of sensation in a body part or in the whole body, generally induced by a drug or drugs that depress the activity of nervous tissue either locally (peripherally) or generally (centrally); the act of producing anesthesia is usually divided into phases that include the preanesthetic and postanesthetic periods (see box)

THE FIVE PHASES OF ANESTHESIA

I. Preanesthetic or Preinduction period
II. Induction to anesthesia
III. Maintenance
IV. Recovery
V. Postanesthetic period

Local anesthesia: Analgesia limited to a local area

Regional anesthesia: Analgesia limited to a local area produced by blocking sensory nerves

General anesthesia: Loss of consciousness in addition to loss of sensation; ideally includes hypnosis, hyporeflexia, analgesia, and muscle relaxation; can be produced with a single drug or by a combination of drugs

Surgical anesthesia: Loss of consciousness and sensation accompanied by sufficient muscle relaxation and analgesia to allow surgery to be performed without pain or movement by the patient

Balanced anesthesia: Surgical anesthesia produced by a combination of two or more drugs or anesthetic techniques, each contributing its own pharmacologic effects; includes tranquilizers, opioids, nitrous oxide, muscle relaxants, and inhalants

Dissociative anesthesia: A central nervous system (CNS) state characterized by catalepsy, analgesia, and altered consciousness; produced by drugs like ketamine, tiletamine

MAC (minimum alveolar concentration): A term used to imply the minimum alveolar concentration of inhalant anesthetic required to prevent movement in response to a noxious stimulus in 50% of anesthetized patients or infrequently, in human outpatient anesthetic practice, as monitored anesthetic care

Antagonist: A drug that occupies a receptor site but produces minimal or no effect (e.g., opioid antagonist naloxone)

Catalepsy: State in which there is malleable rigidity of the limbs. The patient is generally unresponsive to aural, visual, or minor painful stimuli

Central sensitization: An increase in the excitability and responsiveness of nerves in the CNS particularly the spinal cord

Distress: The state produced when the biologic cost of stress negatively affects biologic functions critical to the animal's well-being. To cause pain or suffering or to make miserable

Euthanasia: Loss of consciousness and death without causing pain, distress, anxiety, or apprehension

Homeostasis: A state of equilibrium within the body

Hyperalgesia: An increased or exaggerated response to a stimulus that is normally painful (a heightened sense of pain) either at the site of injury (primary) or in surrounding undamaged tissue (secondary or extraterritorial). Stimulated nociceptors respond to noxious stimuli more vigorously and at a lower threshold

Hypnosis: Artificially induced sleep or a trance resembling sleep from which the patient can be aroused by a sufficient stimulus; patients cannot be aroused during general or surgical anesthesia

Multimodal therapy: The use of multiple drugs with different mechanisms of action to produce optimal analgesia

Narcosis: Drug-induced stupor or sedation with or without hypnosis

Neuroleptanalgesia: Hypnosis and analgesia produced by the combination of a neuroleptic drug (i.e., tranquilizers) and an analgesic drug

Pain: An aversive sensation and feeling associated with actual or potential tissue damage

Pathologic Pain: Pain produced by tissue damage. Usually includes peripheral sensitization, central sensitization, and hypersensitivity resulting in allodynia.

Peripheral sensitization: An increase in the activity, excitability, and responsiveness of peripheral nerve terminals

Physiologic pain: The normal response to a noxious stimulus that produces protective mechanisms causing the animal to minimize tissue damage (fight or flight) or to avoid contact with external stimuli during a reparative phase

Quality of life: The properties or characteristics that define an animal's life; usually assessed subjectively as a degree of excellence. An individual's ability to meet the needs of the environment to which it is accustomed and to do so in such a way as to not deviate from normal behavioral patterns that define the level of satisfaction of that individual

Sedation: CNS depression in which the patient is awake but calm; a term often used interchangeably with tranquilization; with sufficient stimuli the patient may be aroused

Stress: The biologic responses of an animal to cope with a disruption or threat to homeostasis. A stressor is a physical, chemical, or emotional factor (e.g., pain, trauma, fear) to which an individual fails to make a satisfactory adaptation and that causes physiologic tensions that may contribute to the development of disease

Tranquilization, ataraxia, neurolepsis: State of tranquility and calmness in which the patient is relaxed, reluctant to move, awake, and unconcerned with its surroundings and potentially indifferent to minor pain; sufficient stimulation will arouse the patient

V. Clinical jargon

Bag: "The animal was bagged." The rebreathing bag on the anesthetic machine was squeezed to inflate the animal's lungs during anesthesia

Block: "The leg was blocked." Local anesthesia was produced at a specific site, locally or regionally

Bolus: "A bolus of thiobarbiturate was administered." A specified quantity of drug was rapidly administered intravenously

Breathed: "The animal was breathed six times a minute." The lungs were either manually or mechanically inflated

Bucking: "The animal is bucking the ventilator." The patient is resisting being artificially (manually or mechanically) breathed. The patient breathes out during the inspiratory cycle or in during the expiratory cycle

Crashed: "The animal crashed." The patient demonstrated marked CNS and cardiopulmonary depression after the administration of an anesthetic drug. "The animal was crash induced." Anesthesia was rapidly induced with an intravenous (IV) or inhalant anesthetic drug

Deep: "The animal is in a deep stage of anesthesia." The anesthetic drugs produced significant CNS depression. The greater the degree of CNS depression, the deeper the anesthesia. This term is used in direct contrast to the term *light,* which implies minimal CNS depression. Animals that are "light" demonstrate active corneal and palpebral reflexes, may develop nystagmus, and occasionally lift their heads or move a limb

Down: The animal was "knocked down" or "put down." The animal was given a drug or combination of drugs that produced recumbency. The term *put down* is also used to denote euthanasia

Dropped: "The animal was dropped." The animal received drugs that produce recumbency

Extubated: "The animal was extubated." The endotracheal tube was removed from the airway. The term is the opposite of "intubated"

Hit or stick a vein: "I hit the vein on the first attempt." A successful venipuncture was performed

Induced: "The animal was induced." The animal was given a drug or drugs that produced anesthesia

Intubated: "The animal was intubated." An endotracheal tube was placed through the nose or mouth into the trachea

IV drip: "The patient received an IV drip." A fluid with or without added drug(s) was administered intravenously

Mask induced: "The animal was mask induced." A face mask was used to facilitate delivery of inhalant anesthetics for induction of anesthesia

Pre or post: "A preanesthetic was administered." Anything administered or done before anesthesia is considered to be in the preanesthetic period. Occurrences after the discontinuation of anesthetic drugs are considered postanesthetic

Preemptive: "The patient received preemptive analgesia." The deliberate administration of therapy (in this case, analgesia) before the event requiring therapy. A form of prophylaxis

Pushed: "The thiobarbiturate was pushed." An IV drug or fluids were administered either rapidly or in amounts greater than usually given

Ran a strip: "I ran a strip on that animal." An electro-cardiogram was obtained

Reversed: "The animal was reversed." A drug's effects were antagonized by administering a specific antagonist. For example, the opioid antagonist naloxone can be administered to reverse the effects of morphine

Spiked: "The animal spiked a fever" or "The fluids were spiked with potassium." Depending on the clinical situation, *spiked* may mean a sudden rapid increase or that some substance (i.e., K^+) or drug was added to a solution

Stabilized: "The animal is stable" or "The animal has been stabilized." Cardiopulmonary variables or the "depth" of anesthesia have been returned to or are within acceptable limits

TIVA: "The animal was administered TIVA" or total intra-venous anesthesia (inhalants were not used)

Topped-off: "The animal was topped off with a thiobar-biturate." An additional drug was administered to produce the desired effect. The term implies that the original calculated dose was insufficient to produce the desired effect

Tubed: "The animal was tubed." An endotracheal tube was placed in the trachea through either the mouth or nasal cavities (see also intubated)

Weaning: "The animal was weaned off the ventilator." The gradual discontinuation of artificial ventilation so that spontaneous ventilation would resume

USE OF ANESTHETICS

I. Restraint
   A. Diagnostic imaging (ultrasonography, radiography, magnetic resonance imaging)
   B. Cleaning, grooming, dental prophylaxis
   C. Biopsy, radiation therapy, bandaging, splinting, cast application

    D. Capture of exotic and wild animals

    E. Transportation

    F. Manipulation

       1. Catheterization

       2. Wound care

       3. Obstetrics

    G. Assist or control breathing

II. Anesthesia (see Definitions: Anesthesia)

    A. To facilitate or permit medical and/or surgical procedures

III. Control of convulsions

IV. Euthanasia

TYPES OF ANESTHESIA (ACCORDING TO ROUTE OF ADMINISTRATION)

Acupuncture	Infiltration*	Intravenous*
Buccal	Inhalation*	Oral†
Controlled hypothermia	Intramuscular*	Rectal
Electroanesthesia	Intraosseous	Subcutaneous
Epidural*	Intraperitoneal	Topical*
Spinal (subarachnoid)	Intratesticular	Transdermal*
Field block	Intrathoracic	

*Route commonly used in veterinary medicine

EFFECT OF ROUTE AND METHOD OF ADMINISTRATION OF ANESTHETIC DRUG

    I. Given intravenously (Figs. 1-2 and 1-3): onset of action is immediate; peak effect is rapidly obtained; duration of action is short; and effects are generally more intense than with other routes

    II. Given intramuscularly or subcutaneously: onset of action may take 10 to 15 minutes; peak effect may not be obtained for many minutes to hours and depends on the blood supply to the tissues at the site of injection, drug absorption, and the rate of metabolism of the drug; duration of action is more prolonged than by the IV route

    III. Given transdermally: peak systemic effects may not occur for many hours

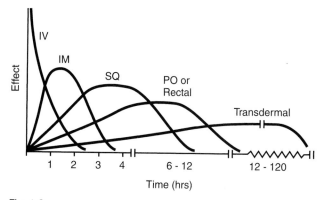

Fig. 1-2

Magnitude of effect and duration of action associated with various routes of administration.

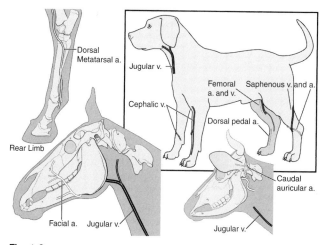

Fig. 1-3

The jugular, cephalic, and saphenous veins can be used to administer intravenous drugs and fluids. The dorsal metatarsal and facial arteries (horses), auricular (cattle, sheep, goats, camelids), and dorsal pedal arteries (dogs) are used to monitor arterial blood pressure and to obtain arterial blood samples when necessary.

IV. Rapidity of injection: rapid injections generally cause more intense effects, especially true when cardiac output is low

V. Concentrations of solutions

    A. Drugs should be administered on a unit/kg basis (e.g., mg/kg); most drugs list concentration as unit/ml (e.g., mg/ml) or percent (%); percent solutions can be converted to unit/ml (a 1% solution contains 10 mg/ml); therefore a 0.5% solution contains 5 mg/ml, and a 3% solution contains 30 mg/ml

    B. Increasing the drug concentration increases the intensity and duration of the immediate drug effect

    C. Increasing concentrations may increase vascular irritation and cause pain on injection

VI. Amount: the amount (dose) of drug administered should be reduced in sick patients

VII. The onset of action of inhalation drugs requires absorption of gas from alveoli into the blood, then diffusion of anesthetic into the CNS

VIII. Duration of drug action is primarily determined by the pharmacokinetic characteristics of the drug (metabolism and elimination), but it is also influenced by the potency of the drug, hemodynamics, and the influence of the drug on cellular function

CHAPTER TWO

Patient Evaluation and Preparation

"For every mistake that is made for not knowing, a hundred are made for not looking."

ANONYMOUS

OVERVIEW

Anesthesia is more than just the delivery of anesthetic drugs to produce anesthesia. Safe anesthesia includes selecting the appropriate drugs for each procedure, assessing the physical status of the patient, noting the administration of concurrent medications, and having a working familiarity with anesthetic drugs, their potential toxicities, and their treatment. This chapter outlines preoperative evaluation as it relates to subsequent anesthetic management.

GENERAL CONSIDERATIONS

I. The preanesthetic evaluation (history, physical condition (see Fig. 2-1) and physical examination) dictates the choice and dose of anesthetics to be used

II. The history and physical examination are the basis of patient evaluation; the need for further workup is indicated by abnormalities found during physical examination *or* historical information that suggests altered bodily functions

III. Laboratory tests are no substitute for a thorough physical examination

IV. A patent airway must be maintained in every patient

V. A patent intravenous route must be maintained for all high-risk patients

11

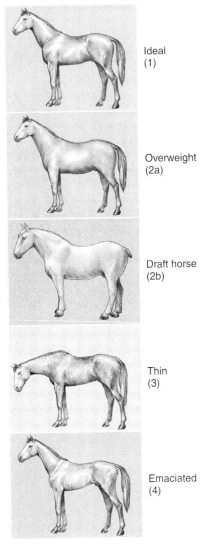

Ideal
(1)

Overweight
(2a)

Draft horse
(2b)

Thin
(3)

Emaciated
(4)

Fig. 2-1
Categoric scoring systems (e.g., horse) can be used to provide information regarding patient status and are helpful in determining total drug dose adjustments.

VI. Anticipate likely untoward events based on patient history and physical status

VII. An emergency cart with appropriate antidotes and antagonists should be maintained (see Chapter 28)

PATIENT EVALUATION

I. Patient identification
- A. Case number or identification
- B. Signalment
  1. Species
  2. Breed
  3. Age
  4. Sex
- C. Body weight

II. Client complaint and anamnesis (history)
- A. Duration and severity of illness
- B. Concurrent symptoms or disease
  1. Diarrhea
  2. Vomiting
  3. Hemorrhage
  4. Seizures
  5. Heart failure (cough, exercise intolerance)
  6. Renal failure
- C. Level of activity (exercise tolerance)
- D. Recent feeding
- E. Previous and current administration of drugs (see Chapter 13)
  1. Organophosphates
  2. Insecticides
  3. Antibiotics
     a. Sulfonamides
     b. Gentamicin, amikacin, polymyxin B
  4. Digitalis glycosides
  5. β-blockers
  6. Calcium channel blockers
  7. Diuretics
  8. Catecholamine-depleting drugs
- F. Anesthetic history and reactions

CURRENT PHYSICAL EXAMINATION

I. General body condition
   A. Obesity
   B. Cachexia
   C. Pregnancy
   D. Hydration
   E. Temperature
   F. Calm or excited
   G. Nervous or apprehensive (stress)
II. Cardiovascular
   A. Heart rate and rhythm (see Table 2-1)
   B. Arterial blood pressure and pulse pressure quality and regularity
   C. Capillary refill time (<1.5 seconds)
   D. Auscultation (cardiac murmurs)
III. Pulmonary
   A. Respiratory rate, depth, and effort
      1. Usually 15 to 25 breath/min for small animals, 8 to 20 for large animals
      2. Tidal volume approximately 14 ml/kg
   B. Mucous membrane color
      1. Pallor (anemia or vasoconstriction)
      2. Cyanosis (>5 g/dl of unoxygenated hemoglobin)
   C. Auscultation (breath sounds)
   D. Upper airway obstruction
   E. Percussion

TABLE 2-1
NORMAL HEART RATE AND MEAN ARTERIAL BLOOD PRESSURE RANGES

ANIMAL	HEART RATE (BEATS/MIN)	MEAN ARTERIAL BLOOD PRESSURE
Dog	70-100	70-100
Cat	100-200	80-120
Cow	60-80	90-140
Horse	30-45	70-90
Foal	50-80	60-80
Sheep, goat	60-90	80-110
Pig	60-90	80-110

IV. Hepatic
    A. Jaundice
    B. Failure of blood to clot
    C. Coma, seizures
V. Renal
    A. Vomiting
    B. Oliguria/anuria
    C. Polyuria/polydipsia
VI. Gastrointestinal
    A. Diarrhea
    B. Vomiting
    C. Distention
    D. Auscultation of intestinal sounds
    E. Rectal palpation when appropriate
VII. Nervous system and special senses
    A. Aggression/depression
    B. Seizures
    C. Fainting
    D. Coma
VIII. Metabolic and endocrine
    A. Temperature (hypothermia, hyperthermia)
    B. Hair loss
    C. Hyperthyroidism/hypothyroidism
    D. Hyperadrenocorticism/hypoadrenocorticism
    E. Diabetes
IX. Integument
    A. Hydration
    B. Neoplasia (pulmonary metastasis)
    C. Subcutaneous emphysema (fractured ribs)
    D. Parasites (fleas, mites); anemia
    E. Hair loss
    F. Burns (fluid and electrolyte loss)
    G. Trauma
X. Musculoskeletal
    A. Muscle mass (% fat)
    B. Weakness
    C. Electrolyte imbalance (hypokalemia, hyperkalemia; hypocalcemia)
    D. Ambulatory or nonambulatory
    E. Fractures

PRESURGICAL LABORATORY WORKUP

I. Minimum laboratory evaluation (see Table 2-2)
  A. Plasma protein (oncotic pressure)
  B. Packed cell volume or hemoglobin
II. Other laboratory tests (see Tables 2-2 through 2-5)
  A. Complete blood count
  B. Blood gases and pH
  C. Hemostasis
  D. Albumin
III. Blood chemistry profile (Table 2-3)
  A. Electrolytes (Na+, K+, Cl-, Ca2+)
  B. Blood urea nitrogen
  C. Creatinine
  D. Aspartate aminotransferase (AST), alanine aminotransferase (ALT)
  E. Bile acids
IV. Urinalysis (normal findings given in parentheses)
  A. Specific gravity (1.010 to 1.030)
  B. Physiochemical evaluation
    1. pH (7.0 to 7.5, meat diet; 7.0 to 8.0, vegetable diet)
    2. Protein (negative)
    3. Acetone (negative)
    4. Bilirubin (negative)
    5. Blood (negative)
  C. Microscopic evaluation of urine sediment
    1. Casts (negative or rare)
    2. Red blood cells (negative); occasional red blood cells are seen depending on how sample is collected
    3. White blood cells (negative)
    4. Epithelial cells (negative)
    5. Bacteria (negative)
    6. Crystals
      a. Oxalate (normal finding)
      b. Triple phosphates (normal finding)
      c. Urates (normal finding)
      d. Calcium carbonate (normally found in horses only)

TABLE 2-2
NORMAL HEMATOLOGIC VALUES

	DOG	CAT	HORSE	COW	SHEEP	PIG
Plasma protein (g/dl)	5.7-7.2	5.6-7.4	6.5-7.8	7.0-9.0	6.3-7.1	6-7.5
PCV (%)	36-54	25-46	27-44	23-35	30-50	30-48
Hb (g/dl)	11.9-18.4	8.0-14.9	9.7-15.6	8.3-12.3	10-16	10-15
RBC ($\times 10^{12}$/L)	4.9-8.2	5.3-10.2	5.1-10.0	5.0-7.5	—	—
Total leukocytes ($\times 10^9$/L)	4.1-15.2	4.0-14.5	4.7-10.6	3.0-13.5	4-12	6.5-20
Neutrophils—segmented ($\times 10^9$/L)	3.0-10.4	3.0-9.2	2.4-6.4	0.7-5.1	1-6	3-15
Neutrophils—band ($\times 10^9$/L)	0.0-0.1	0.0-0.1	0.0-0.1	0.0-0.1	0-0.1	0-0.5
Lymphocytes ($\times 10^9$/L)	1.0-4.6	0.9-3.9	1.0-4.9	1.1-8.2	2-8	2-12
Monocytes ($\times 10^9$/L)	0.0-1.2	0.0-0.5	0.0-0.5	0.0-0.6	0-0.6	0-0.6
Eosinophils ($\times 10^9$/L)	0.0-1.3	0.0-1.2	0.0-0.3	0.0-1.5	0-1	0-0.6
Basophils ($\times 10^9$/L)	0.0	0.0-0.2	0.0-0.1	0.0-0.1	0-0.1	0-0.1

PCV, Packed cell volume; *Hb,* hemoglobin; *RBC,* red blood cells.

TABLE 2-3
SERUM CHEMISTRY

	UNITS	DOG	CAT	HORSE	COW	SHEEP	PIG
Calcium	mg/dl	9.3-11.6	8.4-10.1	11.1-13.0	8.6-10.0	8.1-9.5	—
Phosphorus	mg/dl	3.2-8.1	3.2-6.5	1.2-4.8	3.8-7.7	3.5-6.7	5.3-9.6
Glucose	mg/dl	77-126	70-260	83-114	55-81	50-80	60-100
Creatinine	mg/dl	0.6-1.6	0.9-2.1	0.8-1.7	0.7-1.6	—	1.0-2.7
Bilirubin (T)	mg/dl	0.1-0.4	0.1-0.4	0.6-1.8	0.0-0.4	—	—
Bilirubin (D)	mg/dl	0.0-0.1	0.0-0.1	0.1-0.3	0.0-0.0	—	—
Albumin	g/dl	2.9-4.2	2.5-3.5	2.8-3.6	2.7-4.6	2.4-3	—
Total protein	g/dl	5.1-7.1	5.6-7.6	6.4-7.9	6.4-9.5	6.3-7.1	—
BUN	mg/dl	5-20	13-30	13-27	4-31	5-20	8-24
Cholesterol	mg/dl	80-315	65-200	51-97	40-380	—	—
ALP	IU/L	15-120	15-65	80-187	20-80	—	—
Amylase	IU/L	150-1040	400-1300	—	—	—	—
CK	IU/L	50-400	70-550	150-360	90-310	—	—
SDH	IU/L	—	—	4-13	14-80	—	—
AST	IU/L	12-40	10-35	170-370	50-120	—	—
ALT	IU/L	10-55	20-95	—	—	—	—
Na	mEq/L	143-153	146-156	132-142	133-143	140-145	139-152
K	mEq/L	4.2-5.4	3.2-5.5	2.4-4.6	3.9-5.2	4.9-5.7	4.4-6.7

Cl	mEq/L	109-120	114-126	97-105	98-108	100-105
Ca^{2+}	mg/dl	5.0-6.1	4.9-5.5	6.0-7.2	4.7-5.4	9.5-12.7
Mg	mg/dl	0.53-0.89	0.6-1.0	0.53-0.91	0.6-1.1	—
pH	Units	7.27-7.43	7.25-7.33	7.32-7.45	7.32-7.45	—
P_{O_2} (venous)	mm Hg	25-46	31-49	24-39	24-39	—
P_{CO_2} (venous)	mm Hg	28-49	35-49	34-53	34-53	—
HCO_3	mEq/L	18-25	18-22	23-31	23-31	—
Base excess	mEq/L	-6.0 to 0.5	-6.0 to -3.0	-1.0 to 5.0	-1.0 to 4.2	—
Cortisol 0 hr	µg/dl	1.0-11.0	1.0-13.5	2.0-14.0	0.7-1.4	—
Cortisol 1 hr post ACTH	µg/dl	5.0-26.0	6.8-12.1	2.7-6.0	2.7-6.0	—
T3 (RIA)	ng/dl	30-130	40-75	20-160	60-190	—
T4 (RIA)	µg/dl	0.5-2.1	1.0-3.0	0.6-2.7	1.7-5.8	—

ACTH, Adrenocorticotropic hormone; *ALP,* alkaline phosphatase; *ALT,* alanine aminotransferase; *AST,* aspartate aminotransferase; *BSP,* bromosulphalein; *BUN,* blood urea nitrogen; *CK,* creatine kinase; *LDH,* lactate dehydrogenase; *R,* retention; *SDH,* sorbitol dehydrogenase; *T1/2,* half-life; *T3,* triiodothyronine; *T4,* thyroxine.

TABLE 2-4
ARTERIAL BLOOD GASES

	NORMAL VALUES (21% O_2)	VALUES ROUTINELY OBSERVED DURING ANESTHESIA
pH	7.4 ± 0.2	7.30-7.45
$PaCO_2$ mm Hg	40 ± 3	30-60*
PaO_2 mm Hg	94 ± 3	250 to 500 (100% O_2) up to 250 (50% O_2)
Base excess	0 ± 1	–4 to –10

*The development of respiratory acidosis during anesthesia is common; its degree of severity depends in part on the drugs used, the depth of anesthesia, the duration of anesthesia, the species, and patient status.

FURTHER PRESURGICAL TESTS

  I. Electrocardiography
   A. Traumatized patients (myocardial trauma and arrhythmias)
   B. Irregular rhythm on physical examination
  II. Radiology
   A. Thorax
   B. Abdomen
  III. Ultrasonography

PATIENT PREPARATION

  I. Withhold food
   A. Withholding food is species-dependent (see species-specific recommendations)
   B. Do not withhold food for excessive periods in neonates, toy breeds, animals weighing under 5 kg, or birds
  II. Correct or compensate for
   A. Dehydration (hypovolemia)
   B. Anemia, blood loss, or hypoproteinemia
   C. Acid-base and electrolyte abnormalities
   D. Cardiac dysfunction
   E. Respiratory distress
   F. Renal dysfunction
   G. Hemostatic defects
   H. Temperature

TABLE 2-5
HEMOSTASIS AND TEMPERATURE

	UNITS	DOG	CAT	HORSE	COW	SHEEP	PIG
Platelets	$\times 10^9/L$	106-424	150-600	125-310	192-746	250-800	200-700
PT	sec.	6-7.5	8-11.5	8-10	12-18.5	13-17	—
APTT	sec.	9-21	8-17	30-39	24-57	35-50	—
Normal body temperature	Fahrenheit	101.5-102.5 (small breed) 99.5-101.5 (large breed)	100-102.5	99.5-101.5 (foal) 99-100.5 (adult)	101.5-103.5 (calf up to 1 yr) 100-102.5 (ox)	102-104	102-104 (piglet) 100-102 (adult)
	Celsius	38.5-39.2 (small breed) 37.5-38.6 (large breed)	37.8-39.2	37.5-38.6 (foal) 37.2-38 (adult)	38.6-39.8 (calf up to 1 yr) 37.8-39.2 (ox over 1 yr)	38.9-4	38.9-40 (piglet) 37.8-38.9 (adult)

PT, Prothrombin time; *APTT,* activated partial thromboplastin time.

III. Specific preparation for intended procedure
   A. Thoracic
   B. Abdominal
   C. Orthopedic
   D. Ophthalmologic
   E. Neurologic
IV. Other considerations
   A. Fluid and caloric needs during and after anesthesia
   B. Special medications (inotropes, antiarrhythmics)
   C. Duration of surgery
   D. Needs of the surgeon

PLAN FOR ANESTHETIC MANAGEMENT

I. Formulation of anesthetic care plan
   A. Surgical procedure (special requirements)
   B. Positioning
   C. Selection of drugs: emphasis on the control of pain during all phases of the preoperative, intraoperative, and postoperative periods
   D. Airway management
   E. Fluid management
   F. Body temperature management
   G. Monitoring
   H. Anticipation of possible untoward effects and response problems
II. Assembling of emergency drugs and equipment (see Chapter 28)

PATIENT PHYSICAL STATUS

1. Class I: normal patient with no organic disease
2. Class II: patient with mild systemic disease
3. Class III: patient with severe systemic disease that limits activity but is not incapacitating
4. Class IV: patient with incapacitating systemic disease that is a constant threat to life
5. Class V: moribund patient not expected to live 24 hours with or without intervention
   Designate emergency operation by an "E" after appropriate classification

CHAPTER THREE

Drugs Used for Preanesthetic Medication

"No patient should ever be anesthetized without the benefit of preanesthetic medications."

WILLIAM WALLACE MUIR, III, 1970

OVERVIEW

Preanesthetic medications are an essential part of safe anesthetic management. When used appropriately, they minimize stress, cardiopulmonary depression, and the deleterious effects associated with many intravenous (IV) and inhalation anesthetics. Preanesthetic medications almost always reduce the dose of injectable or inhalant anesthetics.

Routine preanesthetic medications are classified into four categories. *Anticholinergics* limit excessive salivary secretions and prevent bradycardia. *Phenothiazine* and *butyrophenone* (rarely used) *tranquilizers* produce calming and decrease the amount of general anesthetic required to produce anesthesia. α_2-*Agonists* produce sedation, analgesia, and muscle relaxation without producing general anesthesia. *Opioids* produce analgesia; some produce sedation. The combination of an α_2-agonist or tranquilizer with an opioid (neuroleptanalgesia) produces marked calming, muscle relaxation, and analgesia and light stages of anesthesia in young animals.

GENERAL CONSIDERATIONS

Purposes of Preanesthetic Drugs

I. Aid in animal restraint by modifying behavior (Fig. 3-1)
   A. Easier to work with

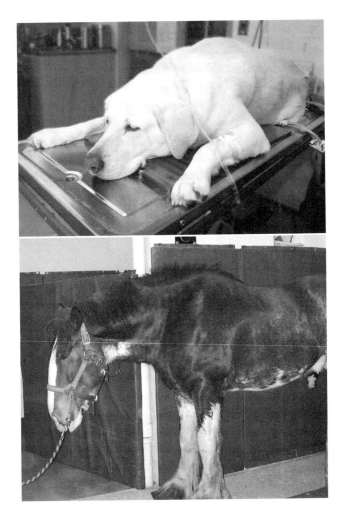

Fig. 3-1
Drugs that are used to produce tranquilization or sedation should make the patient easier to work with, reluctant to move, and uninterested in their surroundings while reducing the amount of drug(s) required to produce anesthesia.

    B. Not interested in its surroundings

    C. Reluctant to move

II. Reduce stress

III. Prevent or reduce pain before, during, and after surgery

IV. Produce muscle relaxation

V. Decrease the amount of potentially more dangerous drugs required to produce sedation, muscle relaxation, analgesia, or general anesthesia

VI. Facilitate safe and uncomplicated induction, maintenance, and recovery from anesthesia

VII. Minimize the adverse and potentially toxic effects of concurrently administered drugs

VIII. Minimize autonomic reflex activity, whether of sympathetic or parasympathetic origin

DRUG CATEGORIES

I. Anticholinergics (e.g., atropine, glycopyrrolate, scopolamine)

    A. Competitively antagonize acetylcholine at sites innervated by postganglionic, parasympathetic (cholinergic) nerve fibers and on smooth muscles that are influenced by acetylcholine but lack innervation; referred to as parasympatholytics, anticholinergics, or antispasmodics

    B. Primarily used to limit salivary secretions, prevent bradycardia, or deliberately increase heart rate. Increases in heart rate generally increase arterial blood pressure (BP) and cardiac output. Heart rate $\times$ stroke volume = cardiac output (HR $\times$ SV = CO)

    C. Atropine and scopolamine may produce drowsiness and potentiate the effects of central nervous system (CNS) depressant drugs; large doses may stimulate cerebral areas, leading to restlessness, disorientation, and delirium, an effect more common in ruminants and elephants

    D. Glycopyrrolate, a quaternary ammonium drug, does not cross the blood-brain or placental barriers

    E. Reduce glandular secretions of the respiratory tract, gastrointestinal tract, oral and nasal cavities

        1. The accumulation of excessive secretions in the oral cavity of small animals (e.g., cats) may predispose to upper airway obstruction or trigger laryngospasm

2. Increased secretory activity may occur after para-sympatholytic drug effects subside; this is known as a *postparasympatholytic rebound phenomenon*
3. Gastric pH is increased (i.e., less acidic); gastrointestinal motility and contractions of the bladder and ureters are reduced; intestinal motility can be decreased for several hours in horses, an effect that could cause colic. Ruminal atony (bloat) can occur in ruminants

F. Produce bronchodilation (increased physiologic dead space) and mydriasis

G. Inhibit bradycardia caused by reflex increases in vagal tone (e.g., laryngeal or ocular stimulation and vasovagal reflexes)
   1. Increasing heart rate generally increases arterial BP and cardiac output ($HR \times SV = CO$)
   2. Parasympatholytics may induce a sinus tachycardia or occasionally precipitate ventricular arrhythmias. Anticholinergic drugs may cause sinus bradycardia to progress through first- and second-degree atrioventricular block before the establishment of a faster sinus rhythm (Fig. 3-2)
   3. Atropine sulfate may stimulate vagal nuclei in the medulla and thus induce an initial sinus bradycardia; not seen with glycopyrrolate
   4. Vagal reflexes produced by traction on visceral organs or during ocular surgery can be but are not always successfully treated with parasympatholytic drugs
   5. General anesthetics, opioids, α_2-agonists, digitalis glycosides, hyperkalemia, acidosis, and injection of calcium salts augment vagal effects and may precipitate bradycardia
      a. Opioids and α_2-agonists increase parasympathetic tone and can produce sinus bradycardia and first- and second-degree atrioventricular block
      b. Isoflurane, sevoflurane, and barbiturates indirectly enhance parasympathetic effects by suppressing sympathetic tone
      c. Phenothiazine tranquilizers rarely produce a CNS-induced cholinergic effect and pronounced sinus bradycardia

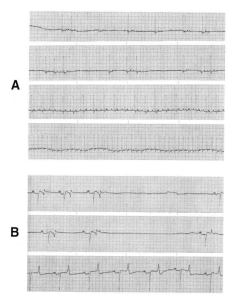

Fig. 3-2

Sinus bradycardia with or without second-degree atrioventricular block (P wave not followed by a QRS) can occur in normal quiet dogs (**A**) and horses (**B**) and is produced by many drugs (opioids, α_2-agonists). Care should be taken not to allow the ventricular rate to become too slow. Atropine or glycopyrrolate are generally effective therapy (second and third tracings in **A**; third tracing in **B**).

USEFUL FACTS ▪ Anticholinergics

- Competitively antagonize acetylcholine (vagal tone)
- Inhibit bradycardia by decreasing vagal tone; may cause sinus tachycardia
- Reduce glandular secretions; increase gastric pH; decrease gastrointestinal motility
- Bronchodilation and mydriasis
- Atropine and scopolamine may produce drowsiness
- Glycopyrrolate does not cross the blood-brain or placental barriers

H. Administer intramuscularly (IM) or subcutaneously (SQ) (IV for emergencies)
   1. Atropine sulfate (20 to 40 μg/kg) or glycopyrrolate (10 μg/kg) increases heart rate and dries secretions in small animals. The duration of action of atropine sulfate is 60 to 90 minutes; the duration of action of glycopyrrolate is 2 to 4 hours
   2. Parasympatholytics are of questionable value in horses and cattle because of side effects (colic) or lack of effect, respectively
      a. Horses: atropine, 20 to 40 μg/kg; glycopyrrolate, 3.3 to 6.6 μg/kg, IV in response to bradycardia
      b. Ruminants: not recommended for decreasing salivation; atropine temporarily decreases secretions, which can become more viscus; proper positioning of the head and neck is of the utmost importance to prevent pooling of saliva in the pharynx and subsequent aspiration
      c. Pigs: atropine (20 to 40 μg/kg); glycopyrrolate (3.3 μg/kg)

DOSES ▪ Anticholinergics			
AGENT	**ANIMAL**	**DOSE**	**DURATION**
Atropine sulfate	Small animals	20-40 μg/kg	60-90 min
	Horses	20-40 μg/kg	
	Pigs	20-40 μg/kg	
Glycopyrrolate	Small animals	5-10 μg/kg	2-4 hr
	Horses	3.3-6.6 μg/kg	
	Pigs	3.3 μg/kg	

I. Untoward reactions
   1. Atropine may slow heart rate temporarily after IV administration
   2. Cardiac arrhythmias: first- and second-degree atrioventricular block progressing to sinus tachycardia can be observed after IV administration of atropine or glycopyrrolate; ventricular arrhythmias may occur after IV atropine administration

3. Sinus tachycardia increases myocardial oxygen consumption and can precipitate heart failure or pulmonary edema in patients with preexisting cardiovascular disease (heart failure)
4. Atropine may cause depression in dogs and cats; it may cause restlessness, delirium, and disorientation in ruminants and elephants
5. Colic in horses caused by ileus

CAUTIONS ▪ Anticholinergics

- Atropine IV may cause an initial bradycardia
- Atropine or glycopyrrolate IV may cause first- and second-degree atrioventricular block before sinus tachycardia
- Atropine IV may cause ventricular arrhythmias
- Atropine may cause depression in dogs and cats, restlessness in ruminants
- Colic in horses, bloat in ruminants

II. Tranquilizers and sedatives (e.g., phenothiazines, butyrophenones, benzodiazepines, and α_2-agonists) (Table 3-1)
   A. Phenothiazines (e.g., acepromazine, promazine), butyrophenones (e.g., droperidol)
      1. Mode of action
         a. Calming and neurologic effects appear to be mediated by depression of the reticular activating system and antidopaminergic actions in the CNS
         b. Suppression of the sympathetic nervous system (depresses mobilization of catecholamines centrally and peripherally)
         c. Phenothiazine tranquilizers may lower seizure threshold in animals with epilepsy; they may inhibit chemically induced seizures (e.g., ketamine)
         d. Phenothiazines and butyrophenones produce antiemetic effects by inhibiting dopamine interaction in the chemoreceptor trigger zone in the medulla
      2. Physical properties
         a. Water soluble
         b. Can be mixed with other water-soluble drugs (e.g., acepromazine and hydromorphone)

TABLE 3-1

INTRAVENOUS DOSES OF COMMONLY USED TRANQUILIZERS AND SEDATIVES

AGENT	DOG	CAT	HORSE	COW	GOAT	PIG
Major tranquilizers						
Acepromazine*	0.05-0.2	0.05-0.2	0.01-0.04	0.01-0.02	0.02-0.04	0.1-0.2
Promazine	0.6-1	1-3	0.2-1	0.2-1	0.2-1	1-3
Minor tranquilizers						
Diazepam	0.2-0.4	0.2-0.4	0.02-0.1	0.02-0.09	0.02-0.09	0.5-2
Midazolam	0.2-0.4	0.2-0.4	0.02-0.1	—	—	0.1-0.5
Sedatives						
Detomidine	—	—	0.01-0.02	2-11 μg/kg	—	—
Medetomidine	0.005-0.02	0.01-0.04	5-20 μg/kg	—	—	—
Romifidine	0.04-0.09	0.09-0.18	0.08-0.12	—	—	—
Xylazine	0.4-1	0.4-1	0.4-1	0.02-0.1	0.02-0.07	1-2
Chloral hydrate	—	—	20-30	40-70	30-60	40-70

Doses are given as mg/kg unless otherwise stated.
*The maximum dose for acepromazine when used as a preanesthetic medication in dogs is 4 mg.

3. Produce mental calming, decrease motor activity, and increase threshold for responding to external stimuli
   a. Not analgesic, but improve the analgesic effects of drugs with analgesic activity
   b. Excessive doses of phenothiazines and butyrophenones can cause apparent involuntary (extrapyramidal) musculoskeletal effects and hallucinatory activity in some animals, particularly horses
   c. The calming effect can be temporarily reversed with an adequate stimulus; larger doses may be required in excitable or apprehensive animals

---

USEFUL FACTS ▪ Phenothiazines, Butyrophenones

- Calming and muscle relaxation
- Antiemetic effects
- Potentiate analgesics
- Antiarrhythmic effects
- Antihistaminic effects
- Metabolized by the liver
- Effective for 4 to 8 hours, up to 48 hours

---

4. Cardiopulmonary effects
   a. α_1-adrenergic blockade results in vasodilation and a decrease in arterial BP (hypotension). Subsequent epinephrine administration may cause a paradoxic drop (β_2 effect) in arterial BP because alpha receptors are blocked
      (1) Hypotension occurs more frequently in excited or apprehensive patients. Reflex tachycardia may occur in response to hypotension. Treat with IV fluids
      (2) Severe reactions include hypotensive crises resulting in fainting and (rarely) bradycardia resulting in death
      (3) Phenylephrine (α_1-agonist) and IV fluids can be used to increase BP if hypotension is severe
   b. Heart rate usually decreases as the patient becomes calm; however, reflex tachycardia may occur if hypotension occurs

    c. Antiarrhythmic effects: phenothiazines block α_1-receptors, produce quinidine-like effects, and decrease central sympathetic, ganglionic, and peripheral (adrenal) activity, reducing the incidence of ventricular arrhythmias

    d. Dose-dependent depression of the myocardium and vascular smooth muscle

    e. Reduces respiratory rate; may decrease tidal volume when administered in large doses; decreases respiratory center sensitivity to increases in CO_2

5. Potentiates the ventilatory and cardiovascular depressant effects of α_2-agonists, opioids, and drugs used to produce general anesthesia

6. Useful as antiemetics

7. Most have antihistaminic properties; phenothiazines and butyrophenones should be avoided when skin testing for allergies

8. Most phenothiazine tranquilizers cross the placental barrier relatively slowly

9. Many phenothiazine tranquilizers, including acepromazine and promazine, may cause erection (priapism) and temporary or permanent prolapse of the penis in stallions or geldings. Potentially reversible by administering benztropine (20 µg/kg, IV)

10. Butyrophenone tranquilizers produce calming and antiemetic effects

11. Primary organ of metabolism is the liver; should be avoided in patients with moderate to severe liver disease or intrahepatic or extrahepatic (porto-caval) shunts

12. Clinical effects are present for 4 to 8 hours but may last up to 48 hours or longer in older animals or animals with liver disease (porto-caval shunts)

13. Commonly used phenothiazines include acepromazine and promazine; butyrophenone tranquilizers are rarely used in veterinary medicine (Tables 3-1 and 3-2)

14. Dose (Table 3-1)

15. Side effects

    a. Tachycardia or (rarely) bradycardia

TABLE 3-2

INTRAVENOUS DOSES OF COMMONLY USED OPIOIDS AND NEUROLEPTANALGESICS

AGENT	DOG	CAT	HORSE	COW	GOAT	PIG
Opioid agonists and partial agonists						
Morphine	0.4-1	0.1-0.2	0.04-0.1	0.04	0.04	0.05-0.1
Meperidine	1-5	0.5-1	2-4	2-4	—	0.4-1
Hydromorphone	0.1-0.2	0.1	0.02-0.1	—	—	—
Oxymorphone	0.1-0.2	0.1	0.02-0.1	—	—	—
Methadone	0.5-1	0.1	0.05-0.1	—	—	0.1-0.2
Fentanyl	2-6 μg/kg	1-3 μg/kg	0.07-0.15	—	—	—
Pentazocine	0.5-2	0.5-1	0.5-3	—	—	0.5-2
Butorphanol	0.2-0.4	0.2-0.4	0.01-0.2	0.1	0.1	0.1-0.2
Buprenorphine	0.02	0.02	0.01	—	—	—
Neuroleptanalgesics						
Acepromazine-Hydromorphone	0.2-0.4 (acepromazine)* 0.1 (hydromorphone)*					
Acepromazine-oxymorphone	0.2-0.4 (acepromazine)* 0.1 (oxymorphone)*					
Xylazine-morphine	0.1-0.5 (xylazine) 0.1-0.3 (morphine)					

Doses are given as mg/kg unless otherwise stated.
IM dose is one to two times the IV dose. Lower drug doses should be used in sick patients.
*Dogs and cats only.

CAUTIONS ▪ Phenothiazines, Butyrophenones

- Hypotension
- Hypothermia
- Inhibit platelet aggregation
- Not analgesic
- Phenothiazines may lower seizure threshold in animals with epilepsy
- Excessive doses of phenothiazines or butyrophenones can cause apparent involuntary musculoskeletal effects and hallucinatory activity, particularly in horses
- Occasional bradycardia (e.g., Boxer dogs)
- Long duration of action (e.g., intrahepatic or extrahepatic shunts)

---

     b. Hypotension

     c. Hypothermia

     d. Akathisia: restless condition in which the patient needs to be in constant motion

     e. Acute dystonic reactions: hysteria, seizures, ataxia

     f. Inhibits platelet aggregation: may promote bleeding. Avoid in dogs with von Willebrand disease or other clotting abnormalities

     g. Tranquilizers (e.g., droperidol) can cause excitement and extrapyramidal effects in old dogs and horses at relatively low doses

B. Benzodiazepines (e.g., diazepam, midazolam, zolazepam) are centrally acting muscle relaxants that are sometimes referred to as *minor tranquilizers* (Table 3-1)

   1. Mode of action

     a. Exert many of their pharmacologic effects by enhancing the activity of CNS inhibitory neurotransmitters (γ-aminobutyric acid, glycine) and opening chloride channels, thereby hyperpolarizing membranes; also produce their effects by combining with CNS benzodiazepine (BZ_1, BZ_2) receptors. Effects can be antagonized by the benzodiazepine antagonist flumazenil

     b. Depress the limbic system, thalamus, and hypothalamus (reducing sympathetic output), thereby inducing a mild calming effect

    c. Reduce polysynaptic reflex activity, resulting in muscle relaxation

    d. Cause minimal CNS depression and produce anticonvulsant effects in most animals; may cause disorientation and agitation after rapid IV administration, particularly in cats

    e. Stimulate appetite and pica

USEFUL FACTS ▪ Benzodiazepines

- Enhance the activity of CNS inhibitory neurotransmitters: γ-aminobutyric acid, glycine; combine with CNS benzodiazepine receptors
- Muscle relaxation
- Anticonvulsant effects
- Mild calming effect; may produce apprehension and nervousness in dogs and cats
- Minimal cardiopulmonary effects in dogs, cats, and horses
- Stimulate appetite and produce pica
- Midazolam and zolazepam are water soluble
- Antagonized by flumazenil

---

2. Physical properties

    a. Diazepam is solubilized by mixing with 40% propylene glycol, ethyl alcohol, sodium benzoate, or benzoic acid; in rare cases produces hypotension, bradycardia, and apnea if administered too rapidly IV

    b. Midazolam and zolazepam are water soluble

3. Recommended doses produce minimal or no calming in normal animals; calming effects are observed in sick, depressed, or debilitated animals

    a. Muscle relaxation

    b. Anticonvulsant

    c. Mild calming

4. Cardiopulmonary effects

    a. Minimal hypotensive effects are observed after IV administration

    b. Bradycardia and hypotension have occurred after rapid IV administration

    c. Respiratory rate and tidal volume are minimally affected

    d. Some antiarrhythmic effects are produced as a result of decreases in sympathetic nervous system activity

5. Produce excellent muscle relaxation in animals and reduce muscle spasms and spasticity; effects are additive or synergistic with other drugs used to produce general anesthesia (e.g., barbiturates, propofol)

6. Increase seizure threshold

7. Effects on gastrointestinal activity undetermined

8. Use in pregnancy not investigated

9. Diazepam is eliminated in the urine and feces after metabolism by the liver; duration of action is 1 to 4 hours

10. Diazepam increases appetite in domestic cats and ruminants (probably in all species)

11. Dose (Table 3-1)

12. Side effects

    a. Ataxia, particularly evident in large animal species

    b. Paradoxic increase in anxiety leading to aggression in cats

    c. Possible CNS depression in neonates

    d. Diazepam is painful if administered IM because of propylene glycol

    e. Bradycardia and hypotension can occur if administered rapidly IV

13. Antagonists: Benzodiazepine antagonist (e.g., flumazenil: 0.01 to 0.1 mg/kg IV; Table 3-3)

CAUTIONS ■ Benzodiazepines

- May cause disorientation and agitation, particularly in cats
- Diazepam painful if administered IM

C. α-2 agonists (i.e., xylazine, detomidine, medetomidine, romifidine) (Table 3-1)

1. Mode of action

    a. Produce CNS depression by stimulating both presynaptic and postsynaptic α_2-adrenoceptors in

TABLE **3-3**
BENZODIAZEPINE, α_2-, AND OPIOID ANTAGONISTS*

AGENT	DOSE
Benzodiazepine antagonist	
Flumazenil	0.01-0.1 IV
α_2-Antagonist	
Yohimbine	0.1-0.3 IV
	0.3-0.5 IM
Tolazoline	0.5-5 slow IV
Atipamezole	0.05 IV
Opioid antagonist	
Naloxone	5-15 µg/kg IV
Nalmefene	0.25-30 µg/kg
Naltrexone	0.05-0.1 SQ
Nalorphine	0.05-0.1 IV

Doses are given as mg/kg unless otherwise stated.
*Antagonists are used whenever drug reversal is desired. Analgesia may be reversed also.

the CNS and peripherally; decreasing norepinephrine release centrally and peripherally and reducing ascending nociceptive transmission; the net result is a decrease in CNS sympathetic outflow and a decrease in circulating catecholamines and other stress-related substances; the CNS effects of α_2-agonists can be antagonized by α_2-receptor antagonists (e.g., yohimbine, tolazoline, atipamezole)
  b. Comparative alpha receptor selectivity for α_2- vs. α_1-receptors

RELATIVE SELECTIVENESS OF α-2 AGONISTS	
DRUG	α_2: α_1-SELECTIVITY
Xylazine	160:1
Detomidine	260:1
Medetomidine	1620:1
Romifidine	340:1
Clonidine	220:1

    c. Polysynaptic reflexes are inhibited; depress internuncial neuron transmission (centrally acting muscle relaxant), but the neuromuscular junction is not influenced

    d. Induce a sleeplike state comparable to phenothiazines, but more pronounced

    e. Produce analgesia by stimulating CNS α_2-receptors

    f. Effects are additive and may be synergistic when combined with other depressants and analgesic drugs (e.g., opioids) used to produce chemical restraint or general anesthesia

2. General properties

    a. Produce calming effect/sedation, muscle relaxation, and analgesia

      (1) Xylazine: 20 to 40 minutes IV

      (2) Detomidine: 90 to 120 minutes IV

      (3) Medetomidine: 45 to 90 minutes IV

      (4) Romifidine: 45 to 90 minutes IV

    b. Can be administered epidurally or subarachnoidally to produce regional or segmental analgesia

---

USEFUL FACTS ▪ α_2-Agonists

- Pronounced sedation
- Muscle relaxation
- Analgesia
- Can be used for epidural or subarachnoid analgesia
- Antagonized by α_2-receptor antagonists: yohimbine, tolazoline, atipamezole

---

3. Cardiopulmonary effects

    a. Decreased heart rate caused by decreased CNS sympathetic outflow and increased parasympathetic activity; may initiate sinus bradycardia, first- or second-degree atrioventricular block; complete (third-degree) atrioventricular block with escape beats occurs rarely

    b. Increased cardiac sensitivity to catecholamine-induced arrhythmias during halothane anesthesia; this effect occurs early, is transient, and is caused by

α_1- and possibly α_2-adrenoceptor stimulation; this effect coincides with the increase in arterial BP and is not observed after detomidine, medetomidine, or romifidine administration

c. Cardiac output may decrease by 30% to 50% and coincides with decreases in heart rate and increases in peripheral vascular resistance

d. Arterial BP increases shortly after drug administration (α_1- and α_2-adrenoceptor stimulatory effect increasing peripheral vascular resistance), then decreases to below control values because of decreases in CNS sympathetic outflow and a decrease in norepinephrine from sympathetic nerve terminals

e. Initial vasoconstriction may cause pale mucous membranes

f. Depress respiratory centers centrally

g. Decrease respiratory center sensitivity to increases in Pco_2; decrease tidal volume and respiratory rate with an overall decrease in minute volume when administered in large doses IV

h. Respiratory threshold to CO_2 increases when large doses are administered, resulting in marked respiratory depression

i. May induce stridor and dyspnea in horses and brachycephalic dogs with upper airway obstruction

4. Other organ systems

a. Suppress salivation, gastric secretions, and gastrointestinal motility; may stimulate pica (abnormal craving) and appetite at low doses

b. Cause vomiting in dogs and cats and are suspected of predisposing to bloat in large-breed dogs

c. Depress swallowing reflex

d. Excellent for treating gastrointestinal pain (colic), although prolonged effects may delay surgery or mask the severity of disease

e. Suppress insulin release by stimulating presynaptic α_2-receptors in the pancreas, resulting in an increase in plasma glucose concentration and glucosuria

f. Promote diuresis with increases in water and sodium excretion

5. Absorption, fate, and excretion
   a. Rapidly absorbed after IM, SQ, or oral administration
   b. Relatively rapidly metabolized by the liver and excreted in the urine
   c. Active metabolites possible; more than 20 identified
6. Other
   a. Produce profound sleep in dogs, cats, foals, and small ruminants
   b. Cross the placenta, but an abortifacient effect has not been noted in pregnant dogs, cats, or mares; no observable effects on gestation or parturition; xylazine may induce premature delivery in cattle
   c. Effect is oxytocin-like in ruminants; this activity has not been reported in dogs, cats, or mares
   d. Highly excited or nervous animals may react adversely by becoming extremely ataxic, reacting violently or viciously when approached or touched, or showing inadequate response
   e. Clinical value of xylazine in pigs is questionable because of relatively rapid metabolism
7. Side effects
   a. Bradyarrhythmias (Fig. 3-3)
   b. Hypotension (long-term effect)
   c. Decreased tissue perfusion
   d. Respiratory depression (respiratory acidosis)

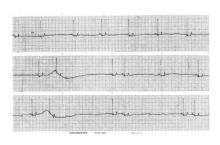

Fig. 3-3
Medetomidine is an α_2-agonist that can produce profound bradycardia. Decreases in heart rate decrease cardiac output (CO) because heart rate × stroke volume = CO.

    e. Ataxia in large animals
    f. Sweating in horses
    g. Diuresis
    h. Occasional unpredictable effects
    i. Xylazine can produce severe inflammatory response if administered SQ in horses or cattle

---

CAUTIONS ■ α_2-Agonists

- Sinus bradycardia, first- or second-degree atrioventricular block
- Xylazine may transiently increase cardiac sensitivity to catecholamine-induced arrhythmias (ventricular arrhythmias) in dogs
- Decrease cardiac output (and tissue perfusion), increase peripheral vascular resistance
- Ileus and "bloat" in dogs; colic in horses
- Pale mucous membrane caused by vasoconstriction
- Respiratory depression
- Ataxia
- Cause vomiting in dogs and cats
- Suppress insulin release
- Oxytocin-like effects in ruminants

---

    8. α_2-Antagonists (Table 3-3)
        a. Yohimbine (0.1 to 0.3 mg/kg IV, 0.3 to 0.5 mg/kg IM)
        b. Tolazoline (0.5 to 5 mg/kg slow IV)
        c. Atipamezole (0.05 mg/kg IV)
        d. Doxapram HCl (0.1 to 0.4 mg/kg), although not a specific antagonist, is useful for reversing respiratory depression and mild sedation
III. Opioids (Table 3-2)
    A. Mode of action
        1. Act by reversible combination with one or more specific receptors (i.e., μ, κ, δ) in the brain and spinal cord to produce a variety of effects including analgesia, sedation, euphoria, dysphoria, and excitement
        2. Referred to as opioid agonists, partial agonists, agonist-antagonists, and antagonists

OPIOID CLASSIFICATIONS

agonist: binds to one or more types of receptor and causes
ain effects (e.g., morphine)
 gonists-antagonists: cause less pronounced effects than that of
. pure agonist (e.g., butorphanol)
Partial agonist: binds to more than one type of receptor and
causes an effect at one but no effect or a less pronounced effect
at another (e.g., buprenorphine)
• Antagonist: binds to one or more types of receptor but causes
no effect at those receptors. By competitively displacing an
agonist from a receptor, the antagonist effectively "reverses"
the agonist's effect (e.g., naloxone)

    a. Represented by a variety of naturally occurring (opiate) derivatives and synthetically manufactured drugs

    b. Classified according to analgesic activity or addiction potential

    c. Commonly used opioid agonists include morphine, methadone, meperidine, hydromorphone, oxymorphone, and fentanyl

    d. Opioid agonist-antagonists (pentazocine, butorphanol) or partial agonists (buprenorphine) produce less sedation than full agonists (e.g., morphine)

    e. Analgesic potency

       (1) Morphine: 1

       (2) Methadone: 1

       (3) Meperidine: 0.5

       (4) Hydromorphone: 7

       (5) Oxymorphone: 5 to 10

       (6) Fentanyl: 100

       (7) Remifentanil: 50

       (8) Butorphanol: 0.5 to 3

       (9) Buprenorphine: 25

  3. Senses are not significantly depressed by opioids

    a. Touch

    b. Vibration

    c. Vision

    d. Hearing

    e. Smell

B. Used before (preemptive), during, or after surgery for analgesia

Fentanyl, sufentanil, hydromorphone, and oxymorphone are generally used during surgery as part of a balanced anesthetic technique

1. Fentanyl patches can be used to provide analgesia. The fentanyl patch is a transdermal drug delivery system. Doses for dogs and cats are 2 to 5 $\mu g/kg/hr$; patch sizes are 25, 50, 75, or 100 $\mu g/hr$
2. Preservation-free morphine (Astramorph®) can be administered epidurally or subarachnoidally to produce regional or segmental analgesia

C. Produce analgesic action at doses lower than needed for sedation (dose tailored to individual animal)

D. Effects in addition to analgesia

1. Behavioral changes (e.g., sedation, euphoria, dysphoria, excitement; animal may not recognize owner)
2. Change in response to external stimuli (e.g., sound)
3. Miosis in dogs and pigs; mydriasis in cats and horses
4. Decreases in body temperature in dogs caused by resetting of the thermoregulatory center and panting in dogs
   a. Hyperthermia in cats; mechanism is uncertain
5. Sweating, particularly in horses
6. Vomiting, constipation, and urine retention

E. May be used in combination with tranquilizers, sedatives, or anesthetics to produce neuroleptanalgesia or balanced anesthesia, respectively (Tables 3-2 and 3-4)

F. Produce excellent sedation in dogs but may cause excitement when given rapidly IV; cats and horses are particularly susceptible to the excitatory effect of opioids; this is typified by increased motor activity and pacing in horses

G. Use is strictly controlled; increased security and accurate record keeping are required

H. Cardiopulmonary effects

1. Bradycardia caused by stimulation of medullary vagal nuclei
2. Possible hypotension caused by release of histamine (morphine, meperidine)
3. Minimal inotropic effect when used in low doses

TABLE 3-4
COMMONLY USED ANALGESIC AND TRANQUILIZER COMBINATIONS FOR IV USE*

ANIMAL	DRUGS	RECOMMENDED IV DOSES	UNTOWARD EFFECTS
Dog	Acepromazine-meperidine	0.1-0.2	Hypotension
	Acepromazine-hydromorphone	0.1-0.2	Hypotension
		0.1-0.2	
	Acepromazine-oxymorphone	0.1-0.2	Hypotension
		0.1-0.2	
	Acepromazine-butorphanol	0.1	Bradycardia
		0.2-0.4	Hypotension
	Diazepam-fentanyl	0.2-0.4	Bradycardia
		0.01	
Cat	Acepromazine-hydromorphone	0.2 (IM)	Excitement
		0.05	
	Acepromazine-oxymorphone	0.2 (IM)	Excitement
		0.05	
	Acepromazine-butorphanol	0.1	Bradycardia
		0.2-0.4	Hypotension

Horse	Xylazine-morphine†	0.6	Bradycardia
		0.2-0.6	Hypotension
	Xylazine-meperidine	0.6	Hypotension
		1	
	Xylazine-butorphanol	0.6	Ataxia
		0.02	
	Xylazine-acepromazine	0.6	Hypotension
		0.05	
	Meperidine-acepromazine	0.5	Hypotension
		0.5	
Ruminants			
Cow	Xylazine	0.04-0.1	Respiratory depression, bradycardia
Sheep	Xylazine	0.1-0.2	
Goat‡	Xylazine	0.01-0.1*	

Doses are given as mg/kg unless otherwise stated.

*Lower doses should be used in sick patients.

† Detomidine (2 to 10 µg/kg IV) can be substituted for xylazine in horses; medetomidine (7-20 µg/kg IV) or romifidine (0.02 to 0.09 mg/kg IV) can be substituted for xylazine in dogs and cats.

‡ Variable response.

> **USEFUL FACTS ▪ Opioids**
>
> - Produce analgesia without loss of proprioception or consciousness
> - Produce excellent sedation in dogs, but excitement occurs in some species, especially cats and horses
> - Metabolized by the liver and eliminated in the urine
> - Controlled substances

      4. Respiratory depression (rate and tidal volume) is dose-dependent and rarely observed unless the patient is already depressed or unconscious; raises the threshold of the respiratory center to increases in Pco_2

I. Gastrointestinal effects
1. Salivation
2. Nausea
3. Vomiting in dogs and cats
4. Nonpropulsive gastrointestinal hypermotility ("ropy guts"), increases in sphincter tone
5. Initially defecation followed by constipation

J. Urine retention and decreases in urine production as a result of increased ADH release

K. Cross the placental barrier relatively slowly; useful for cesarean section because depressant effects can be antagonized

L. Rapid absorption; can be given by IV, IM, SQ, oral, transdermal (fentanyl patches [Fig. 3-4]), or rectal routes. Wide distribution; kidney, liver, and lungs; the majority in skeletal muscle, lower levels in the CNS; low bioavailability with oral or rectal administration because of high first-pass effect. Extensively metabolized by the liver, and metabolites are eliminated in the urine; the opioid agonists vary in biologic half-life, most with durations of action ranging from 30 minutes to 3 hours in most species; morphine may produce effects lasting 6 to 8 hours in horses

M. Tolerance develops with continued use

N. Opioid antagonists (Table 3-3)
1. Mechanism of action

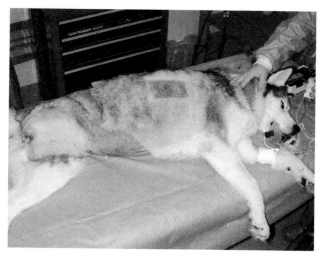

Fig. 3-4
Some drugs can be administered transcutaneously. Fentanyl is an opioid analgesic that can be absorbed transcutaneously. This dog has had a fentanyl patch placed on its lateral thorax.

        a. Opioid antagonists compete with opioid drugs for specific receptor sites
        b. Partial antagonists act in a fashion similar to opioid antagonists
           (1) Can produce autonomic, endocrine, analgesic, and respiratory depressant effects
           (2) Are less potent than morphine as analgesics
           (3) May add to existing respiratory depression
    2. Metabolized in the liver
    3. Dose (Table 3-3)
        a. Naloxone: 5 to 15 μg/kg IV
        b. Nalmefene: 0.25 to 30 μg/kg IV
        c. Naltrexone: 0.05 to 0.1 mg/kg SQ
        d. Nalorphine: 0.05 to 0.1 mg/kg IV
  O. Side effects
    1. Excitement, dysphoria
    2. Apnea

3. Bradycardia
4. Ataxia and incoordination
5. Excessive vomiting
6. Excessive sweating in horses

CAUTION ▪ Opioids

- Morphine and meperidine IV can produce histamine release
- Bradycardia
- Dose-dependent respiratory depression
- Vomiting
- Constipation
- Defecation
- Increase ADH release
- Tolerance can occur

IV. Neuroleptanalgesia
   A. A state of CNS depression and analgesia produced by the combination of a tranquilizer or sedative and analgesic drug; useful in dogs, cats, horses, and pigs (see Definitions, Chapter 1; Table 3-4)
   B. The animal may or may not remain conscious and be responsive to auditory stimuli; many animals defecate, some vomit
   C. Results of the drug combination
      1. Sedation-analgesia, ataxia, and/or recumbency
      2. Depression of ventilation (apnea may occur)
      3. Bradycardia
      4. Defecation and flatulence
      5. Analgesia for periods up to 40 minutes
   D. Overdoses usually result in profound bradycardia and respiratory depression; respiratory depression can generally be reversed by an opioid antagonist (e.g., naloxone)
   E. Most animals are premedicated with a parasympatholytic (e.g., atropine or glycopyrrolate) to prevent bradycardia and excessive salivation
   F. Neuroleptanalgesics are used in combination with barbiturates in dogs to eliminate the stimulatory effect of loud noises and to produce better muscle relaxation

1. Thiopental (2.2 mg/kg) after acepromazine-hydomorphone

PRINCIPAL POINTS ▪ Neuroleptanalgesics

- Hypnosis and analgesia
- May or may not remain conscious and respond to stimuli
- Useful for short operative procedure and cesarean section

G. Opioids and tranquilizers have been used to produce sedation and analgesia
   1. Acepromazine (0.2 to 0.4 mg/kg) in combination with morphine (0.4 to 0.8 mg/kg IV or SQ), meperidine (1 to 2 mg/kg IV), hydromorphone (0.1 to 0.2 mg/kg IV), or oxymorphone (0.1 to 0.2 mg/kg IV) is used to produce neuroleptanalgesia in dogs; diazepam (0.2 mg/kg IV) and hydromorphone (0.1 to 0.2 mg/kg IV) or oxymorphone (0.1 to 0.2 mg/kg IV), or acepromazine (0.2 mg/kg IM) and butorphanol (0.2 to 0.4 mg/kg IM) are used in dogs and cats
   2. α_2-Agonists (xylazine, medetomidine) combined with opioids (morphine, butorphanol) and/or dissociative anesthetics (ketamine) are also used to produce neuroleptanalgesia in dogs and cats
      a. Medetomidine (2 to 10 µg/kg IM) combined with morphine (0.2 mg/kg IM) in dogs
      b. The combination of morphine (0.2 mg/kg IM), medetomidine (60 µg/kg IM), and ketamine (5 mg/kg IM) in cats
   3. The combination of xylazine (0.6 mg/kg IV) or detomidine (20 to 60 µg/kg IV) and morphine (0.2 to 0.6 mg/kg IV) or butorphanol (0.2 to 0.4 mg/kg IV) is commonly used for horses
H. Useful for short operative procedures and for cesarean section in small animals
I. Side effects
   1. Respiratory depression
   2. Bradycardia
   3. Ataxia

4. Excitement
5. CNS and behavioral abnormalities in some breeds of dogs or old dogs (e.g., Doberman pinschers)

CAUTION ▪ Neuroleptanalgesics

- Respiratory depression
- Bradycardia

TREATMENT OF EMERGENCIES · Neuroleptanalgesics

- Severe respiratory depression can generally be reversed by an opioid antagonist

---

V. Nonsteroidal anti-inflammatory drugs; see Chapter 18)

CHAPTER FOUR

Local Anesthetic Drugs and Techniques

"And don't give me any of those local anesthetics. Get me the imported stuff."

FROM THE CARTOON "HERMAN" UNIVERSAL PRESS SYNDICATE

OVERVIEW

Local anesthetics produce desensitization and analgesia of skin surfaces (topical anesthesia), tissues (infiltration and field blocks), and regional structures (conduction anesthesia, intravenous regional anesthesia). Local anesthetic techniques are an alternative or adjunct to intravenous and inhalation anesthesia. A number of anesthetic drugs are available; they vary in potency, toxicity, and cost. The most commonly used local anesthetic drugs are lidocaine, mepivacaine, and bupivacaine hydrochloride. Vasoconstrictors (epinephrine) are occasionally incorporated with or added to lidocaine to increase the intensity of effect and prolong anesthetic activity. Adding hyaluronidase increases tissue penetration in the region of infiltration and hastens the onset of analgesic activity.

GENERAL CONSIDERATIONS

   I. Use sterile solutions, equipment, and techniques
  II. Avoid injection into inflamed areas (if possible)
 III. Use as small a gauge of needle as practical
  IV. Aspirate for blood before injecting
   V. Use lowest effective concentration of local anesthetic drug to produce the desired effect. Wait for onset of analgesia before proceeding

LOCAL ANESTHETICS

I. Mechanism of membrane and impulse conduction
   A. Local anesthetics are membrane-stabilizing agents
   B. The drugs enter and occupy (by polar association) the membrane channels through which sodium (Na^+) ions normally move
   C. The most immediate and apparent effect is the prevention of the inflow of Na^+ blocking subsequent ionic flow
   D. Nerve cell depolarization is prevented, thus retarding or stopping the conduction of nerve impulses

II. Uptake
   A. The salt of the local anesthetic base is an ionizable quaternary amine with little or no anesthetic properties of its own
      1. Salts are not lipid soluble
      2. Salts are not absorbed into the nerve cell membrane
   B. Once the salt of the anesthetic base is deposited into tissues, it dissociates, and the anesthetic base (B) is liberated as follows:

$$BH^+Cl^- \Leftrightarrow Cl^- + BH^+ \Leftrightarrow B + H^+ + Cl^-$$

    Salt   anion cation base

   C. The free anesthetic base is absorbed at the outer lipid nerve membrane. The anesthetic base combines with a hydrogen ion inside the nerve cell and blocks Na^+ channels (Fig. 4-1)
   D. Effect of tissue pH; the acid ionization constant (pK_a) values of local anesthetics are usually between 8 and 9 (except for benzocaine: 2.9)
      1. Local anesthetics become more ionized (more poorly absorbed) the lower (more acid) the pH
      2. Infected or inflamed tissues are more acidic and lack buffering capacity; smaller amounts of the free base are produced, resulting in poor local anesthesia

III. Absorption
   A. Local anesthetics are poorly absorbed through intact skin
   B. Local anesthetics are absorbed from:
      1. Mucous membranes

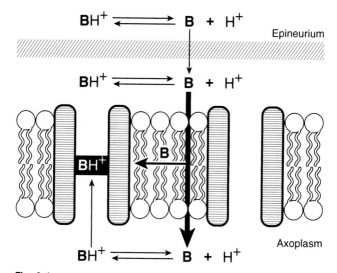

Fig. 4-1
The uncharged (unionized) local anesthetic (B) is absorbed and responsible for producing local anesthetic effects. Increases in tissue acidosis (decreased tissue pH) decrease local anesthetic effect.

      2. Serosal surfaces
      3. Respiratory epithelium
      4. Intramuscular deposition
      5. Subcutaneous deposition
      6. Injured skin
IV. Classification and function of nerve fibers (Table 4-1)
    A. Myelinated A-fibers
      1. α (Alpha): motor, proprioception
      2. β (Beta): motor, touch
      3. γ (Gamma): muscle spindles
      4. δ (Delta): pain, temperature
    B. Myelinated B-fibers: preganglionic sympathetic
    C. Nonmyelinated C-fibers transmit
      1. Pain, temperature
      2. Postganglionic sympathetic

TABLE 4-1
CLASSIFICATION OF NERVE FIBERS

	ANATOMIC LOCATION	FIBER TYPE AND DIAMETER (μm)	FUNCTION	SENSITIVITY TO BLOCK
A-fibers		**Myelinated**		
Aα	Efferent and afferent to muscles and joints	6-22 μm	Motor, proprioception	+
Aβ	Efferent and afferent to muscles and joints	6-22 μm	Motor, touch, proprioception	++
Aγ	Efferent to muscle spindle	3-6 μm	Pain, temperature, muscle tone	++
Aδ	Sensory roots	1-4 μm	Pain, temperature, muscle tone	+++
B-fibers	Preganglionic sympathetic	< 3 μm myelinated	Vasomotor, visceromotor	++++
C-fibers	Postganglionic sympathetic, sensory roots	0.4-1.2 μm nonmyelinated	Vasomotor, visceromotor, pain, temperature, touch	++++

V. Sensitivity to local anesthetic effects (least resistant to most resistant)
   A. C-fibers >Aδ-fibers > Aα-fibers
   B. Sensation disappears in the following order: pain, cold, warmth, touch, joint, deep pressure
   C. Motor function can be maintained after all sensation is lost

VI. Blocking quality
   A. Potency is related to lipid solubility: local anesthetics with high lipid solubility have more potent effects
   B. Latency is the time between injection and the peak effect
   C. Duration of action
      1. Binding affinity to receptor protein; local anesthetics with greater protein-binding ability have a longer duration of action; can bind to the receptors in Na$^+$ channel reliably (bupivacaine, ropivacaine > tetracaine > lidocaine > procaine)
      2. Doubling the concentration of local anesthetic increases the duration of analgesia by approximately 30% (proportional to the logarithm of the concentration)
   D. Recovery time is the time it takes for normal sensation to return
      1. Dependent on outflow diffusion and gradual release of local anesthetic from the nerve membrane
      2. It may be 2 to 200 times longer than the onset time

VII. Ampules of hydrochloride salts can be autoclaved at 120° C for 20 to 30 minutes without affecting potency

DRUGS USED FOR VASOCONSTRICTION

I. Effects of vasoconstriction
   A. Vasoconstrictors delay absorption—reducing toxicity and increasing the margin of safety
   B. Vasoconstrictors increase intensity and prolong anesthetic activity (up to 5 times)
   C. Use of vasoconstrictors may cause disturbances of the circulation (e.g., toes, penis)
   D. Vasoconstrictors can increase risk of cardiac arrhythmias and ventricular fibrillation
   E. Dose: epinephrine 5 μg/ml (1: 200,000)

DRUGS USED TO HASTEN THE TIME OF ONSET OF ANESTHESIA

   I. Hyaluronidase
      A. Increases tissue penetration (may double), resulting in a larger total area being desensitized
      B. Often produces a rapid onset of analgesia
      C. Usually shortens anesthesia time because of increased absorption, unless a vasoconstrictor is also used
      D. May enhance systemic absorption and toxicity
      E. Is not a substitute for precise, accurate technique; fascial planes are barriers to diffusion
      F. Dose: use five turbidity-reducing units per milliliter of local anesthetic solution

SPECIFIC LOCAL ANESTHETIC DRUGS

   I. Ester-linked drugs (Table 4-2)
      A. Cocaine (alkaloid of the leaf of *Erythroxylon coca*)
      B. Procaine hydrochloride (Novocaine)
         1. Prototype of all local anesthetics
         2. Standard drug for comparison of anesthetic effects
         3. Hydrolyzed in plasma by pseudocholinesterase
         4. Less potency and shorter duration than most local anesthetics but minimal toxicity
         5. Not recommended for topical administration because of poor absorption
      C. Tetracaine hydrochloride (Pontocaine)
         1. 10 to 15 times more potent than procaine
         2. 1.5 to 2 times longer duration than procaine
         3. Relatively toxic
         4. Prolonged anesthetic effect
         5. Hydrolyzed by pseudocholinesterase
         6. Useful for topical anesthesia
      D. Benzocaine/butamben/tetracaine (Cetacaine)
         1. Benzocaine blocks Na^+ channels with pressure caused by membrane expansion, not by a direct inhibition of the channel
         2. pK_a: 2.9 (benzocaine), 2.5 (butamben)
         3. Rapid onset (approximately 30 seconds) and short duration (approximately 30 to 60 minutes)

TABLE 4-2
LOCAL ANESTHETICS

AGENT (GENERIC NAME)	TRADE NAME (REGISTERED BY)	CHEMICAL NAME	POTENCY RATIO (PROCAINE = 1)
Esters			
Procaine	Novocain (Winthrop Stearns)	Para-aminobenzoic acid ester of diethylaminoethanol	1 : 1
Tetracaine	Pontocaine (Winthrop Laboratories)	Parabutylamino benzoyl-dimethylaminoethanol-HCl	12 : 1
Benzocaine + Butamben + Tetracaine	Cetacaine (Cetylite)	Ethyl 4-aminobenzoate (benzocaine) 4-aminobenzoic acid butyl (butamben)	
Amides			
Lidocaine	Xylocaine (Astra Pharmaceutical)	Diethylaminoacet-2,6 xylidide	2 : 1
Mepivacaine	Carbocaine (Winthrop Laboratories)	1-methyl-2',6'-pipecoloxylidide monohydrochloride	2.5 : 1
Bupivacaine	Marcaine (Breon Laboratories)	1-butyl-2',6'-pipecoloxylidide-HCl	8 : 1
Ropivacaine	Naropin (Astra)	S-(-)-1-propyl-2',6'-pipecoloxylidide-HCL monohydrate	8 : 1
Lidocaine + Prilocaine	EMLA cream (AstraZeneca)	Propylamine-2-methyl-propionanilidehydrochloride (prilocaine)	

Continued

TABLE 4-2
LOCAL ANESTHETICS—cont'd

DRUG	TOXICITY RATIO (PROCAINE = 1)	DOSE (%)	STABILITY	COMMENTS
Esters				
Procaine	1:1	1-2 for infiltration and nerve block	Aqueous solutions are heat resistant, decomposed by bacteria	Hydrolyzed by liver and plasma esterase
Tetracaine	10 : 1	0.1 for infiltration and nerve block; topically 0.2	Crystals and solutions should not be autoclaved	Slow onset of anesthesia (5-10 min); 2 hr duration; for eye instillation
Benzocaine + Butamben + Tetracaine			Keep away from flames, high temperature, alkali or alkaline earth metals, oxidizing agents	Never use for injection; rapid onset (30 sec); 30-60 min duration; may cause methemoglobinemia

Amides

Lidocaine	0.5% 1 : 1 1% 1.4 : 1 2% 1.5 : 1	0.5-2 for infiltration and nerve block; topically 2-4	Aqueous solutions are thermostable; multiple autoclaving possible	Excellent penetrability; rate of onset twice as fast as procaine; 2 hr duration with epinephrine
Mepivacaine	Less toxic than lidocaine	1-2 for infiltration and nerve block	Resistant to acid and alkaline hydrolysis; multiple autoclaving possible	Absence of vasodilator effects makes addition of a vasoconstrictor unnecessary
Bupivacaine	Greater margin of safety than lidocaine	0.25 for infiltration; 0.5 for nerve block; 0.75 for epidural block	Stable compound	Intermediate onset, lasting 4-6 hr
Ropivacaine	Greater margin of safety than bupivacaine	0.2 for infiltration; 0.5 for nerve block; 0.75 and 1.0 for epidural block	Stable compound	Intermediate onset, lasting 4-6 hr
Lidocaine + Prilocaine		(Do not spread out; apply a thick layer of medicine)		Possibility of skin trouble, deterioration of methemoglobinemia

4. Use on larynx or pharynx may cause methemoglobinemia
5. Metabolized by plasma cholinesterase
6. Used for surface anesthesia
7. Localized allergic reactions may occur (e.g., erythema, pruritus)

II. Amide-linked drugs
   A. Lidocaine hydrochloride (Xylocaine, Lignocaine, Lidoderm)
      1. Most stable drug in this group; not decomposed by boiling, acids, or alkali
      2. Superior penetration compared with procaine: fast onset (effects are evident in one-third the time); effects persist 1.5 times longer; spread over a wider field
      3. Minimal tissue damage or irritation
      4. No allergy or hypersensitivity
      5. Mild sedative effects when administered intravenously (IV) (anesthetic sparing)
      6. Antiarrhythmic
      7. Gastrointestinal promotility effects when administered IV
      8. Antiinflammatory effects
      9. Antishock effects but potentially can induce hypotension when administered IV in some animals
      10. Metabolized in the liver
      11. Can be infused IV continuously with inhalation anesthesia to augment analgesia
   B. Mepivacaine hydrochloride (Carbocaine)
      1. Similar to lidocaine
      2. No irritation or tissue damage
      3. Metabolized in the liver
      4. Should be avoided in pregnant animals; may have toxic effects in infants
   C. Bupivacaine (Marcaine)
      1. Longer time to onset of analgesic effects than lidocaine
      2. Anesthetic effect is longer than procaine (3 to 10 hours)
      3. Metabolized in the liver
      4. May produce central nervous system and cardiac toxicity

D. Ropivacaine (Naropin)
   1. Similar to bupivacaine; slow onset and long duration
   2. Less cardiotoxic

TOPICAL ANESTHETICS

I. Commonly used topicals
   A. Butacaine (Butya sulphate)
   B. Tetracaine (Pontocaine)
   C. Piperocaine (Metycaine)
   D. Proparacaine (Ophthaine)
   E. Benzocaine/butamben/tetracaine (Cetacaine)
   F. EMLA Cream (lidocaine and prilocaine mixture)
II. Vascular effect: local anesthetic drugs are local and occasionally systemic vasodilators, with the exception of cocaine (a vasoconstrictor)
III. Toxicity (Table 4-3) dependent on:
   A. Rate of absorption
   B. Rate of metabolism

METHODS OF LOCAL ANESTHETIC APPLICATION

I. Surface anesthesia
   A. Sprayed or brushed on mucous membranes (mouth, nose, larynx)
   B. Dropped into the eye
   C. Infused into the urethra
   D. Injected subsynovially (synovial membranes)
   E. Injected intrapleurally

TABLE 4-3
TOXIC REACTIONS OF LOCAL ANESTHETICS

SYSTEMIC
Central nervous system (seizures)
Cardiac/vascular (hypotension, arrhythmia)
Respiratory (apnea)
Methemoglobinemia (benzocaine, prilocaine)
Localized or systemic
Allergic reaction (procaine)

II. Infiltration anesthesia
   A. Diffuse infiltration of operative area
      1. Sensitive tissues: skin, nerve trunks, blood vessels, periosteum, synovial membranes, mucous membranes near orifices (mouth, nose, rectum, anus)
      2. Insensitive tissues: subcutis, fat, muscles, tendons, fascia, bone, cartilage, visceral peritoneum
   B. Infiltration techniques
      1. Bleb (very localized deposition of a small quantity)
      2. Tissue layer by tissue layer
   C. Uses
      1. Minimize or prevent pain
      2. Facilitate surgery
         a. Skin incision
         b. Surgical removal of superficial tumors
         c. Wound repair
III. Regional (perineural) anesthesia
   A. Linear block
   B. Field block
   C. Peripheral nerve block
   D. Paravertebral block
   E. Nerve block: injection in neuroplexus, ganglia, nerve trunks
   F. Epidural block
   G. Spinal anesthesia: injection in subarachnoid space
IV. Intraarticular anesthesia
V. Subsynovial anesthesia
VI. Intravenous regional anesthesia
VII. Refrigeration or hypothermic anesthesia

ANALGESIC ACTIVITY OF EPIDURALLY ADMINISTERED α_2-ADRENOCEPTOR AGONISTS

α_2-Adrenoceptor agonists such as clonidine, xylazine, detomidine, medetomidine, dexmedetomidine, and romifidine are used for their sedative, analgesic, anxiolytic, anesthetic sparing, and hemodynamic stability properties; xylazine, detomidine, medetomidine, or romifidine injected epidurally in cattle and horses can produce caudal (S3 to coccyx) localized analgesia with minimal impairment of motor function.

> **NOTE**
>
> Opioids and ketamine are also administered epidurally to enhance analgesic activity.

I. Site of action
   A. The antinociceptive effects of epidurally and intrathecally (subarachnoid) administered α_2-adrenoceptor agonists are primarily the result of:
      1. Stimulation of α_2-adrenoceptors in the spinal cord inhibits the release of norepinephrine, hyperpolarizing dorsal horn neurons and inhibiting substance P (a pain-related neurotransmitter) release, thereby producing analgesia
      2. Inhibition of impulse conduction in primary afferent nerve fibers; C-fibers (pain, reflex responses, and post-sympathetic transmission) are blocked to a greater extent than A-fibers (somatic motor function and proprioception)
   B. The antinociceptive effects of epidurally and intrathecally (subarachnoid) administered α_2-adrenoceptor agonists are independent of opioid receptor mechanisms
   C. The addition of xylazine to an epidural solution containing lidocaine prolongs the duration of analgesia
II. Epidural xylazine
   A. Xylazine is the most commonly used α_1-and α_2-agonist for epidural injection in cattle, horses, and pigs (Table 4-4)
      1. Xylazine has a high affinity and selectivity for α_1- and α_2- receptors
      2. Xylazine has local anesthetic properties that are independent of α-adrenergic stimulation
   B. Clinical use of epidural xylazine
      1. Cattle: xylazine (0.05 mg/kg expanded to a 5 ml volume with sterile saline solution) given in the epidural space at the first coccygeal intervertebral or the sacrococcygeal space produces anesthesia in the anal and perineal region for surgery and obstetric procedures (Table 4-4)

TABLE 4-4

EPIDURAL ANALGESIA: XYLAZINE-, XYLAZINE/LIDOCAINE-, DETOMIDINE-, MEDETOMIDINE-, MORPHINE-, DETOMIDINE/MORPHINE-, AND KETAMINE-INDUCED ANALGESIA IN CATTLE, GOAT, PONY, HORSE, PIG, LLAMA, DOG, AND CAT

SPECIES	AGONIST	DOSE (MG/KG)	VOLUME OF DILUENT (ML)
Cattle	Xylazine	0.05	5 ml of 0.9% NaCl
	Medetomidine	15 µg/kg	5 ml with sterile water
Goat	Xylazine	0.15	5 ml with sterile water
	Medetomidine	20 µg/kg	5 ml with sterile water
Pony	Xylazine	0.35	
Horse	Xylazine	0.17	6 ml/450 kg with sterile water
	Xylazine	0.17	5 ml/450 kg with 2% lidocaine (0.22 mg/kg)
	Xylazine	0.25-0.35	8 ml of 0.9% NaCl or
			6 ml/450 kg
	Xylazine	0.17	6 ml/454 kg with sterile water
	+ Lidocaine	0.22	
	Detomidine	0.06	10 ml/500 kg with sterile water
	Morphine	0.05	10 ml/450 kg with 0.9% NaCl
	Morphine	0.2	8 ml/450 kg with 0.9% NaCl
	+ Detomidine	0.03	
	Ketamine	2	10 ml/450 kg with 0.9% NaCl

Pig	Xylazine	2	5 ml of 0.9% NaCl
	Xylazine	1 in large sows >180 kg	10 ml of 2% lidocaine
		2 in small pigs <50 kg	
Llama	Detomidine	0.5	5 ml of 0.9% NaCl
	Xylazine	0.17	2 ml/150 kg of sterile water
	Xylazine	0.17	1.7 ml/150 kg with 2% lidocaine (0.22 mg/kg)
Dog	Medetomidine	15 µg/kg	0.1 ml/kg with 0.9% sterile saline
Cat	Medetomidine	10 µg/kg	1 ml physiological saline

TABLE 4-4

EPIDURAL ANALGESIA: XYLAZINE-, XYLAZINE/LIDOCAINE-, DETOMIDINE-, MEDETOMIDINE-, MORPHINE-, DETOMIDINE/MORPHINE-, AND KETAMINE-INDUCED ANALGESIA IN CATTLE, GOAT, PONY, HORSE, PIG, LLAMA, DOG, AND CAT—cont'd

| SPECIES | SITE OF INJECTION | SPREAD OF ANALGESIA | ANALGESIA | | SIDE EFFECTS |
			ONSET (MIN)	DURATION (MIN)	
Cattle	$C_0 1$-$C_0 2$	S3 to coccyx	10	>120	Sedation, ataxia, cardiopulmonary depression, ruminal hypomotility, diuresis
	$C_0 1$-$C_0 2$	Tail, perineum, pelvic limbs	5-10	00	Mild-moderate sedation, moderate ataxia, salivation, diuresis, occasional recumbency
Goat	Lumbosacral	Flank, perineum, forelimbs, head	5	>180	Marked sedation, variable cardiopulmonary depression, lateral recumbency
	Lumbosacral	Perineum, thorax, forelimbs, neck, head	3-6	40	Sedation, cardiopulmonary depression, recumbency
Pony	$C_0 1$-$C_0 2$	S3 to coccyx	20-30	240	Mild ataxia

Species	Site	Area affected			Effects
Horse	S5-C₀1	S3 to coccyx	30	200	—
	S5-C₀1	S3 to coccyx	5	300	Mild ataxia
	C₀1-C₀2	S3 to coccyx	13	160-180	Minimal cardiovascular and respiratory depression, head ptosis
	C₀1-C₀2	Tail, perineum	20	240	Mild transient ataxia
	S5-C₀1	Bilateral cauda	5	300	Mild sedation, sweating
	C₀1-C₀2	S3-T15 to coccyx	10-15	130-150	Sedation, ataxia, cardiopulmonary depression, diuresis
	C₀1-C₀2	S3 to coccyx	20	180	—
	C₀1-C₀2	S3 to coccyx	<5	330	Mild sedation, occasional recumbency
	C₀1-C₀2	Lumbosacral	20-480	480-780	Mild sedation, hypotension, occasional urticaria
Pig	L6-S1 (via catheter)	Entire pelvic limbs	60	>360	Marked sedation, mild ataxia, bradycardia, bradypnea
	Midsacral (S2-S3), via catheter	Tail, perineum, upper pelvic limbs	5-15	80	Mild sedation, mild ataxia
Llama	Lumbosacral	Umbilicus to coccyx	5	>120	Sedation, immobilization
	Lumbosacral	Umbilicus to coccyx	5-10	300-480	—
	Lumbosacral	Umbilicus to coccyx	10	<30	Atipamezole (0.2 mg/kg IV) reverses sedation
Dog	Lumbosacral	—	—	7 hr.	Bradycardia, increase in blood pressure
Cat	Lumbosacral	Hindlimbs, forelimbs	15	Forelimbs: 120 Hindlimbs: 240	Sedation, emesis

a. Xylazine-induced caudal epidural anesthesia in cattle is associated with these side effects:
   1) Marked sedation (head drop)
   2) Mild ataxia
   3) Bradycardia
   4) Hypotension
   5) Respiratory depression and subsequent respiratory acidosis
   6) Hypoxemia
   7) Transient ruminal amotility (in cattle)
   8) Diuresis
   9) Salivation (in cattle)
b. The side effects in cattle are dose-dependent and partially reversed by administration of tolazoline (Tolazine) (0.3 mg/kg slowly IV)

2. Horses: xylazine (0.2 to 0.4 mg/kg expanded to a 6 ml to 10 ml volume with sterile saline solution) given in the epidural space at the first coccygeal intervertebral space produces anesthesia in the anal and perineal region for surgery and obstetric procedures, with minimal ataxia (Table 4-4)
   a. Side effects (see above)

3. Pigs: xylazine (2 mg/kg expanded to a 0.5 to 1.0 ml/kg volume with sterile saline solution) given in the epidural space at the lumbosacral, the sacrococcygeal, or first intercoccygeal space produces bilateral surgical anesthesia of the trunk caudal to the umbilicus and analgesia and paralysis of rear limbs, with minimal cardiovascular depression (Table 4-4)
   a. Smaller doses of epidural xylazine (<1 mg/kg) do not produce surgical anesthesia
   b. Larger doses of epidural xylazine (>3 mg/kg) induce weakness of rear limbs for 36 hours or longer

4. Adult goats: xylazine (0.15 mg/kg expanded to a 5 ml volume with sterile saline solution) given in the epidural space at the lumbosacral space produces analgesia of the flank and perineum, which extends to the head and forelimb. Frequently produces lateral recumbency

C. Onset and duration of epidural analgesia
1. Signs of analgesia develop within 10 to 30 minutes (compared with 5 to 10 minutes after epidural lidocaine)
2. A mixture of xylazine and lidocaine can be used to shorten the onset of analgesia to approximately 5 minutes and prolong analgesia up to approximately 5 hours (Table 4-4)
   a. Duration of analgesia is longer for the xylazine-lidocaine combination than for either drug used alone
   b. Duration of analgesia after epidural drug administration is highly variable (Table 4-4)
      1) 110 minutes after lidocaine
      2) 220 minutes after xylazine
      3) 330 minutes after xylazine-lidocaine combination
   c. Surgical and obstetric procedures can commence after injection without the need for additional anesthetic
D. α-Antagonists
1. Atipamezole (0.2 mg/kg), a potent α_2-adrenoceptor antagonist, when injected IV does not abolish the analgesic or immobilizing effects of epidurally administered xylazine in pigs
2. Tolazoline (0.3 mg/kg), an α_1- and α_2-adrenoceptor antagonist, when injected IV does not reverse xylazine-induced epidural analgesia in cattle

III. Epidural detomidine
A. Horses: detomidine (0.06 mg/kg expanded to a 10 ml volume with sterile saline solution) given in the epidural space at the first coccygeal intervertebral space produces variable analgesia. Analgesia may extend from the coccyx to the third sacral (S3) and coccyx to the fourteenth thoracic (T14) spinal cord segment (Table 4-4)
1. Detomidine-induced caudal epidural analgesia in horses is associated with side effects
   a. Marked sedation, head drop
   b. Bradycardia with second-degree, atrioventricular heart block
   c. Hypotension

        d. Hypercarbia (respiratory depression with subsequent respiratory acidosis)

        e. Diuresis

    2. These side effects are dose-dependent and can be partially antagonized by atipamezole (0.2 mg/kg IV)

IV. Epidural medetomidine

    A. Cattle: medetomidine (15 µg/kg expanded to a 5 ml volume with sterile saline solution) given in the epidural space at the second coccygeal space produces variable analgesia (Table 4-4)

        1. Onset of analgesia is 5 to 10 minutes and maintained up to 7 hours

        2. Medetomidine-induced caudal epidural analgesia in cattle is associated with side effects

            a. Mild to moderate sedation

            b. Moderate ataxia

            c. Salivation

            d. Diuresis

    B. Goats: medetomidine (20 µg/kg expanded to a 5 ml volume with sterile saline solution) given in the epidural space at the lumbosacral space produces adequate analgesia of the flank and perineum

        1. Analgesia extends to the thorax, forelimbs, neck, and head, with variable cardiopulmonary depression

        2. The duration of analgesia is 2 hours

        3. Analgesia and cardiopulmonary depression are reversed by atipamezole (80 µg/kg IV)

    C. Dogs: medetomidine (15 µg/kg) given in the epidural space at the lumbosacral space produces variable analgesia

        1. Medetomidine-induced caudal epidural analgesia in dogs may be associated with side effects such as bradycardia with second-degree atrioventricular heart block

        2. The duration of analgesia is 7 hours

    D. Cats: medetomidine (10 µg/kg in 1 ml saline solution) given in the epidural space at the lumbosacral space produces variable analgesia

        1. The pain threshold for the hindlimbs increases from 20 to 245 minutes after injection

2. The pain threshold for the forelimbs also increases from 15 to 120 minutes after injection
3. Produces mild sedation for a short period (3 to 10 minutes)

NOTE

Restraint: movements of head, shoulder, and forelimbs are not suppressed by epidural analgesia/anesthesia and should be controlled by physical or chemical restraint.

V. Subarachnoid xylazine
    A. Goats: xylazine (50 $\mu g/kg$) given into the lumbosacral subarachnoid space produces moderate analgesia of hind quarter, perineum, and flank, mild ataxia, and sedation
        1. Minimum effects in hemodynamic, hematologic, physiological, and biochemical parameters
        2. The onset of analgesia is within 10 minutes and the duration is 2 hours
VI. Subarachnoid detomidine
    A. Horses: detomidine (30 $\mu g/kg$ expanded to a 3 ml volume with cerebrospinal fluid) given into the subarachnoid space at midsacral vertebrae (catheter technique) produces analgesia and side effects similar to those produced by epidural administration of detomidine (60 $\mu g/kg$)
        1. Most of the side effects, except bradycardia and bradypnea, are reversed by atipamezole (0.1 mg/kg IV)
        2. The duration of analgesia is shorter than that after epidural administration; 2 hours and 2.5 hours, respectively
VII. Subarachnoid medetomidine
    Goats: medetomidine (10 $\mu g/kg$) given into the lumbosacral subarachnoid space produces similar effects to xylazine (50 $\mu g/kg$)

CHAPTER FIVE

Local Anesthesia in Ruminants and Pigs

"The pain of the mind is worse than pain of the body."
PUBLILIUS SYRUS

OVERVIEW

The most commonly used local anesthetic techniques in ruminants are surface (topical) anesthesia, infiltration anesthesia, nerve block (conduction) anesthesia, epidural anesthesia, and intravenous regional anesthesia. The standing position is optimal for surgery in ruminants because it reduces the problems associated with bloating, salivation, recumbency-related regurgitation, and nerve or muscle damage.

The most commonly used local anesthetic techniques in appropriately tranquilized pigs are infiltration anesthesia, lumbo-sacral epidural anesthesia, and intratesticular injection.

RUMINANTS: LOCAL ANESTHESIA FOR STANDING LAPAROTOMY

  I. There are four techniques for producing local anesthesia of the paralumbar fossa in ruminants:
    A. Infiltration anesthesia
    B. Proximal paravertebral anesthesia
    C. Distal paravertebral anesthesia
    D. Segmental dorsolumbar epidural anesthesia
  II. Abdominal surgeries in which these anesthetic techniques may be used:
    A. Rumenotomy
    B. Cecotomy

      C. Correction of gastrointestinal displacement

      D. Intestinal obstruction

      E. Volvulus

      F. Cesarean section

      G. Ovariectomy

      H. Liver or kidney biopsy

III. Infiltration anesthesia

    A. Line block

        1. Area blocked: skin and muscle layers of the flank, and parietal peritoneum along the line of incision

        2. Needle: 18-gauge, 7.6- to 10.2-cm

        3. Anesthetic: 10 to 100 ml of 2% lidocaine

        4. Method: make multiple subcutaneous injections of 0.5 to 1 ml of anesthetic, 1 to 2 cm apart with a 20-gauge, 2.54-cm needle; then infiltrate the muscle layers and parietal peritoneum through the desensitized skin

        5. Advantages

          a. Easiest technique

          b. Use of routinely sized needles (2.5-cm, 20-gauge or smaller for skin block; 7.6- to 10.2-cm, 18-gauge for infiltrating the muscle layers and peritoneum)

        6. Disadvantages

          a. Large volume of anesthetic

          b. Lack of muscle relaxation

          c. Incomplete block of deeper layers of the abdominal wall

          d. Formation of hematomas along the incision line

          e. Increased cost due to larger amounts of anesthetic use and time required

        7. Complications

          a. Toxicity can occur if a significant amount of anesthetic of 2% lidocaine hydrochloride (i.e., 250 ml [5 g]) is inadvertently administered intraperitoneally to a 450 kg cow or 10 ml [200 mg] is administered intraperitoneally to an adult goat)

          b. Interference with healing

    B. Inverted L block (Fig. 5-1)

        1. Area blocked: flank caudal and ventral to site of injection

        2. Site: a line along the caudal border of the last rib and along a line ventral to the lumbar transverse

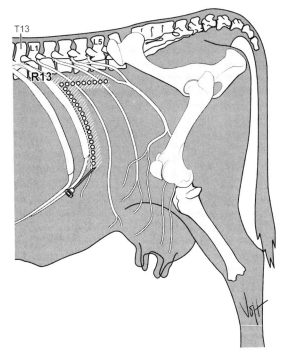

Fig. 5-1
Regional anesthesia of the cow's left flank using inverted L infiltration pattern.

    processes from the last rib to the fourth lumbar vertebra (inverted L)
3. Needle: 18-gauge, 7.6-cm
4. Anesthetic: up to 100 ml of 2% lidocaine in adult cattle, evenly distributed
5. Method: inject drug into the tissues bordering the dorsocaudal aspect of the last rib and ventrolateral aspect of the lumbar transverse processes, creating a wall of anesthetic enclosing the incision site
6. Advantages
    a. Similar to line block

      b. Absence of anesthetic agent from the incision line minimizes edema, hematoma, and possible interference with healing

   7. Disadvantages

      a. Large volume of anesthetic required

      b. Length of time required to infiltrate such a long line

      c. Incomplete block of the deep layers of the abdominal wall (particularly the peritoneum)

   8. Complications: similar to line block

V. Specific nerve anesthesia

  A. Proximal paravertebral anesthesia (Farquharson, Hall, or Cambridge technique)

    1. Area blocked: flank of side on which technique is performed

    2. Nerves blocked: dorsal and ventral branches of T13, L1, and L2 and occasionally L3 and L4 (desensitization of L3 and L4 produce analgesia of the caudalmost part of the paralumbar fossa for cesarean section or ipsilateral fore-teat and mammary gland; if L3 and L4 are blocked, the animal may become unable to stand)

    3. Site: 2.5 to 5 cm from midline (Fig. 5-2); T13 immediately in front of transverse process of L1; L1 immediately in front of transverse process of L2; L2 immediately in front of transverse process of L3

    4. Needle: 14-gauge, 1.3-cm needle, creating passage for a 16- or 18-gauge, 3.81- to 15.2-cm needle

    5. Anesthetic: 20 ml of 2% lidocaine at each site

    6. Method: the skin overlying the spinal column on the side to be desensitized is clipped, surgically scrubbed, and disinfected; palpate the lumbar transverse processes, starting from L5 and moving forward; L1 may be difficult to feel; measure 5 cm from midline; palpate the lumbar dorsal processes; injection site is at a 90-degree angle to the spaces between the dorsal processes; pass the needle vertically down until hitting the cranial edge of the transverse process and proceed down through the intertransverse ligament; inject 10 to 15 ml of 2% lidocaine below the ligament to block the ventral branch of the nerve

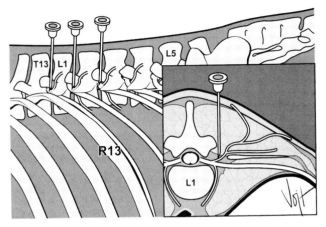

Fig. 5-2
Needle placement for proximal paravertebral nerve block in cattle. Left lateral aspect and cranial view of a transection of the first thoracolumbar vertebra at the location of the intervertebral foramen. *R13* is the last rib, *T13, L1,* and *L5* are the spinous processes of the last thoracic and the first and fifth lumbar vertebrae.

(there should be minimal resistance to injection); withdraw the needle 1 to 2.5 cm sufficiently to inject 5 ml of 2% lidocaine above ligament, level with dorsal surface of transverse process to block the dorsal branch (resistance to injection); if the first lumbar transverse process cannot be palpated, anesthetize the other nerves first and then measure the distance between injection sites to find the site for blocking nerve T13

7. In sheep and goats, T13, L1, and L2 are desensitized similarly to the cattle method, but 2.5 to 3 cm off the midline and with less anesthetic (2 to 3 ml per site)

8. Advantages over local block
   a. Anesthesia of skin, musculature, and peritoneum; wide and uniform area of analgesia and muscle relaxation
   b. No additional restraint required

      c. Large quantities of local anesthetic not required

      d. Shorter postsurgical convalescent period; incision site avoided

   9. Disadvantages

      a. Procedure difficult in fat cattle and some beef cattle

      b. Arching of the spine caused by paralysis of back muscles

      c. No anesthesia of abdominal viscera

      d. Bowing out toward the area of incision (after unilateral blockade), making the closure of the incision more difficult

  10. Complications

      a. Possible penetration of the aorta

      b. Possible penetration of the thoracic longitudinal vein (posterior) or vena cava

      c. Loss of motor control of the pelvic limb caused by caudal migration of drug (femoral nerve block)

B. Distal paravertebral anesthesia (Magda, Cakala, or Cornell technique)

   1. Area blocked: flank of side on which technique is performed

   2. Nerves blocked: dorsal and ventral rami of T13, L1, and L2

   3. Site: distal ends of lumbar transverse processes of L1, L2, and L4 (Fig. 5-3)

   4. Needle: 18-gauge, 7.6-cm

   5. Anesthetic: 10 to 20 ml of 2% lidocaine at each site

   6. Method: the skin overlying the spinal column on the side to be desensitized is clipped, surgically scrubbed, and disinfected; insert the needle ventral to the tips of the respective transverse process; inject anesthetic (up to 20 ml) in a fan-shaped infiltration pattern; withdraw the needle a short distance, reinsert it dorsal and caudal to the transverse process, and inject approximately 5 ml of the anesthetic

   7. Advantages of distal paravertebral nerve block over proximal paravertebral block

      a. Use of routinely sized needles

      b. Minimizes risk of penetrating a major blood vessel

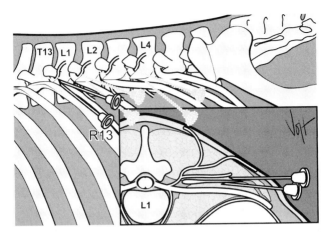

Fig. 5-3

Needle placement for distal paravertebral nerve blockades in cattle. Left lateral aspect and cranial view of a transection of the first lumbar vertebra at the location of the intervertebral foramen. *R13* is the last rib, and *T13, L1, L2,* and *L4* are the spinous processes of the last thoracic and first, second, and fourth lumbar vertebrae.

     c. Lack of scoliosis

     d. Minimal ataxia or weakness in the pelvic limb

   8. Disadvantages

     a. Larger volume of anesthetic

     b. Variations in efficacy, particularly if the nerves follow a variable anatomic pathway

   9. Complications: none

C. Segmental dorsolumbar epidural block (Arthur block)

   1. Area blocked: the skin area caudal to the T13 or L1 spinous process and flank on both sides

   2. Nerves blocked: T13 and anterior lumbar nerves, depending on the total dose administered

   3. Site: epidural space between L1 and L2 vertebrae (Fig. 5-4)

   4. Needle: spinal, preferably 18-gauge, 12.7-cm

   5. Anesthetic: 8 ml of 2% lidocaine in an 500-kg cow, no more than 1 ml/50 kg of 2% lidocaine in sheep and goats

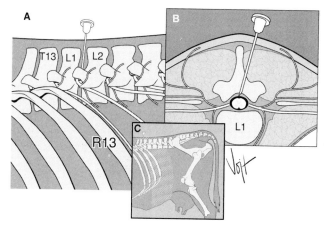

Fig. 5-4

Needle placement for segmental dorsolumbar epidural block. **A,** Left lateral aspect. **B,** Cranial view of a transection of the first lumbar vertebra at the location of the intervertebral foramen. **C,** *(inset)* Desensitized area of skin after segmental epidural anesthesia. *R13* is the last rib; and *T13, L1,* and *L2* are the spinous processes of the last thoracic and first and second lumbar vertebrae.

6. Method: the skin overlying the spinal column is clipped, surgically scrubbed, and disinfected; to reach the epidural space, insert the spinal needle 8 to 12 cm ventral and cranial at an angle of 10 to 15 degrees from vertical; piercing of the interarcuate ligament is felt as slight resistance during the insertion process; no blood or cerebrospinal fluid (CSF) can be aspirated, and also no resistance to the injection of anesthetic results after correct needle placement; if bleeding occurs, the stylet is placed into the needle and the needle is withdrawn after 2 to 3 minutes

7. Advantages over proximal or distal paravertebral anesthesia
   a. Only one injection
   b. Small quantity of anesthetic
   c. Uniform anesthesia and relaxation of the skin, musculature, and peritoneum (begins 10 to 20 minutes

after administration and continues for 45 to 120 minutes)

8. Disadvantages
   a. Difficult technique to perform
   b. Potential for trauma to the spinal cord or venous sinuses
9. Complications
   a. Loss of motor control of the pelvic limbs caused by overdose or subarachnoid injection
   b. Physiologic disturbance caused by overdose or subarachnoid injection
   c. Potential for trauma to the spinal cord or venous sinuses

ANESTHESIA FOR OBSTETRIC PROCEDURES AND RELIEF OF RECTAL TENESMUS

I. Caudal epidural anesthesia and desensitization of the internal pudendal nerve are commonly used in ruminants for obstetric manipulations, caudal surgical procedures, and as an adjunct treatment for control of rectal tenesmus; these techniques are not effective in pigs

II. Cattle
   A. Low posterior or caudal epidural anesthesia
      1. Area blocked: anus, perineum, vulva, and vagina
      2. Nerves blocked: coccygeal and posterior sacral nerves
      3. Site: first intercoccygeal space (Co1-Co2: Fig. 5-5, *A*; more commonly and easily) or sacrococcygeal space (S5-Co1)
      4. Needle: 18-gauge, 3.8- to 5.1-cm (average dairy cow)
      5. Anesthetic: 5 to 6 ml of 2% lidocaine or other drugs (Table 4-2)
      6. Method: the skin overlying the spinal column is clipped, surgically scrubbed, and disinfected; locate the sacrococcygeal joint by moving the tail up and down; this joint moves very little and is located just anterior to the anal folds; the first intercoccygeal joint is easily located by its movement; it is much wider and is posterior to the anal folds; insert the needle exactly

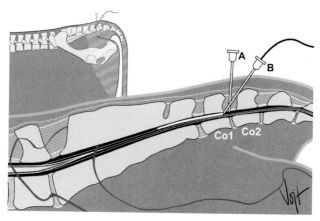

Fig. 5-5
Needle placement for **A,** caudal epidural anesthesia and **B,** continuous caudal epidural anesthesia in cattle. *Co1* is the first coccygeal vertebra, and *Co2* is the second coccygeal vertebra. Desensitized area of skin is patterned in diagonals.

at the midline of the first intercoccygeal space at a right angle (approximately 10 degrees to vertical) to the skin surface; push the needle ventrally through the interarcuate ligament to the floor of the neural canal, which is at approximately 2 to 4 cm; withdraw the needle slightly (approximately 0.5 cm) into epidural space and test by injecting 1 ml of air; no resistance should be felt

7. Advantages
   a. Minimal effect on cardiovascular and respiratory systems
   b. Little effect on organ systems
   c. Little problem with toxicity
   d. Good muscle relaxation
   e. Good postoperative analgesia
   f. Rapid recovery
   g. Relatively simple
   h. Inexpensive

8. Disadvantages
   a. Technically difficult if Co1-Co2 interspace is not identified
   b. Technically difficult if the sacrococcygeal interspace is ossified in older cows
9. Complications
   a. Rare
   b. Infection resulting in draining tracts or permanently paralyzed tail
   c. Possible ataxia and collapse caused by overdose
   d. Hemorrhage caused by puncture of a venous sinus

B. Continuous caudal epidural anesthesia
   1. Indications: painful prolapse of the vagina and/or rectum that provokes severe continuous straining
   2. Nerves blocked: coccygeal and posterior sacral nerves
   3. Site: first intercoccygeal space; Co1-Co2 (or sacrococcygeal space; S5-Co1) (Fig. 5-5, *B*)
   4. Needle: 16- or 17-gauge, 7.6-cm, thin-walled, Huberpoint directional needle or Hustead needle
   5. Catheter: 30-cm, medical-grade vinyl catheter (0.036 cm outside diameter) or a commercially available epidural catheter with graduated markings
   6. Anesthetic: 3 to 5 ml of 2% lidocaine every 4 to 6 hours
   7. Method: the skin overlying the spinal column is clipped, surgically scrubbed, and disinfected; identify the first intercoccygeal joint as previously described; desensitize the skin and needle tract; with stylet in place and bevel directed cranial, advance the spinal needle 5 to 8 cm approximately 45 degrees to vertical, until an abrupt reduction in resistance to needle passage is noted; remove the stylet from the needle and inject 3 ml (test dose) of 2% lidocaine with minimal resistance; the test dose ensures proper placement of the needle in the vertebral canal; place the catheter aseptically, introduce into the canal through the needle, and advance it cranially approximately 3 to 4 cm beyond the tip of the needle (Fig. 5-5, *B*); withdraw the needle, leaving the catheter in

position; inject local anesthetic solution into the catheter at 4- to 6-hour intervals or as needed; place a catheter adapter on the free end of the catheter; secure the catheter at the entrance into the skin with adhesive tape sutured to the skin; place a protective sterile gauze over the free end of the catheter to allow the catheter to be used for many hours of infusion in the field

8. Advantages
   a. Similar to caudal epidural anesthesia
   b. Repeated administration of small fractional doses of local anesthesia
   c. No fibrosis of the extradural space from repeated standard epidural blocks
9. Disadvantages
   a. Similar to caudal epidural anesthesia
   b. Greater cost of equipment
   c. Acute tolerance to repeated injections
10. Complications
   a. Similar to caudal epidural anesthesia
   b. Kinking and curling of the catheter and occlusion of the tip with fibrin

C. Internal pudendal nerve block
   1. Indications
      a. Analgesia and relaxation of the penis for examination
      b. Relief of tenesmus associated with vaginal and uterine prolapse
   2. Nerves blocked: internal pudendal (fibers of the ventral branches of S3 and S4), caudal rectal (fibers of the ventral branches of S4 and S5), and pelvic splanchnic nerves
   3. Site: identified by rectal palpation (Fig. 5-6)
   4. Needle: spinal, preferably 18-gauge, 10.2-cm
   5. Anesthetic: up to 35 ml of 2% lidocaine per side
   6. Method: use rectal palpation to locate the lesser sciatic foramen, a soft, circumscribed depression in the sacrosciatic ligament; find the nerve a finger's width dorsal to the pudendal artery present in the fossa; pass the needle through the disinfected skin in the

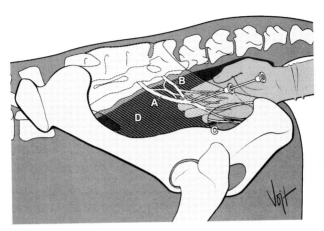

Fig. 5-6
Right hand and needle placement at the internal pudendal nerve on the medial side of the left pelvis. **A,** Internal pudendal nerve. **B,** Pelvic splanchnic nerves. **C,** Pudendal artery. **D,** Sacrosciatic ligament.

ischiorectal fossa; deposit up to 25 ml of 2% lidocaine around the nerve; withdraw and direct the needle 2 to 3 cm caudodorsally and inject another 10 ml of the anesthetic in the area of the pelvic splanchnic nerve; repeat the procedure on the opposite side of the pelvis

7. Advantages
   a. No loss of tail tone
   b. No sciatic nerve involvement
   c. Ballooning of the vagina may aid in retention of the vagina after it is repositioned in a cow with prolapse

8. Disadvantages
   a. Technical difficulty and necessity of identifying the injection sites by rectal palpation
   b. Lack of cervical anesthesia
   c. Anesthesia duration of 3 to 6 hours
   d. Larger volume of anesthetic

9. Complications: injury to the bull's penis, which must be protected from injury by replacing it into the prepuce

III. Sheep and goats: low posterior or caudal, epidural anesthesia
  A. Similar to that used in cattle
  B. Excellent for tail docking in lambs and intravaginal obstetric procedures
  C. Alcohol-epidural injection for continuous caudal epidural anesthesia
     1. Can be used for long-term demyelinization
     2. First, 0.5 to 1 ml/50 kg of 2% lidocaine hydrochloride is injected epidurally as a test; after full sensation has returned, a mixture of equal volumes of 70% to 95% ethyl or isopropyl alcohol and 2% lidocaine solution is injected; analgesia of the pelvic and perineal area and paralysis of the tail lasts from a few days to several months
     3. Inflammation, necrosis, and purulence can occur because of fly strike
  D. Internal pudendal nerve block
     1. Needle: spinal, 18-gauge, 3.8-cm
     2. Anesthetic: 3 to 5 ml of 2% lidocaine per site
     3. Method: A gloved finger is placed into the rectum to locate the slitlike sciatic foramen; insert a needle through the corresponding skin site while advancing its point to the foremen and inject 3 to 5 ml of the anesthetic; withdraw the needle and massage the injection site; repeat the procedure on the opposite side of the pelvis

ANTERIOR EPIDURAL ANESTHESIA

I. Anterior epidural anesthesia can be used for all procedures caudal to the diaphragm; the lumbosacral space is commonly used in calves, sheep, and goats because the injection sites are usually palpable; this space is the only practical injection site for producing anterior anesthesia in pigs. The sacrococcygeal or first intercoccygeal space is the injection site of choice in adult cattle for producing anterior anesthesia, because the technique is relatively simple and avoids trauma to the spinal cord and meninges; proper techniques should provide anesthesia of the following areas:
  A. Perineal region

    B. Inguinal region

    C. Flank

    D. Abdominal wall caudal to the umbilicus

II. Increasing the dose (volume × concentration) of the anesthetic increases the area of blockade

    A. Increasing the volume improves segmental spread

    B. Increasing the concentration produces a more rapid onset, greater effects, and longer duration of analgesia and motor blockade

III. Rapid epidural injections must be avoided to prevent complications

    A. Discomfort to the patient

    B. Increased rate of vascular absorption, which can result in less drug for neural uptake; reduced neural uptake can result in the following:

        1. Reduced duration of action

        2. Higher incidence of incomplete anesthesia

        3. Only a slight increase in segmental spread

IV. The technique is contraindicated in animals with certain known conditions:

    A. Severe cardiovascular disease

    B. Bleeding disorders

    C. Shock or toxemic syndromes because of sympathetic block and resulting depression of blood pressure

V. The following complications may result from overdose or subarachnoid injection

    A. Transient loss of consciousness

    B. Flexor spasm

    C. Rapid muscular contractions

    D. Convulsions

    E. Respiratory paralysis

    F. Hypotension

    G. Hypothermia

    H. Possibly headache after dural puncture (changes in CSF pressure)

VI. Small ruminants (sheep and goats)

    A. Landmarks and techniques for injection at the lumbosacral space are similar to those used in dogs (Fig. 5-7, *C*); the site for needle placement is usually palpable as a

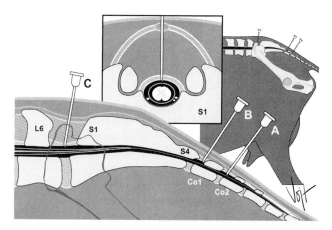

Fig. 5-7
Needle placement for caudal epidural anesthesia (**A** and **B**) and anterior epidural anesthesia (**C**) in the goat. **A,** Lateral aspect and cranial view of a transection to the first sacral vertebra. A needle is placed into **A,** the first intercoccygeal vertebral space; **B,** the sacrococcygeal space; and **C,** the lumbosacral space.

depression on the midline just caudal to a line joining the anterior border of the ilium on each side

B. Dose: 0.2 ml/kg of 2% lidocaine

C. Effect
  1. Onset of posterior paralysis occurs in 2 to 15 minutes
  2. Anesthesia generally reaches three fourths of the distance from pubis to umbilicus
  3. Duration of action is 1 to 2 hours
  4. Similar extent and duration of anesthesia can be achieved if only half the dose (0.1 ml/kg) is injected subarachnoidally (the space from which spinal fluid is aspirated into the syringe) at a rate of 1 ml every 2 to 3 seconds; true CSF anesthesia results with the onset of posterior paralysis within 1 to 3 minutes and lasts 60 to 90 minutes; anesthesia may extend to the last rib
  5. Gravity, not diffusion of drug in the CSF, determines the spread of anesthesia

6. Morphine (0.1 mg/kg) diluted with saline solution to a volume of 5 ml can be injected epidurally after orthopedic procedures to produce 9 or more hours of analgesia and sedation with minimal cardiopulmonary complications

VII. Pigs

A. Used for
   1. Cesarean section
   2. Repair of rectal, uterine, or vaginal prolapses
   3. Repair of umbilical, inguinal, or scrotal hernias
   4. Surgery of scirrhous cord
   5. Surgery of the prepuce, penis, or rear limbs

B. Landmarks and techniques for injection at the lumbosacral space are similar to those used in dogs and small ruminants (Fig. 5-8)

C. Dose when using 2% lidocaine: calculated by either weight or length of the pig
   1. By weight
      a. 1 ml/5 kg
      b. 1 ml/7.5 kg for pigs up to 50 kg and an additional 1 ml/10 kg

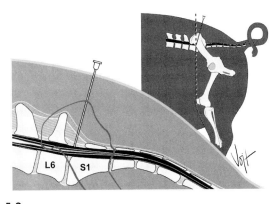

Fig. 5-8

Needle placement for epidural anesthesia in the pig. *L6* is the sixth lumbar vertebra, and *S1* is the first sacral vertebra.

2. By length
   a. 1 ml for the first 40 cm of back length from the base
   of the tail and an additional 1.5 ml/10 cm

LUMBOSACRAL EPIDURAL ANESTHESIA IN PIGS	
STANDING CASTRATION	**CESAREAN SECTION**
4 ml/100 kg	10 ml/100 kg
6 ml/200 kg	15 ml/200 kg
8 ml/300 kg	20 ml/300 kg

D. Effect
   1. Onset of anesthetic action generally occurs within
   5 minutes
   2. Maximum effect is within 15 to 20 minutes
   3. Duration of action is 120 minutes
   4. Most pigs develop posterior paresis

LOCAL ANESTHESIA FOR DEHORNING

I. Cattle
   A. Area blocked: horn and base of the horn
   B. Nerves blocked: cornual branch of zygomaticotemporal
      (lacrimal) nerve, a portion of the ophthalmic division of
      the trigeminal nerve
   C. Site: temporal ridge, 2 to 3 cm from the base of horn
      (Fig. 5-9); needle penetration is from 1 cm in small cattle
      to 2.5 cm in large bulls
   D. Needle: 18-gauge, 2.54-cm
   E. Anesthetic: 5 to 10 ml of 2% lidocaine
   F. Method: palpate the lateral temporal ridge of the frontal
      bone; the nerve is relatively superficial, 7 to 10 mm deep
      on the upper third of the ridge, lying between the thin
      frontalis muscle and the temporal muscle, and can usually
      be palpated between these muscles; aspiration ensures
      that the needle point is not inadvertently intravascular;
      inject 2 to 3 cm in front of the base of the horn

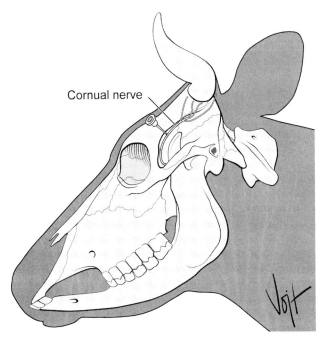

Cornual nerve

Fig. 5-9
Needle placement for desensitizing the cornual branch of the zygomati-cotemporal nerve in the cow.

G. Advantages
1. Minimal systemic effects on the cardiopulmonary system
2. Relatively simple procedure
H. Disadvantages
1. Cornual anesthesia does not result if the anesthetic is injected too deeply in the aponeurosis of the temporal muscle
2. A second injection posterior to the horn may be required in adult cattle with well-developed horns
3. Anesthesia of a fractured horn involving the frontal bone or sinuses may require a Peterson eye block
I. Complications: none

II. Goats
   A. Area blocked: horn and base of the horn
   B. Nerves blocked: cornual branch of the zygomaticotemporal (lacrimal) nerve and cornual branch of the infratrochlear nerve
   C. Site: halfway between lateral canthus of the eye and lateral base of the horn (lacrimal nerve) (Fig. 5-10, *A*) and halfway between medial canthus of the eye and medial base of the horn (cornual branch of infratrochlear nerve) (Fig. 5-10, *B*)

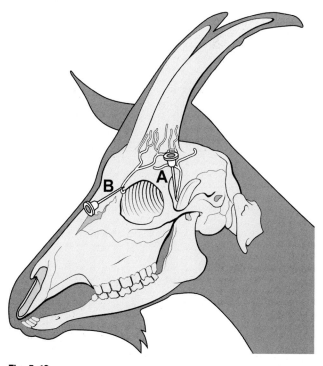

Fig. 5-10
Needle placement for desensitizing **A,** the cornual branch of the zygomaticotemporal (lacrimal) nerve; and **B,** the cornual branch of the infratrochlear nerve in the goat.

D. Needle: 22-gauge, 2.54-cm
E. Anesthetic: 2 to 3 ml of 2% lidocaine at each site in the adult goat; no more than 0.5 ml of 2% lidocaine per site (or 1 ml of 1% lidocaine) for ring block at the horn base in young kids 7 to 14 days of age
F. Method: to reach the cornual branch of the zygomaticotemporal nerve, insert the needle as close as possible to the caudal ridge of the supraorbital process and 1 to 1.5 cm deep (Fig. 5-10, *A*); to reach the cornual branch of the infratrochlear nerve, insert the needle dorsal and parallel to the dorsomedial margin of the orbit; inject the anesthetic in a line, because this nerve is frequently branched (Fig. 5-10, *B*)
G. Advantages
   1. Alleviation of pain during dehorning
   2. Alleviation of pain during disbudding
H. Disadvantages
   1. Sedation of the animal is required if the frontal sinus will be entered during horn removal
   2. A total dose of 10 mg/kg (0.5 ml of 2% solution per kilogram or 1 ml of a 1% solution per kilogram) must not be exceeded to minimize adverse reactions
 I. Complications: toxicity caused by overdose of lidocaine and any of the following clinical signs:
   1. Excitation
   2. Lateral recumbency
   3. Muscular twitching
   4. Generalized tonic-clonic convulsions
   5. Opisthotonus
   6. Coma
   7. Respiratory depression
   8. Cardiac arrest

LOCAL ANESTHESIA FOR THE EYE

I. Topical and regional anesthetic techniques are used for surgery of the eye and its associated structures; paralysis of the eyelids (without analgesia) is accomplished by selectively desensitizing the auriculopalpebral branch of the facial nerve (producing akinesia); anesthesia of the eye and orbit and immobilization of the globe are commonly achieved by the Peterson technique (Fig. 5-11)

A. Area blocked: eye and orbit, orbicularis oculi muscle, *except* the eyelids

B. Nerves blocked: oculomotor, trochlear, and abducens nerves and the three branches of the trigeminal nerve (ophthalmic, maxillary, and mandibular)

C. Sites: the points at which these nerves emerge from the foramen orbitorotundum

D. Needle: 14-gauge, 2.5-cm to serve as a cannula; 18-gauge, 10.2- to 12.7-cm

E. Anesthetic: 7 to 15 ml of 2% lidocaine at the foramen orbitorotundum; 5 to 10 ml of 2% lidocaine for desensitizing the auriculopalpebral nerve

F. Method

   1. Fully extend cow's head in a standing position with frontal and nasal bones parallel to the ground

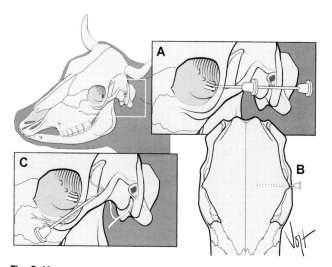

Fig. 5-11
Needle placement for Peterson eye block, with needle tip at the foramen orbitorotundum. **A,** Craniolateral aspect. **B,** Dorsal aspect. **C,** Needle placement for akinesia of the eyelids in the cow.

2. Surgically prepare area posterior and ventral to the eye
3. Inject several milliliters of anesthetic with a small-gauge needle into the skin and subcutaneously into the notch formed by the zygomatic and temporal process of the malar bone (where the supraorbital process of the frontal bone meets the zygomatic arch) (Fig. 5-11)
4. Place a 14-gauge, 1.3- to 2.54-cm needle (to serve as a cannula) through the skin as far anterior and ventral as possible in the notch
5. Direct a straight, 18-gauge, 12.7-cm needle with no syringe attached (to feel the bony landmarks) through the cannula in a horizontal and slightly posterior direction, until it strikes the coronoid process of the mandible
6. Reposition the point of the needle anteriorly until it passes medially around this bone
7. Advance needle slightly posteriorly and somewhat ventrally until it strikes a solid bony plate, which is at a depth of between 7.6 to 10.2 cm
8. Inject 15 ml of 2% lidocaine anterior to the foramen orbitorotundum
9. Block the auriculopalpebral branch of the facial nerve (Fig. 5-11, *C*)
   a. Fill a 10-ml syringe with local anesthetic, attach it to the needle, and partially withdraw the cannula
   b. Withdraw the needle until it almost leaves the skin and direct it posteriorly for 5 to 7.5 cm lateral to the zygomatic arch while injecting lidocaine
   c. If the upper lid is involved in the surgical procedure, make a line of infiltration with local anesthetic subcutaneously approximately 2.5 cm from the margin of the lid

G. Advantages
   1. Technique is useful for surgery of the cornea, enucleation of the eyeball, and removal of tumors from the eye and eyelids
   2. Technique is quick, safe, and effective if done properly
   3. Less edema and inflammation result than when the eyelids and the orbit are infiltrated

4. Surgery of the cornea (removal of tumors and dermoids) can be done easily without retraction or fixation forceps if the eyeball is proptosed
5. Peterson eye block is safer than retrobulbar injections of local anesthetic, which often lead to orbital hemorrhage, direct pressure on the globe, penetration of the globe, damage to the optic nerve, or injection into the optic nerve meninges

H. Disadvantages
1. Technique is difficult
2. The cow's head is difficult to keep horizontal when the animal is in a chute or stanchion with the head tied to one side; this makes the landmarks difficult to locate
3. If the needle point strikes the pterygoid crest, the anesthetic drug will be deposited at the wrong site; therefore no anesthesia results after injection of the local anesthetic
4. In 50% of cases incomplete anesthesia of the upper eyelid results because of sensory innervation from other nerves
5. Blinking is prevented for several hours
6. Sterile saline solution should be applied to the eye frequently during surgery to keep the cornea moist
7. Antibiotic eye ointments should be applied to the cornea after orbital replacement of the globe
8. Sunlight, dust, and wind in the eye must be avoided to prevent keratoconjunctivitis
9. The lids may be sutured together until motor activity of the lids returns

I. Complications
1. In procedures other than enucleation, keratitis may result from postoperative drying of the cornea because effective block prevents blinking for several hours
2. Penetration of the turbinates and injection with local anesthetic into the nasopharynx and optic nerve meninges can cause severe central nervous system toxicity, including certain clinical signs:
   a. Hyperexcitability
   b. Lateral recumbency

c. Tonic-clonic convulsions
d. Opisthotonus
e. Respiratory arrest
f. Cardiac arrest

LOCAL ANESTHESIA OF THE FOOT: THREE METHODS

I. Infiltrating the tissues around the limb with local anesthetic solution (ring block)
II. Desensitizing specific nerves (regional anesthesia)
   A. Brachial plexus block
   B. Epidural anesthesia
III. Injecting local anesthetic solution into an accessible superficial vein in an extremity isolated from circulation by placing a tourniquet on an animal's leg (intravenous regional anesthesia)
   A. Area blocked: extremity distal to tourniquet
   B. Veins used: *A*, Common dorsal metacarpal vein; *B*, radial vein; *C*, plantar metacarpal vein in the thoracic limb; *D*, cranial branch of the lateral saphenous vein, lateral plantar digital vein in the pelvic limb (Fig. 5-12)
   C. Needle: 20- to 22-gauge, 2.54- to 3.81-cm
   D. Anesthetic: 10 to 30 ml of 2% lidocaine (without epinephrine) in adult cattle; 3 to 10 ml lidocaine in small ruminants and pigs
   E. Method: place rubber tourniquet (inflation pressure >200 mm Hg) proximal to the metatarsal or metacarpal region for foot surgery or at a more proximal position for surgery of the carpal or tarsal region; rapidly inject local anesthetic into the prominent vein, directing the needle either proximally or distally
   F. Advantages
      1. Technique is simple and safe
      2. Can be used for the analgesia of the digit in cattle, small ruminants, and pigs; ideal for digital surgery because the amount of bleeding at the surgical site is decreased
      3. No special skill or knowledge of anatomy of the limb is needed

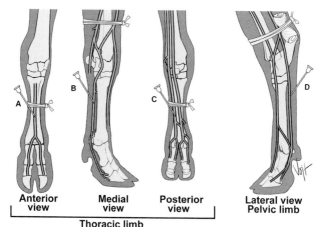

Anterior view	Medial view	Posterior view	Lateral view Pelvic limb

Thoracic limb

Fig. 5-12

Tourniquet and needle placement for intravenous regional anesthesia of the cow. In the thoracic limb, the needle tip is placed at **A,** the common dorsal metacarpal vein; **B** the radial vein; or **C,** the plantar metacarpal vein. In the pelvic limb, the needle tip is placed at **D,** the cranial branch of the lateral saphenous vein.

    4. Only one injection is required, with little risk of introducing bacteria

    5. Onset of anesthesia distal to the tourniquet is rapid (5 to 10 minutes); anesthesia occurs last in the interdigital region

    6. Recovery is rapid after removal of the tourniquet (5 to 10 minutes)

  G. Disadvantages

    1. Inexplicable failure rate of 7%

    2. Occasional hematoma at the injection site

    3. Failure of anesthesia caused by tourniquet slipping or extravascular injection

  H. Complications: ischemic necrosis, severe lameness, and edema if the tourniquet is left in place longer than 2 hours

TEAT AND UDDER ANESTHESIA OF CATTLE

I. Techniques for surgical procedures on the forequarters and foreteats
   A. Paravertebral anesthesia of L1, L2, and L3 spinal nerves
   B. Segmental lumbar epidural anesthesia of L1, L2, and L3 spinal nerves
   C. Both techniques are difficult and often result in cows lying down

II. Techniques for surgical procedures of the caudal-most teats and escutcheon areas of the udder
   A. Desensitization of the perineal nerve in the standing cow
   B. High caudal epidural anesthesia in recumbent ruminants
   C. Lumbosacral epidural anesthesia in recumbent ruminants

III. Most surgical procedures on the teat (e.g., repair of a stenotic teat sphincter, repairs of teat fistulae, lacerations, and injuries) are generally performed with the animal under local anesthesia
   A. Needle: 25-gauge, 1.3-cm or teat cannula
   B. Anesthetic: 4 to 10 ml of 2% lidocaine
   C. Methods
      1. Inverted V block: line infusion of the anesthetic using an inverted V pattern, which encloses the teat skin defect (Fig. 5-13, *A*)
      2. Ring block: local anesthetic infused into the skin and muscular tissue of base of the teat, after thorough cleaning of the external surface of the teat and quarter (Fig. 5-13, *B*)
      3. Teat infusion block
         a. Teat opening is cleaned
         b. Tourniquet is placed at the base of the teat
         c. 10 ml of 2% lidocaine is infused into the teat cistern (Fig. 5-13, *C*)
         d. Mucous membrane of the teat cistern is anesthetized within 5 minutes; the muscular and skin layers remain sensitive; thereafter the remaining lidocaine is milked out, and the tourniquet is removed

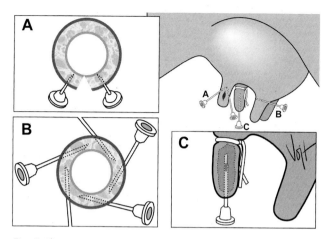

Fig. 5-13
Needle placement in the cow's teat. **A,** Inverted V block. **B,** Teat ring block. **C,** Tourniquet and cannula placement for teat cistern infusion.

CHAPTER SIX

Local Anesthesia in Horses

"A horse is dangerous at both ends and uncomfortable in the middle."

IAN FLEMING

OVERVIEW

Many diagnostic and surgical procedures can be performed safely and humanely on horses by coupling physical restraint and sedation with surface (topical) anesthesia, infiltration anesthesia, nerve block (regional) anesthesia, or epidural anesthesia. Peripheral nerve blocks, intraarticular and intrabursal injections, and local infiltrations (ring block) are used to diagnose equine lameness and to anesthetize surgical sites. Desensitization of the auriculopalpebral nerve is most frequently used to prevent voluntary closure of the eyelids during examination and treatment of the eye. Although regional anesthesia of the head can be induced by various techniques, the most frequently desensitized nerves are the supraorbital, infraorbital, and mandibular alveolar.

Caudal epidural anesthesia is used to facilitate surgery involving the tail, perineum, anus, rectum, vulva, vagina, and urethra and for symptomatic relief of painful conditions during obstetric manipulations.

Improper injection techniques contribute to inadequate anesthesia. Overdosing potentially leads to more serious complications including ataxia of hindlimbs, hindlimb motor blockade, recumbency, and respiratory depression.

REGIONAL ANESTHESIA OF THE HEAD

The Most Frequently Desensitized Nerves of the Head

  I. Supraorbital (frontal)
  II. Auriculopalpebral

III. Infraorbital
IV. Mandibular alveolar

ANESTHESIA OF THE UPPER EYELID AND FOREHEAD

I. Area blocked: upper eyelid except medial and lateral canthi
II. Nerve blocked: supraorbital (or frontal) nerve
III. Site: supraorbital foramen (Fig. 6-1, *A*)
IV. Needle: 22- to 25-gauge, 2.54-cm
V. Anesthetic: 5 ml of 2% lidocaine
VI. Method: palpate the supraorbital foramen approximately 5 to 7 cm above the medial canthus where it perforates the supraorbital process of the frontal bone; insert the needle into the foramen to a depth of 1.5 to 2 cm; inject 2 ml of lidocaine into the foramen; 1 ml as the needle is withdrawn and 2 ml subcutaneously over the foramen
VII. Use
    A. Desensitization of the upper eyelid
    B. Palpebral motor supply is derived from the auriculopalpebral nerve

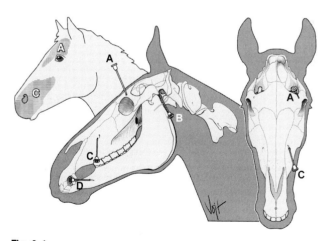

Fig. 6-1
Needle placement for nerve blocks on the head. **A,** Supraorbital (or frontal). **B,** Auriculopalpebral. **C,** Infraorbital. **D,** Mandibular alveolar nerves.

AKINESIA OF THE EYELIDS

I. Area blocked: paralysis of orbicularis oculi muscles; no desensitization
II. Nerve blocked: auriculopalpebral nerve (Fig. 6-1, *B*)
III. Site: caudal to posterior ramus of the mandible
IV. Needle: 22- to 25-gauge, 2.54-cm
V. Anesthetic: 5 ml of 2% lidocaine
VI. Method: insert the needle into the depression caudal to the mandible at the ventral edge of the temporal part of the zygomatic arch; inject local anesthetic subfascially as the needle is withdrawn
VII. Use: examination of the eye; successful blockade of the motor nerve supply prevents the horse from closing the eyelids

ANESTHESIA OF THE UPPER LIP AND NOSE

I. Area blocked: upper lip and nostril, roof of nasal cavity, and related skin up to the infraorbital foramen
II. Nerve blocked: infraorbital nerve
III. Site: external opening of the infraorbital canal (Fig. 6-1, *C*)
IV. Needle: 20- to 25-gauge, 2.54-cm
V. Anesthetic: 5 ml of 2% lidocaine
VI. Method: halfway along the bony lip of the infraorbital foramen, about 2.5 cm dorsal to a line connecting the nasomaxillary notch and the rostral end of the facial crest; push the flat levator labii superioris muscle, which runs over the foramen, upward with the fingertips and place the needle tip at the foramen opening
VII. Use: simple lacerations in quiet or sedated horses

ANESTHESIA OF THE LOWER LIP AND PREMOLARS

I. Area blocked: lower lip, all parts of mandible rostral up to and including the third premolar tooth (PM3)
II. Nerve blocked: mandibuloalveolar nerve
III. Site: within mandibular canal (Fig. 6-1, *D*)
IV. Needle: 20-gauge, 7.6-cm
V. Anesthetic: 10 ml of 2% lidocaine

VI. Method: palpate the lateral border of the mental foramen as a ridge along the lateral aspect of the ramus in the middle of the interdental space; insert the needle into the foramen as far as possible in a ventromedial direction; injection requires pressure, and fluid might partially drain back from the canal under the skin

VII. Use: simple lacerations in quiet or sedated horses. The technique is difficult so tooth extraction is better done with the animal under general anesthesia

CAUDAL EPIDURAL ANESTHESIA

I. Area blocked: tail, perineum, anus, rectum, vulva, vagina, urethra, and bladder

II. Nerves blocked: coccygeal and last three pairs of sacral nerves

III. Site: epidural space in the first intercoccygeal space (Co1-Co2) (Fig. 6-2)

IV. Needles: spinal with stylet (spinal: 18-gauge, 5.1- to 7.6-cm)

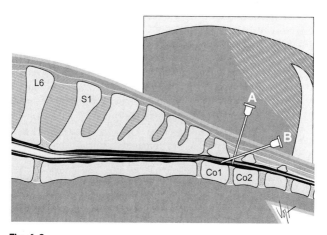

Fig. 6-2

Needle placement into **A** or **B,** caudal epidural space at the first intercoccygeal space (Co1-Co2). Stippled markings indicate desensitized subcutaneous area after caudal blockade.

V. Anesthetic: 6 to 10 ml of 2% lidocaine; other drugs can be considered (see Table 4-2)

VI. Method

A. Use proper restraint, depending on the horse's temperament; clip, surgically scrub, and disinfect the injection site; make a skin wheal and infiltrate the tissues down to the interarcuate ligament with 1 to 3 ml of 2% lidocaine to minimize movement during insertion of the spinal needle

B. Method A (see Fig. 6-2, *A*): insert the spinal needle into the epidural space in the center of the first intercoccygeal space (approximately 5 cm cranial to the origin of the first tail hairs and the caudal fold of the tail) at a right angle to the general contour of the croup and press the needle ventrally in a median plane until it strikes the floor of the vertebral canal; withdraw the needle approximately 0.5 cm

C. Method B (see Fig. 6-2, *B*): insert the spinal needle approximately 2.5 cm caudal to the first intercoccygeal space and slide its point ventrocranially at an angle of approximately 30 degrees to the horizontal plane and to its full length into the vertebral canal

D. Test with a syringe of air for resistance to the injection; alternatively, fill the needle hub with isotonic saline solution and manipulate slightly until the solution is aspirated from the needle by subatmospheric epidural pressure (hanging drop technique); inject local anesthetic; needle can be left in place with stylet reinserted; maximum blockade may require 10 to 30 minutes, and it is not advisable to redose during this time if surgery is to be done with the horse standing

VII. Use

A. Anesthesia of pelvic viscera without loss of hind leg motor control during obstetric manipulations

B. Anesthesia of genitalia without loss of hind leg motor control during obstetric manipulations

C. For standing surgical procedures of viscera and genitalia
1. Caslick procedure (for pneumovagina)
2. Rectovaginal fistula repair
3. Prolapsed rectum repair

      4. Urethrostomy

      5. Tail amputation

      6. Tenesmus prevention

VIII. Common causes for inadequate anesthesia or incomplete block

    A. Improper injection technique

      1. Use of solutions of diminished potency

      2. Inadequate dispersal of anesthetic

    B. Inappropriate angulation of the spinal needle

      1. Needle point strikes the dorsal aspect of the vertebral arch

      2. Deviation of the needle from the midline

    C. Horses that have fibrous connective tissue from previous epidural injections, which limits diffusion of anesthetic agent

    D. Anatomic peculiarities

      1. Presence of septa within the epidural space

      2. Presence of patent intervertebral foramina

IX. Potential complications

    A. Trauma to coccygeal nerve(s)

    B. Infection of the neural canal

    C. Extensive cranial migration of local anesthetic solution causing the following:

      1. Ataxia

      2. Staggering

      3. Excitement

      4. Recumbency

REGIONAL ANESTHESIA OF THE LIMB

I. Begin by blocking the most distal branches of the nerve trunks to most effectively localize potential sites of lameness. If lameness is not resolved, continue the examination by injecting local anesthetics more proximally, increasing the size of the desensitized area

II. The palmar (volar) digital nerves of the forelimb or the plantar digital nerves of the hindlimb branch dorsal to the fetlock at the level of the sesamoids, forming three digital nerves

    A. The dorsal digital nerve supplies sensory fibers to the anterior two thirds of the hoof

B. The middle digital nerve (relatively unimportant)
C. The low palmar or plantar digital nerve, which is the most important clinically, supplies sensory fibers to the distal palmar or plantar third of the hoof, including portions, if not all, of the navicular area

PALMAR (VOLAR) OR PLANTAR DIGITAL NERVE BLOCK (Figs. 6-3, *A* and 6-4, *A*)

I. Area blocked: distal palmar or plantar third of the foot, including the navicular bursa
II. Nerves blocked: digital nerves
III. Site: palmar (volar)/plantar region of the pastern joint
IV. Needle: 20- to 25-gauge, 2.54-cm
V. Anesthetic: 1 to 2 ml of 2% lidocaine at each site
VI. Method: palpate the palmar (volar) or plantar nerve just palmar/plantar to the digital vein and artery, dorsal to the flexor tendon; insert the needle in the palmar/plantar region

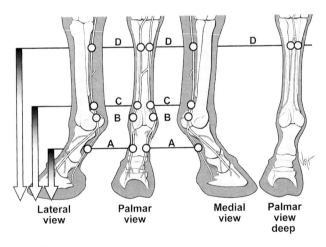

Fig. 6-3
Injection sites for nerve blocks on the left forelimb in the horse. **A,** Palmar (digital). **B,** Abaxial sesamoidean. **C,** Low palmar. **D,** High palmar metacarpal nerves.

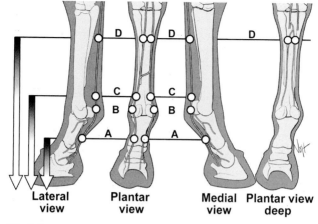

Fig. 6-4
Injection sites for nerve blocks on the left hindlimb in the horse. **A,** Plantar digital. **B,** Abaxial sesamoidean. **C,** Low plantar. **D,** High plantar metatarsal nerves.

of the pastern joint, medially and/or laterally with the leg elevated or bearing weight
VII. Use: diagnosis of equine lameness

ABAXIAL (BASILAR) SESAMOIDEAN NERVE BLOCK
(Figs. 6-3, *B* and 6-4, *B*)

I. Area blocked: entire foot distal to the injection site, including the back of the pastern area and distal sesamoidean ligaments
II. Nerves blocked: anterior and posterior digital nerves
III. Site: palmar region of the fetlock joint over abaxial surface of proximal sesamoids
IV. Needle: 20- to 25-gauge, 2.54-cm
V. Anesthetic: 3 ml of 2% lidocaine at each site
VI. Method: palpate the digital nerve in the palmar region of the fetlock joint over the abaxial surface of proximal sesamoids, just palmar/plantar to the digital artery and vein; insert the needle subcutaneously at this site
VII. Use: diagnosis of equine lameness

PALMAR (VOLAR) OR PLANTAR NERVE BLOCK

I. The palmar (volar) or plantar nerves can be desensitized at either a low site (low palmar/volar or low plantar nerve block) or a high site (high palmar/volar or high plantar nerve block)

II. Midregion blocks (midmetacarpal or midmetatarsal) should be avoided because of the location of the anastomotic branch, which traverses downward from medial to lateral

LOW PALMAR (VOLAR) OR PLANTAR NERVE BLOCK
(Figs. 6-3, C and 6-4, C)

I. Area blocked: almost all structures distal to the fetlock and fetlock joint, except for a small area dorsal to the fetlock joint supplied by sensory fibers of the ulnar (Fig. 6-5) and musculocutaneous nerves (Fig. 6-6)

II. Nerves blocked: palmar metacarpal or plantar metatarsal nerves (medial/lateral: four-point block)

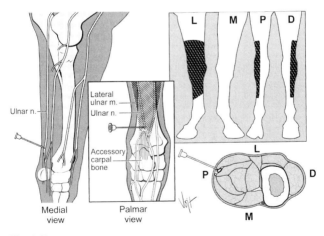

Fig. 6-5
Needle placement for ulnar nerve block: lateral, palmar, and cross-sectional views. Stippled markings indicate desensitized area (L, lateral; M, medial; P, palmar; and D, dorsal views) after ulnar nerve block of the left forelimb.

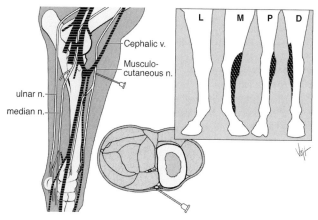

Fig. 6-6

Needle placement for median nerve block: medial and cross-sectional views. Stippled markings indicate desensitized area (*L*, lateral; *M*, medial; *P*, palmar; and *D*, dorsal views) after median nerve block of the left forelimb.

III. Site: medially and laterally at the level of the distal enlargements of metacarpals II and IV and metatarsals II and IV (splints)
IV. Needle: 20- to 25-gauge, 2.54-cm
V. Anesthetic: 2 to 3 ml of 2% lidocaine at each site
VI. Method
    A. Location: just distal to the buttons of the splint bones
    B. Desensitize the palmar nerves (medial/lateral) by injecting the anesthetic between the flexor tendon and suspensory ligament
    C. Desensitize the palmar metacarpal and metatarsal nerves (medial/lateral) by injecting the anesthetic between the suspensory ligament and the splint bone
    Use: diagnosis of equine lameness

HIGH PALMAR (VOLAR) OR PLANTAR NERVE BLOCK
(Figs. 6-3, *D* and 6-4, *D*)

I. Area blocked: palmar (volar) metacarpal or plantar metatarsal region and all of the digit distal to the fetlock

II. Nerves blocked: palmar or plantar nerves (medial/lateral)
III. Site: proximal quarter of the metacarpus or metatarsus proximal to the communicating branch of the medial and lateral palmar (volar) or plantar nerves
IV. Needle: 22-gauge, 3.81-cm
V. Anesthetic: 5 ml of 2% lidocaine at each site
VI. Method: desensitize the medial and lateral palmar (volar) and plantar nerves by injecting anesthetic subfascially into the groove between the suspensory ligament and the deep flexor tendon on both the medial and lateral sides
VII. Use
    A. Diagnosis of equine lameness
    B. The ulnar, median, and musculocutaneous nerves must be desensitized to produce complete anesthesia of the forelimb from the carpus distally

ULNAR NERVE BLOCK (Fig. 6-5)

I. Area blocked: lateral, or dorsal and palmar skin areas
II. Nerve blocked: ulnar nerve
III. Site: 10 cm proximal to the accessory carpal bone
IV. Needle: 22-gauge, 2.54-cm
V. Anesthetic: 5 to 10 ml of 2% lidocaine
VI. Method: the nerve is desensitized 1.5 cm deep beneath the fascia between the flexor carpi ulnaris and ulnaris lateralis muscle
VII. Use: anesthesia of part of the forelimb

MEDIAN NERVE BLOCK (Fig. 6-7)

I. Area blocked: lateral, medial, palmar, and dorsal skin areas
II. Nerve blocked: median nerve
III. Site: medial aspect of the forelimb 5 cm ventral to the elbow joint
IV. Needle: 20- to 22-gauge, 3.81-cm
V. Anesthetic: 10 ml of 2% lidocaine
VI. Method: the median nerve is desensitized between the posterior border of the radius and the muscular belly of the internal flexor carpi radialis
VII. Use: anesthesia of part of the distal limb

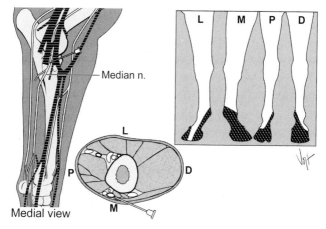

Median n.

Medial view

Fig. 6-7
Needle placement for musculocutaneous nerve block: medial and cross-sectional views. Stippled markings indicate desensitized area (L, lateral; M, medial; P, palmar; and D, dorsal views) after musculocutaneous nerve block of the right forelimb.

MUSCULOCUTANEOUS NERVE BLOCK (FIG. 6-6)

  I. Area blocked: medial, palmar, and dorsal skin areas
 II. Nerve blocked: cutaneous branch of the musculocutaneous nerve
III. Site: anteromedial aspect of the forelimb halfway between the elbow and carpus
 IV. Needle: 22-gauge, 2.54-cm
  V. Anesthetic: 10 ml of 2% lidocaine
 VI. Method: the musculocutaneous nerve is desensitized subcutaneously, where it is easily palpated just cranial to the cephalic vein
VII. Use: anesthesia of part of the forelimb

INTRAARTICULAR INJECTIONS

  I. General considerations
     A. Intraarticular injections require hair clipping and a surgical scrub to reduce the risk of introducing contaminants

B. Use surgical gloves when performing joint blocks
C. Arthrocentesis implies aspiration of synovial fluid but is usually done to allow for instillation of diagnostic and therapeutic agents
  1. Local anesthetic
    a. Adequate amount of local anesthetic should be administered
    b. Enough time should be given for maximal effect and postblock examination
  2. Saline flush
  3. Antibiotics
  4. Hyaluronic acid
  5. Antiinflammatory drugs
II. Common intraarticular and bursal injections at the most distal digit (Fig. 6-8)
  A. Podotrochlear (navicular) bursa
  B. Coffin joint
  C. Pastern joint
  D. Fetlock joint
  E. Distal flexor tendon sheath

INTRAARTICULAR PODOTROCHLEAR (NAVICULAR) BURSA BLOCK

I. Site: podotrochlear (navicular) bursa (Fig. 6-8, *A*)
II. Needle: 18-gauge spinal needle, 5.1- to 7.6-cm
III. Anesthetic: 2 to 5 ml of 2% lidocaine
IV. Method: introduce the needle through the digital pad between the bulbs of the heel at the level of the coronary band until it strikes the bone along the midline while the limb is bearing weight; withdraw the needle until synovial fluid is aspirated, and then inject anesthetic

INTRAARTICULAR COFFIN BLOCK

I. Site: distal interphalangeal (coffin) joint (P2-P3) (Fig. 6-8, *B*)
II. Needle: 18- to 20-gauge, 3.81-cm
III. Anesthetic: 5 to 10 ml of 2% lidocaine
IV. Method: insert the needle 1.5 cm proximal to the coronary band approximately 2 cm lateral to the vertical center of the

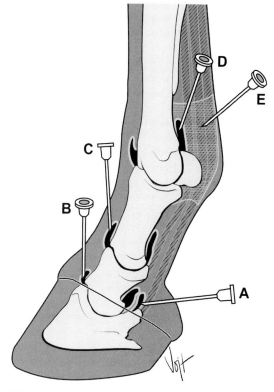

Fig. 6-8
Needle placement. **A,** Podotrochlear (navicular) bursa. **B,** Coffin joint. **C,** Pastern joint. **D,** Fetlock joint. **E,** Distal flexor tendon sheath.

pastern and direct it obliquely ventral to the tendon toward the extensor process

INTRAARTICULAR PASTERN BLOCK

I. Site: proximal interphalangeal (pastern) joint (P1-P2) (Fig. 6-8, *C*)
II. Needle: 20- to 22-gauge, 3.81-cm
III. Anesthetic: 5 to 8 ml of 2% lidocaine

IV. Method: insert the needle medially or laterally to the midline on the palpable epicondyles of P2 for approximately 2.5 cm in a vertical direction

INTRAARTICULAR FETLOCK BLOCK

I. Site: metacarpophalangeal or metatarsophalangeal (fetlock) joint (Fig. 6-8, *D*)
II. Needle: 20- to 22-gauge needle, 3.81-cm
III. Anesthetic: 5 to 10 ml of 2% lidocaine
IV. Method: insert the needle into the lateral pouch distal to the splint bone and dorsal to the annular ligament of the fetlock to a depth of approximately 0.5 to 1 cm

DIGITAL FLEXOR TENDON SHEATH BLOCK

I. Site: digital flexor tendon sheath (Fig. 6-8, *E*)
II. Needle: 18- to 20-gauge, 3.81-cm
III. Anesthetic: 10 ml of 2% lidocaine
IV. Method: insert the needle at the distal end of the splint ("button"), either medially or laterally, cranial to the deep and superficial flexor tendons and caudal to the suspensory ligament

INTRAARTICULAR RADIOCARPAL BLOCK

I. Site: radiocarpal (antebrachial carpal) joint (Fig. 6-9, *A*)
II. Needle: 20-gauge, 3.81-cm
III. Anesthetic: 5 to 10 ml of 2% lidocaine
IV. Method: with the carpus flexed, insert the needle between the radiocarpal joint space on either side of the palpable extensor carpi radialis tendon

INTRAARTICULAR INTERCARPAL BLOCK

I. Site: intercarpal (middle carpal) joint (Fig. 6-9, *B*)
II. Needle: 20-gauge, 3.81-cm
III. Anesthetic: 5 to 10 ml of 2% lidocaine
IV. Method: with the carpus flexed, insert the needle between the

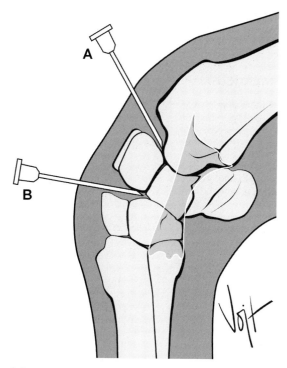

Fig. 6-9
Needle placement. **A,** Radial carpal joint spaces. **B,** Intercarpal joint spaces.

intercarpal joint space on either side of the palpable extensor carpi radialis tendon

CUNEAN BURSA BLOCK

I. Site: cunean bursa on the medial aspect of the tarsus (Fig. 6-10, *A*)
II. Needle: 22-gauge, 2.54-cm
III. Anesthetic: at least 10 ml of 2% lidocaine
IV. Method: insert the needle approximately 1.5 cm distal to the cunean tendon (medial branch of the cranial tibial muscle)

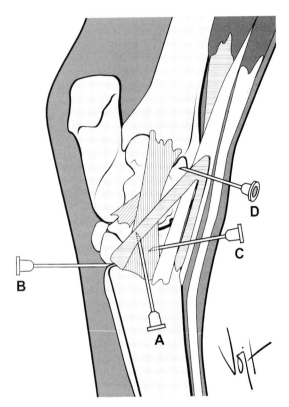

Fig. 6-10
Needle placement. **A,** Cunean bursa. **B,** The tarsometatarsal joint spaces.
C, Intertarsal joint spaces. **D,** Tibiotarsal joint spaces.

and advance it between the cunean tendon and the tarsal bone
to penetrate the bursa distally; at least 20 minutes is required
for maximum anesthetic effect

INTRAARTICULAR TARSOMETATARSAL BLOCK

I. Site: tarsometatarsal joint at the caudal lateral aspect of
the hock over the lateral head of the splint (metatarsal IV)
(Fig. 6-10, *B*)

II. Needle: 22-gauge, 2.54-cm
III. Anesthetic: 6 to 8 ml of 2% lidocaine
IV. Method: the needle is most easily inserted into the tarsometatarsal joint on the caudal lateral aspect of the hock proximal to the palpable lateral head of the splint; the bevel of the needle must be turned away from the bone to allow injection of the anesthetic solution

INTRAARTICULAR INTERTARSAL BLOCK

I. Site: distal intertarsal joint on the medial aspect of the tarsus (Fig. 6-10, *C*)
II. Needle: 22-gauge, 2.54-cm
III. Anesthetic: 6 ml of 2% lidocaine
IV. Method: insert the needle into the joint at a right angle to the skin ventral to the cunean tendon; inject local anesthetic using considerable pressure while turning the needle bevel

INTRAARTICULAR TIBIOTARSAL BLOCK

I. Site: tibiotarsal (tarsocrural) joint at the craniomedial aspect of the tibia (Fig. 6-10, *D*)
II. Needle: 18-gauge, 3.81-cm
III. Anesthetic: 15 ml of 2% lidocaine
IV. Method: the needle is easily inserted less than 2 cm deep into the skin and superficial capsule, 2 to 3 cm ventral to the medial malleolus of the tibia on either the medial or lateral side of the saphenous vein; inject local anesthetic after synovial fluid is recovered on aspiration

CHAPTER SEVEN

Local Anesthesia in Dogs and Cats

"Think globally, act locally."
OLIVER WENDELL HOLMES, JR.

OVERVIEW

Local anesthetic techniques can be used in small animals to perform medical and surgical procedures and avoid the depressant effects of general anesthesia. Local anesthesia is usually administered in combination with sedation or tranquilization to produce a pain-free, cooperative patient. Local analgesic techniques can also be used to produce postoperative analgesia in patients undergoing surgery. Commonly used techniques in small animals include infiltration anesthesia, nerve blocks (e.g., selected nerve blocks), brachial plexus block, intravenous (IV) regional anesthesia, and continuous epidural anesthesia. Epidural opioid, α_2-agonist, or ketamine analgesia, intercostal nerve blocks, and intrapleural analgesia can provide long-lasting postoperative pain relief.

REGIONAL ANESTHESIA OF THE HEAD (Figs. 7-1, 7-2)

The following regional anesthetic techniques, when combined with sedatives or tranquilizers and appropriate physical restraint, can be used to desensitize nerves of the head:

   I. Infraorbital
  II. Maxillary
 III. Ophthalmic
  IV. Mental
   V. Mandibuloalveolar

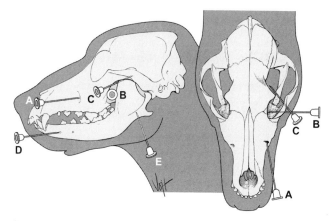

Fig. 7-1
Needle placement for nerve blocks on the head in the dog. **A,** Infraorbital.
B, Maxillary. **C,** Ophthalmic. **D,** Mental. **E,** Mandibuloalveolar.

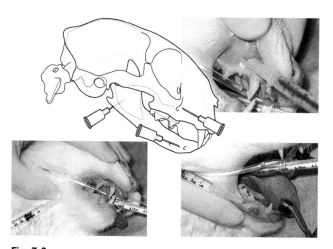

Fig. 7-2
Needle placement for nerve blocks on the head in the cat. **A,** Mandibuloalveolar. **B,** Mental. **C,** Infraorbital.

ANESTHESIA OF THE UPPER LIP AND NOSE

I. Area blocked: upper lip and nose, roof of nasal cavity, and related skin ventral to the infraorbital foramen
II. Nerve blocked: infraorbital
III. Site: point of emergence of the nerve from the infraorbital canal (Figs. 7-1, *A* and 7-2, *A*)
IV. Needle: 22- to 25-gauge, 2.5- to 5-cm
V. Anesthetic: 1 to 2 ml of 1% lidocaine
VI. Method: insert the needle either intraorally or extraorally approximately 1 cm cranial to the bony lip of the infraorbital foramen; advance the needle to the infraorbital foramen, which can be felt between the dorsal border of the zygomatic process and the gingiva of the canine tooth

ANESTHESIA OF MAXILLA, UPPER TEETH, NOSE, AND UPPER LIP

I. Area blocked: maxilla, upper teeth, nose, and upper lip
II. Nerve blocked: maxillary
III. Site: perpendicular portion of the palatine bone between the maxillary foramen and foramen rotundum (Figs. 7-1, *B* and 7-2, *B*)
IV. Needle: 22- to 25-gauge, 2.5- to 5-cm
V. Anesthetic: 1 to 2 ml of 1% lidocaine
VI. Method: insert the needle through the skin at a 90-degree angle, in a medial direction, ventral to the border of the zygomatic process and approximately 0.5 cm caudal to the lateral canthus of the eye; advance the needle in close proximity to the pterygopalatine fossa; local anesthetic is administered where the maxillary nerve courses perpendicular to the palatine bone between the maxillary foramen and foramen rotundum

ANESTHESIA OF THE EYE

I. Area blocked: eye, orbit, conjunctiva, eyelids, and forehead skin
II. Nerves blocked: lacrimal, zygomatic, and ophthalmic (i.e., ophthalmic division of the trigeminal nerve)

   III. Site: at the orbital fissure (Figs. 7-1, *C* and 7-2, *C*)
   IV. Needle: 22- to 25-gauge, 2.5-cm
   V. Anesthetic: 2 ml of 1% lidocaine
   VI. Method: insert the needle ventral to the border of the zygomatic process at the lateral canthus of the eye; the needle point should be approximately 0.5 cm cranial to the anterior border of the vertical portion of the ramus of the mandible; advance the needle medial to the ramus of the mandible in a mediodorsal and somewhat caudal direction until it reaches the orbital fissure

ANESTHESIA OF THE LOWER LIP

   I. Area blocked: lower lip
   II. Nerve blocked: mental
   III. Site: rostral to the mental foramen (Figs. 7-1, *D* and 7-2, *D*)
   IV. Needle: 22- to 25-gauge, 2.5-cm
   V. Anesthetic: 1 to 2 ml of 1% lidocaine
   VI. Method: insert the needle over the mental nerve, rostral to the middle mental foramen at the level of the lower second premolar tooth

ANESTHESIA OF THE MANDIBLE AND LOWER TEETH

   I. Area blocked: cheek teeth, canine, incisors, skin, and mucosa of the chin and lower lip
   II. Nerve blocked: inferior alveolar branch of the mandibular nerve
   III. Site: point of entry of the nerve into the mandibular canal at the mandibular foramen (Figs. 7-1, *E* and 7-2, *E*)
   IV. Needle used: 22- to 25-gauge, 2.5-cm
   V. Anesthetic: 1 to 2 ml of 1% lidocaine
   VI. Method: insert the needle at the lower angle of the jaw approximately 0.5 cm rostral to the angular process; advance the needle 1.5 cm dorsally against the medial surface of the ramus of the mandible to the palpable lip of the mandibular foramen

ANESTHESIA OF THE FOOT

I. Anesthesia of the foot may be induced by the following techniques:

A. Infiltration of the tissues around the limb with local anesthetic solution (ring block) (Fig. 7-3)

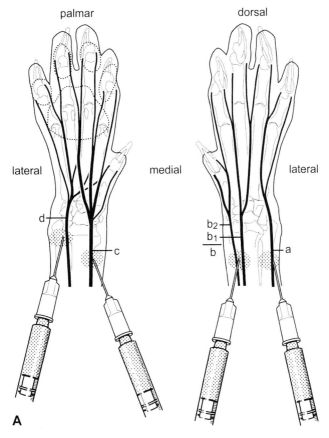

Fig. 7-3
Branches of the ulnar (*a, d*), radial (*b, b1, b2*), and median (*c*) nerves are infiltrated with local anesthetic before a declaw procedure of the front limbs in a cat.

B. Infiltration of the brachial plexus by local anesthetic (brachial plexus block)
C. IV injection of anesthetic into an accessible superficial vein in a distal extremity that is isolated from circulation by placing a tourniquet on the animal's leg (IV regional anesthesia)
D. Injection of local anesthetic into the lumbosacral epidural space (anesthesia of the hind legs)
E. Perineural infiltration of sensory nerves in the limbs (nerve block)

BRACHIAL PLEXUS BLOCK

I. Area blocked: distal foot, up to the elbow region
II. Nerves blocked: radial, median, ulnar, musculocutaneous, and axillary nerves
III. Site: medial to the shoulder joint (Fig. 7-4)
IV. Needle: 20- to 22-gauge, 7.5-cm (3.75-cm in cats); a spinal needle or catheter stylet works well
V. Anesthetic: 10 to 15 ml (in a larger dog) of 2% lidocaine
VI. Method: insert the needle medial to the shoulder joint toward the costochondral junction and parallel to the vertebral column; inject the anesthetic slowly as the needle is withdrawn; anesthesia can be obtained within 20 minutes and for up to 2 hours (total recovery requires approximately 6 hours)
VII. Advantages
  A. Relatively simple and safe to perform
  B. Produces selective anesthesia and relaxation of the limb distal to the elbow joint
VIII. Disadvantages
  A. Relatively long waiting period (15 to 30 minutes) required
  B. Occasional failure to obtain complete anesthesia, particularly in overweight dogs
IX. Complications
  A. Toxic symptoms after intravascular administration of the local anesthetic
  B. Lack of anesthesia after inadvertent intravascular injection

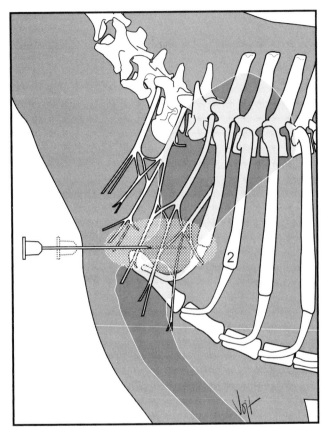

Fig. 7-4
Needle placement for brachial plexus block, lateral aspect of left thoracic limb in the dog.

INTRAVENOUS REGIONAL ANESTHESIA (BIER BLOCK)

  I. Area blocked: extremity distal to tourniquet
 II. Nerves blocked: nerve endings in peripheral tissues
III. Site: any superficial vein distal to tourniquet
 IV. Needle: 22- to 23-gauge, 2.5-cm; place an IV catheter to ensure

V. Anesthetic: 2.5 to 5 mg/kg of 1% lidocaine (without epinephrine)

NOTE

Do not use bupivacaine for intravenous regional anesthesia because of the potential for cardiovascular collapse and death.

VI. Method: the limb is first desanguinated by wrapping it with an Esmarch bandage; a rubber tourniquet is placed around the limb just proximal to the elbow for thoracic limb surgery or proximal to the hock for pelvic limb surgery; the tourniquet must be tight enough to exceed blood pressure; once the tourniquet is secured, the Esmarch bandage is unwrapped, and local anesthetic is injected with light pressure

VII. Advantages
  A. Safe and simple technique
  B. Lack of toxicity to organs if the occlusion of blood supply is limited to 2 hours
  C. Blood-free surgery site is ideal for taking biopsies and removing foreign bodies from the paws

VIII. Disadvantages: limited to 2 hours

IX. Complications
  A. Shock can occur if tourniquet is left on more than 4 hours (reversible)
  B. Sepsis, endotoxemia, and death can occur if tourniquet is left on more than 8 to 10 hours

LUMBOSACRAL EPIDURAL ANESTHESIA

I. Indications
  A. Animals that are severely depressed, are in shock, or require immediate surgery of the rear quarters
  B. Animals that are at high risk, are aged, or in which the use of other analgesic or anesthetic agents is contra-indicated
  C. Opioids are used to provide analgesia after abdominal surgery or surgery of the rear limbs; paralysis is not produced

II. Specific procedures
   A. Surgery
      1. Tail amputation
      2. Anal sac therapy or perianal surgery
      3. Rear limb lacerations or fractures
      4. Urolithiasis therapy
      5. Abdominal surgery
      6. Cesarean section
      7. Obstetric manipulations
      8. Surgical procedures of the tail, perineum, vulva, vagina, rectum, and bladder
   B. Postoperative analgesia
III. Landmarks and anatomy (Figs. 7-5 and 7-6)
   A. Right and left cranial dorsal iliac wings of the ilium
   B. Spinous process of the seventh lumbar vertebra and the median sacral crest
   C. Important anatomic features
      1. Shape of lumbar and sacral spinous processes

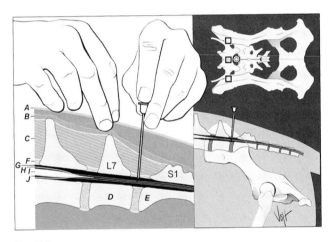

Fig. 7-5
Needle placement for lumbosacral epidural (between L7 and S1) anesthesia in the dog, lateral and dorsal aspects. *A*, Skin; *B*, supraspinous ligament; *C*, interspinous ligament; *D*, seventh lumbar vertebra; *E*, sacrum; *F*, interarcuate ligament (ligamentum flavum); *G*, epidural space; *H*, dura mater spinalis; *I*, spinal cord; *J*, subarachnoid space containing CSF.

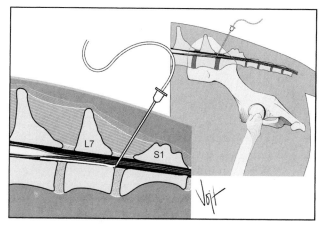

Fig. 7-6
Needle placement for continuous epidural anesthesia or opioid analgesia in the dog, shown in the lateral aspect. *L7* and *S1* are the spinous processes of the seventh lumbar and the first sacral vertebrae.

2. Interspinous ligament
3. Ligamentum arcuatum (ligamentum flavum)
4. Terminal portion of the dural sac
5. Filum terminale
6. Intervertebral disk
D. The spinal cord usually ends at vertebral body L6 to L7 in dogs and L7 to S3 in cats; therefore the procedure is more hazardous when performed on cats

IV. Equipment
   A. 18- or 22-gauge, 5- to 10-cm (22-gauge, 2.5- to 3.75-cm in cats), beveled spinal needle with stylet (disposable needle preferred)
   B. One 3-ml and one 6-ml syringe
   C. A thin-walled, 18-gauge, 7.5-cm needle (Tuohy needle, Crawford needle) is used if a polyethylene catheter is to be placed for continuous epidural anesthesia

V. Procedure
   A. Clip and perform a surgical scrub; this is a sterile procedure

B. Place the spinal needle perpendicular to the skin surface at the midline of the lumbosacral space; this space can be palpated halfway between the dorsoiliac wings and just caudal to the dorsal spinous process of the seventh lumbar vertebra (Figs. 7-5 and 7-6)
   1. Infiltration of the area with 2% lidocaine may facilitate placement of the spinal needle
   2. Push the spinal needle ventrally in a slight cranial or caudal angle as needed
C. Resistance is encountered when the ligamentum flavum is reached; a distinct "pop" is usually felt when the needle is advanced through this ligament
D. On penetrating the ligamentum flavum, the needle is in the epidural space
   1. Needle depth may vary from 1 to 4 cm, depending on animal size
   2. Remove the stylet and examine the needle for blood or cerebrospinal fluid (CSF); if no blood or CSF is observed, the needle should be aspirated for blood or CSF
   3. Inject 1 to 2 ml of air to check for proper needle placement
      a. If subcutaneous crepitus is felt, the needle is incorrectly placed and should be repositioned
      b. No resistance should be felt to the injection of air or local anesthetic agent

VI. Doses
   A. A test dose of 0.5 to 1 ml of 2% lidocaine produces almost immediate dilation of the external anal sphincter, followed by relaxation of the tail and ataxia of pelvic limbs within 3 to 5 minutes
   B. The required dose varies depending on the desired effect
      1. 1 ml/4.5 kg of 2% lidocaine or 0.75% bupivacaine; this will produce anesthesia as far cranial as L1
      2. 1 ml/5 kg 2% lidocaine or 0.75% bupivacaine if anesthesia is required up to T5
      3. 1 ml/6 kg of 2% lidocaine or 0.75% bupivacaine; satisfactory for cesarean section
   C. Small amounts of 1:200,000 epinephrine can be added to lidocaine to delay the rate of absorption, thus prolonging anesthetic action by 30 minutes (total of 2 hours)

D. Bupivacaine with epinephrine (Marcaine) or ropivacaine (Naropin) produces 4- to 6-hour periods of anesthesia

VII. Continuous epidural anesthesia in dogs

A. Procedure
1. The procedure is similar to that previously described, except that a curved bevel spinal needle (Tuohy) is used, through which a catheter is passed (Fig. 7-7)
2. The Tuohy needle is inserted into the epidural space with the needle bevel directed cranially
3. Only 2 to 3 cm of catheter should be advanced into the epidural space
4. Withdraw the needle, but leave the catheter in place

B. Advantages
1. Ability to tailor the duration of anesthesia to the length of operation
2. Route for injecting epidural opioids during and after surgery (see epidural opioid analgesia)

C. Disadvantages
1. Technically difficult

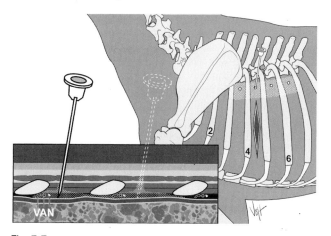

Fig. 7-7
Needle placement for intercostal nerve blocks in the dog, shown in the lateral aspect and the sagittal section. *2, 4, 6* are the second, fourth, and sixth rib; *VAN* is the intercostal vein, artery, and nerve.

2. Potential for damage to the spinal cord, meninges, and nerves
3. Risk of infection
4. Catheter-related problems (e.g., kinks, displacement, clotting with fibrin)

VIII. Factors influencing cranial level of blockade
A. Size of patient
B. Conformation of patient
C. Volume of drug injected
D. Drug mass (volume × concentration)
E. Rate of injection
F. Direction of needle bevel
G. Age of patient
H. Obesity
I. Intraabdominal pressure attributable to presence and size of abdominal mass (e.g., pregnancy)
1. The volume of the epidural space in pregnant animals is decreased because of distention of epidural veins/engorgement
2. Neural tissue sensitivity to drug effects is increased during pregnancy
J. Position of patient: gravity has a more definite role in the spread of subarachnoid anesthesia than in epidural anesthesia; however, with both techniques, a more rapid onset to maximal segmental anesthesia (unilateral anesthesia), a longer duration of anesthesia, and a more intensive motor blockade are achieved in the dependent side than in the upper side

IX. Proposed site of action after epidural injection (Table 7-1)

X. Possible complications
A. Injection of local anesthetic into the vertebral sinuses
1. Vomiting, tremors
2. Decreased blood pressure caused by peripheral vasodilation
3. Convulsions
4. Paralysis
B. Respiratory depression and paralysis in dogs and cats caused by drug overdose
1. The drug must migrate to approximately C5 or C7 to produce complete respiratory paralysis from blockade of the phrenic nerves

TABLE 7-1
PROPOSED SITE OF ACTION AFTER EPIDURAL INJECTION

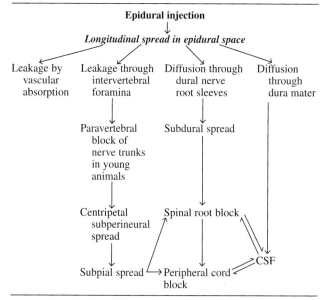

CSF, Cerebrospinal fluid.

2. The cephalad spread of anesthesia after epidural or subarachnoid injection (of specifically prepared hyperbaric solution [e.g., "heavy nupercaine"] in 6% glucose) is limited in an animal that is kept in a sitting position

C. Temperature may fall in small animals because they are unable to shiver; the patient's rear quarters should be kept warm by wrapping them in a towel or a heated water blanket

D. Administer a sedative or tranquilizer for patient cooperation

EPIDURAL OPIOIDS AND α_2-ADRENOCEPTOR OR LOCAL ANESTHETIC ANALGESIA

I. Indications
  A. Intraoperative analgesia
  B. Postoperative analgesia
  C. Critical care patients
II. Site of opioid injection
  A. Lumbosacral epidural space (single-dose injection) (Figs. 7-5 and 7-6)
  B. Anterior lumbar epidural space (catheter technique) (Fig. 7-7)
III. Drugs
  A. Epidural morphine (0.1 mg/kg diluted in 0.1 to 0.3 ml/kg of 0.9% NaCl solution) produces pain relief 30 to 60 minutes after injection and for as long as 6 to 24 hours
  B. Epidural morphine (0.1 mg/kg) alone or combined with xylazine (0.02 mg/kg) or medetomidine (2 to 5 µg/kg) produces minimal cardiovascular changes in dogs anesthetized with 1.5 minimum alveolar concentration (MAC) of isoflurane
  C. Epidural morphine (0.1 mg/kg) with medetomidine (5 µg/kg) produces pain relief for at least 13 hours
  D. Epidural morphine (0.1 mg/kg) with bupivacaine (0.5%, 1 ml/10-cm distance from the occipital protuberance to the lumbosacral space) decreases the required isoflurane delivery more and provides longer lasting analgesia (more than 24 hours) than morphine alone (5.5 hours) or bupivacaine alone (9 hours)
  E. Epidural oxymorphone (0.05 to 0.1 mg/kg diluted in 0.3 ml/kg of 0.9% NaCl solution) produces pain relief 20 to 40 minutes after injection and for an approximate duration of 10 to 15 hours
  F. Epidural fentanyl (1 to 10 mg/kg diluted in 0.2 to 0.3 ml/kg of 0.9% NaCl solution) produces pain relief 15 to 20 minutes after administration, with analgesia lasting 3 to 5 hours
  G. Epidural fentanyl (0.1 mg/kg) with lidocaine (0.3 ml/kg, 2% solution 1:200,000 epinephrine) produces scrotal

anesthesia in 2 minutes after administration, with anesthesia lasting 2 to 2.5 hours

H. Epidural xylazine (0.1 to 0.4 mg/kg) decreases the isoflurane MAC in a dose-dependent manner and is associated with few cardiopulmonary effects in anesthetized dogs

I. Epidural medetomidine (15 µg/kg, diluted in 0.1 ml/kg of 0.9% NaCl solution) produces pain relief for 7 hours in dogs

J. Epidural medetomidine (10 µg/kg) increases the pain threshold for the hindlimb from 20 to 240 minutes after administration and for the forelimb from 15 to 120 minutes after administration; mild sedation can occur; there is occasional emesis in cats

IV. Advantages

A. Small doses produce relief of somatic and visceral pain that is more profound and prolonged than that produced by comparable parenterally administered (intramuscular, IV) opioids with less sedation

B. No interference with sensory function

C. No interference with motor function

D. Minimal depression of the sympathetic nervous system

E. Modification of the endocrine-metabolic stress response, improvement in pulmonary function, decreased morbidity, and a comparatively short recovery

F. Reversal of side effects by low-dose IV infusion of opioid antagonists (e.g., naloxone)

V. Potential side effects (rare)

A. Respiratory depression

B. Urinary retention

C. Delayed gastrointestinal motility

D. Vomiting

E. Pruritus

VI. Complications

A. Respiratory depression after large doses (>1 mg/kg) of epidural morphine

B. Catheter-related problems

1. Catheter displacement

2. Occlusion

3. Infection

EPIDURAL KETAMINE ANALGESIA

I. Mechanism of action
  A. The precise mechanism of analgesic action after epidural or subarachnoid administration of ketamine has not been clearly defined
  B. Hypothetically, ketamine acts as an antagonist at the N-methyl-D-aspartate receptors, preventing the development of neural changes involved in hyperesthesia
  C. N-methyl-D-aspartate receptors play an important role in spinal neural plasticity, such as central sensitization, wind-up, and hyperalgesia
  D. Ketamine may possess some δ opiate agonist activity in addition to being a phencyclidine agonist

II. Indication
  A. Preemptive (postoperative) analgesia when administered epidurally in the preoperative period
  B. Intraoperative analgesia lessens the cardiovascular depressant effects of inhalation anesthesia as a result of MAC-sparing effect
  C. Postoperative analgesia with minimal respiratory depression and cardiovascular changes (e.g., blood pressure, heart rate)

III. Method
  A. Epidural ketamine (2 mg/kg, diluted to a volume of 1 ml of sterile 0.9% NaCl/4.5 kg) produces analgesia for 2 hours
  B. Epidural ketamine (1 mg/kg) can provide pain relief with few cardiopulmonary effects but with occasional salivation
  C. Epidural ketamine (0.5 mg/kg or 1 mg/kg) combined with morphine (0.05 mg/kg or 0.025 mg/kg) can provide pain relief with few cardiopulmonary effects and sedation; ketamine (1 mg/kg) combined with morphine (0.025 mg/kg) may produce salivation
  D. Epidural meperidine may interact antagonistically rather than synergistically with epidural ketamine

IV. Advantages
  A. Local anesthetic effects

    B. Alternative method to epidural opiate administration in dogs anesthetized with isoflurane or sevoflurane

    C. Minimal changes in cardiovascular parameters such as heart rate, blood pressure, central venous pressure, cardiac index, systemic and pulmonary vascular resistance, and rate-pressured product in isoflurane-anesthetized dogs (MAC 1.2% to 1.6%)

V. Potential side effects

    A. Differences in the analgesic response to epidurally administered ketamine have been observed; attributable to anatomic differences, dose regimen, and inhalation anesthesia

INTRAARTICULAR BUPIVACAINE OR MORPHINE

I. Indication: local analgesia for stifle, elbow, hock, and more distal joints

II. Method: an intraarticular injection of bupivacaine or morphine is given after surgery (e.g., surgical repair of ruptured cranial cruciate ligaments) and before skin closure

    A. 0.5 ml of bupivacaine HCl (0.5%)/kg body weight or 0.1 mg morphine (preservative-free morphine, Duramorph, or Astramorph) diluted with 0.9% NaCl to a volume of 0.1 ml/kg

III. Results

    A. Intraarticular bupivacaine and morphine provide postoperative analgesia without adverse reactions

    B. Intraarticular bupivacaine produces the greatest local anesthetic effect, lasting up to 24 hours after administration, allowing dogs to recover completely while alert

    C. Intraarticular morphine provides some analgesia lasting at least 6 hours, but not to the extent of intraarticular bupivacaine

    D. Intraarticular morphine provides effective analgesia comparable to epidural morphine (0.1 mg/kg) in dogs

    E. Inflammation is needed for morphine to produce its antinociceptive effect; inflammation may cause activation of receptors already present within peripheral tissues

IV. Advantages

    A. Easy to perform

B. Local analgesia provides pain relief without the need for systemic administration of analgesic/sedative drugs, allowing systemic functions to be undisturbed

C. Local analgesia allows local inflammation to proceed while providing symptomatic relief of pain

INTERCOSTAL NERVE BLOCKS

I. Indications
   A. Relief of pain during thoracotomy
   B. Analgesia after thoracotomy
   C. Pleural drainage
   D. Rib fractures

II. Nerves blocked: intercostals both cranial and caudal to the incision or injury site because of overlap of nerve supply

III. Site: a minimum of two adjacent intercostal spaces near the intercostal foramen (Fig. 7-8)

IV. Needle: 22- to 25-gauge, 2.5-cm

V. Anesthetic: 0.25 to 1 ml of 0.25% or 0.5% bupivacaine, or 0.2% or 0.5% ropivacaine/site, with or without epinephrine

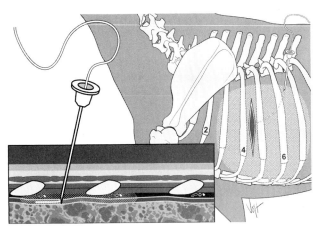

Fig. 7-8
Needle and catheter placement for intrapleural regional analgesia in the dog, shown in the left lateral aspect and the sagittal section. *2, 4, 6* are the second, fourth, and sixth rib.

1:200,000; total dose should not exceed 3 mg/kg (the technique produces high blood concentrations of the anesthetic)
   A. Small dog: 0.25 ml/site
   B. Medium dog: 0.5 ml/site
   C. Large dog: 1 ml/site
VI. Method: insert the needle through the skin at a 90-degree angle caudal to the rib near the intervertebral foramen; inject small volumes and/or diluted anesthetic solutions into a minimum of two adjacent intercostal spaces
VII. Advantages
   A. Selective intercostal nerve block is easily performed because of the proximity of each nerve to its adjacent rib
   B. The intercostal nerves can be visualized beneath the pleura during thoracotomy
   C. The technique provides consistent analgesia for 3 to 6 hours without respiratory depression
VIII. Complications
   A. Pneumothorax after faulty technique
   B. Impaired blood-gas exchange (hypercarbia, hypoxemia) in dogs with pulmonary diseases if ventilatory efforts are reduced

INTRAPLEURAL REGIONAL ANALGESIA

I. Indications
   A. Relief of pain originating from the following conditions:
      1. Thoracotomy
      2. Rib fractures
      3. Mastectomy
      4. Chronic pancreatitis
      5. Cholecystectomy
      6. Renal surgery
      7. Abdominal cancer
      8. Metastasis of the chest wall, pleura, and mediastinum
II. Nerves blocked: mechanisms of pain relief are not fully understood
   A. Retrograde diffusion of local anesthetic through the parietal pleura, causing intercostal nerve block
   B. Desensitization of the thoracic sympathetic chain and splanchnic nerves

   III. Site: place a catheter into the pleural space either percutaneously or before closure of a thoracotomy (Fig. 7-8)

   IV. Equipment: 17-gauge, 5-cm, Huber-point (Tuohy) needle; medical grade silastic tubing, 5 to 10 cm, 2 mm inside diameter; sterile sets for single, continuous interpleural analgesia are available

   V. Anesthetic: approximately 1 to 2 mg of 0.5% bupivacaine/kg or 0.2% ropivacaine/kg (0.5%, with or without 1:200,000 epinephrine)

   VI. Method: in a well-sedated animal, desensitize the skin, subcutaneous tissue, periosteum, and parietal pleura over the caudal border of the rib with 1 to 2 ml of 2% lidocaine with the use of a 22-gauge, 2.5-cm needle; then use the Huber-point needle to place the catheter with minimal resistance into the subatmospheric pleural space, 3 to 5 cm beyond the needle tip (Fig. 7-9); withdraw the needle over the catheter and leave the catheter in place; catheter placement in the open chest is accomplished by inserting the Tuohy needle through the skin at least two intercostal spaces caudal to the incision and passing the catheter through the needle subpleurally under direct vision; inject local anesthetic over 1 to 2 minutes after negative aspiration of air or blood through the catheter; then clear the catheter with 2 ml of physiologic saline solution

   VII. Advantages

      A. The procedure is simple to perform

      B. One needlestick is needed in contrast to multiple intercostal nerve blocks

      C. Post-thoracotomy pain relief lasts longer (3 to 12 hours) than analgesia produced by subcutaneous morphine (0.5 mg/kg) or selective intercostal nerve blocks with bupivacaine (0.5 ml of 0.5% bupivacaine per site)

      D. Long-term use (over several weeks) of an interpleural catheter is possible

   VIII. Complications

      A. Lung trauma

      B. Infection

      C. Phrenic nerve paralysis or paresis; paradoxic respiration with negative intraabdominal pressure

D. Tachyphylaxis to local anesthetic
E. High anesthetic blood concentration
F. Systemic toxicity after excessive doses of the local anesthetic (>3 mg bupivacaine/kg)
G. Catheter-related complications (e.g., pneumothorax)
H. Bleeding
 I. Minimal pain relief
  1. Misplaced catheter
  2. Excessive bleeding into the pleural space
  3. Pleural effusion

CHAPTER EIGHT

Specific Intravenous Anesthetic Drugs

"To sleep: perchance to dream."
WILLIAM SHAKESPEARE

OVERVIEW

Intravenous (IV) and intramuscular (IM) anesthetic drugs can be used to induce chemical restraint and general anesthesia. Proper use of preanesthetic medication (tranquilizers, sedatives, analgesics) is imperative if anesthetic drugs are to produce the desired effect and if side effects are to be avoided. Injectable anesthetic drugs are often more convenient and economical than inhalation anesthetic drugs. Their principal disadvantage is that once administered, they cannot be controlled and are not immediately eliminated. Several injectable drugs (thiopental, methohexital, propofol, etomidate) have a very short duration of action.

GENERAL CONSIDERATIONS

I. Increasing degrees of central nervous system (CNS) depression can be produced, from drowsiness and mild sedation to anesthesia and coma

II. Factors that determine rate of onset, amount of depression, and duration of anesthesia
   A. Type of anesthetic drug used
   B. Dose
   C. Rate of drug administration when administered IV
   D. Route of administration (IV, IM, subcutaneous, intraperitoneal)
   E. Animal's level of consciousness (excited versus depressed) when the drug is administered

140

      F. Acid-base and electrolyte balance; acidosis enhances barbiturate anesthesia

      G. Animal's cardiac output

      H. Drug tolerance (age, breed, obesity)

       I. Interactions with other drugs

III. Most injectable anesthetic drugs produce unconsciousness by depressing the cerebral cortex

      A. Many are used to control convulsions (barbiturates; propofol)

      B. Barbiturates increase the threshold of spinal reflexes and can be used clinically for the treatment of strychnine poisoning

IV. Routes of administration

      A. Most injectable drugs are administered IV; ketamine and tiletamine-zolazepam can be administered IM

      B. Sodium salts of barbiturates can be injected in a solution of up to 10%, guaifenesin in a solution of up to 10%, and chloral hydrate in a solution of up to 7%

      C. Because of the extreme alkalinity of barbiturate solutions, perivascular injection results in necrosis and sloughing; barbiturates are not injected IM or subcutaneously

V. Dose should be calculated on the basis of lean body mass (body weight minus fat) (Table 8-1)

BARBITURATE ANESTHESIA

   I. Barbiturates are categorized according to their duration of action

      A. Long: 8 to 12 hours

      B. Intermediate: 2 to 6 hours

      C. Short: 45 to 90 minutes

      D. Ultrashort: 5 to 15 minutes

 II. Nonproprietary drug names

DRUG	APPROPRIATE DURATION OF ACTION
Phenobarbital sodium	Long
Pentobarbital sodium	Short
Thiopental sodium	Ultrashort
Methohexital	Ultrashort

TABLE 8-1

INTRAVENOUS DRUGS COMMONLY USED TO PRODUCE ANESTHESIA OF SHORT DURATION (MG/KG)

	AGENT	HORSE	DOG	CAT	PIG	COW	GOAT
1	Thiopental	up to 7	8-20	8-20	10-20	7-13	4-10
2	Etomidate	—	0.5-2	0.5-2	0.5-2	—	—
3	Propofol	2-8	4-10	3-10	4-13	—	—
4	Guaifenesin	50-100	40-90	—	40-90	100	100
5	Chloral hydrate	—	—	—	6-9 g/45 kg	6-10 g/45 kg	6-10 g/45 kg
6	Chloral hydrate (7% solution)	10 ml/45 kg*	—	—	20-30 ml/45 kg	20-30 ml/45 kg	20-30 ml/45 kg
7	Chloropent	10 ml/45 kg	—	—	—	10 ml/45 kg	—
	Thiopental	4-6	—	—	5.5-11	4-6	—
8	Ketamine	1.5-2	5-10	2-6	2-6	Up to 2	2-6
9	Telazol®	0.5-1.5	2-10	2-8	4-10	1-4	2-10
10	Guaifenesin	50-100	30-90	—	30-90	50-100	30-90
	Thiopental	4-6	4-9	—	4-9	4-6	—
11	Guaifenesin	50-100	30-90	—	—	50-100	—
	Ketamine	1.2-2.2	1	—	1-2	0.6-1.1	0.6-1.1
12	Acepromazine	—	0.2	0.2	0.4	—	—
	Ketamine	—	10	10	2-7	—	—
13	Xylazine†	1	0.7-1	0.7-1.1	1-2	0.04	0.04
	Ketamine	2.2	10	10-11	6-8	2	2-7

14	Xylazine	1.0-1.1	0.4	0.7	0.7	0.05	0.09
	Telazol®	1.0-2.2	7	2-7	2-7	1	1
15	Diazepam‡	0.1	0.25	0.2	0.2	0.25-0.5	—
	Ketamine	1.5-2	5	5	4	5-10	—
16	Midazolam	—	—	0.4	—	—	—
	Ketamine	—	—	7.5	—	—	—
17	Midazolam	0.02	—	—	—	—	—
	Xylazine	1	—	—	—	—	—
	Propofol	3	—	—	—	—	—
18	Oxymorphone	—	—	—	0.08	—	—
	Xylazine	—	—	—	2	—	—
	Ketamine	—	—	—	2	—	—
19	Xylazine, guaifenesin, ketamine	(500 ml 5% guaifenesin + 500 mg ketamine + 30-50 mg xylazine [ruminants 1-2 ml/kg]; 500 ml 5% guaifenesin + 500 mg ketamine + 500 mg xylazine [horses, pigs]; approximately 3-5 ml/min to effect					

* Sedative dose.
† Detomidine, 2 to 10 µg/kg IV, can be used in xylazine drug combinations.
‡ Midazolam, 0.2 to 0.6 mg/kg IV, can be used in diazepam drug combinations.

III. General anesthetic actions of barbiturates
  A. Effects on the CNS
   1. CNS depression ranging from drowsiness and mild sedation to coma results from interaction with the CNS inhibitor/gamma aminobutyric acid A ($GABA_A$) receptors
   2. Response to barbiturate anesthesia
     a. Pentobarbital sodium and ultrashort-acting barbiturates decrease cerebral blood flow (CBF), cerebral metabolic rate of oxygen ($CMRO_2$), and neuronal activity of the brain (e.g., dogs); the $CBF/CMRO_2$ ratio is unchanged or increased; there are minimal changes in CSF pressure if ventilation is normal
     b. Anesthetic concentrations of barbiturates depress arterial blood pressure (BP) transiently, decrease intracranial pressure, and increase cerebral perfusion pressure
     c. Barbiturates are used to produce a general anesthesia (short-acting) or to induce a patient to surgical anesthesia (ultrashort-acting)
     d. Barbiturates are poor analgesics at subhypnotic doses
   3. Anticonvulsant effects
     a. Long- or intermediate-acting barbiturates are used for control of convulsions
     b. The distinction between an anesthetic and an anticonvulsant barbiturate depends on the concentration at which amino acid modulation and GABA-mimetic activities occur

---

USEFUL FACTS ▪ Barbiturates

- Short- or ultrashort-acting barbiturates are used for anesthesia
- Long- or intermediate-acting barbiturates are used as anticonvulsants
- Decrease CBF and $CMRO_2$; useful for brain surgery

  B. Organ system effects and responses
   1. Effects on the respiratory system
     a. Barbiturates are respiratory depressants

(1) They depress respiratory centers in the medulla and the areas of the brain responsible for the characteristic rhythmic pattern of respiratory movement (apneustic and pneumotaxic centers)

(2) The degree of respiratory depression is related to the dose and rate of drug administration

b. Coughing, sneezing, hiccoughing, and laryngospasm occur frequently; these effects are caused by excessive salivary secretion and are minimized by preanesthetic medication (atropine, glycopyrrolate)

(1) Laryngospasm is a common complication of barbiturate anesthesia in dogs and cats

(2) A short period of apnea frequently occurs after IV bolus administration of barbiturates

c. When respiratory arrest occurs, attention should be directed toward establishing an airway and ventilating the patient; respiratory stimulants (doxapram) may be necessary if the animal does not begin to ventilate spontaneously

2. Effects on the cardiovascular system

a. Barbiturates produce significant cardiovascular depression, both centrally and peripherally, with a transient fall in blood pressure when administered rapidly as a bolus or in large doses

b. Cardiac arrhythmias may occur (Fig. 8-1)

(1) Thiobarbiturates (thiamylal, thiopental, thialbarbitone) sensitize the heart to epinephrine and induce autonomic imbalance; arrhythmias,

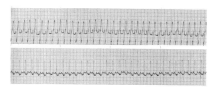

Fig. 8-1

Monomorphic ventricular tachycardia in a dog (top trace). After conversion to sinus tachycardia by administering lidocaine IV (bottom trace).

particularly ventricular extrasystoles and ventricular bigeminy, can occur after thiopental administration

(2) Thiobarbiturates increase both parasympathetic and sympathetic tone; this may lead to atrial or ventricular arrhythmias; sinus bradycardia; or first-, second-, or third-degree heart block and cardiac arrest

c. Barbiturates may cause a transient drop in BP; if the patient is already in a state of surgical anesthesia, small doses of a barbiturate may cause dramatic decreases in cardiac contractility and arterial BP

(1) Barbiturates should be administered slowly and in reduced doses to sick, debilitated, or depressed animals

(2) Concentrations greater than 2.5% are toxic to tissues and may injure the capillary musculature, causing capillary dilation and thrombophlebitis; injection into artery may cause severe pain, vasoconstriction, and tissue necrosis

(3) Induction doses of thiobarbiturates may prompt an initial increase in BP caused by tachycardia and an increase in peripheral vascular resistance caused by increases in sympathetic tone

3. Actions on the gastrointestinal (GI) tract

a. Depress intestinal motility; thiobarbiturates may depress GI tract motility initially, then increase both tone and motility

b. Diarrhea and intestinal stasis are generally not observed at recommended doses

4. Kidney and liver

a. No direct effect on the kidney has been observed, unless a large dose is given, in which case a decrease in renal blood flow occurs; systemic hypotension may cause a cessation in urine production

b. Single administrations at therapeutic doses have no effect on liver function; large or repetitive doses of barbiturates may cause injury in patients with liver damage

5. Effects on the uterus and fetus
   a. The short-acting barbiturate, pentobarbital, is contraindicated in near-term animals
   b. Barbiturates readily diffuse across the placenta into the fetal circulation; thiopental reaches mixed fetal cord blood within 45 seconds
   c. Doses of barbiturates that do not produce anesthesia in the mother can completely inhibit fetal respiratory movements

IV. Absorption, elimination, and excretion
   A. Absorption
      1. IV administration
         a. Adequate provisions should be available to support respiration and circulation
         b. Short-acting barbiturates (pentobarbital) require approximately 5 to 10 minutes to produce maximal CNS effect
         c. Ultrashort-acting barbiturates (thiopental, methohexital) reach maximal effect within 30 seconds of administration
      2. Barbiturates are absorbed from the GI tract after oral administration
   B. Elimination
      1. Redistribution: ultrashort-acting barbiturates (thiopental, methohexital) rely on redistribution to lean body tissues (muscle) for their duration of action (Fig. 8-2)
         a. Emergence from sleep depends on a shift of the drug from the brain to lean body tissues
         b. Concentrations in muscle and skin peak approximately 15 to 30 minutes after thiobarbiturate injection
         c. Concentrations in fat peak in several hours
         d. Repeated doses have a cumulative effect
         e. Extremely thin, heavily muscled animals (e.g., greyhounds, whippets) demonstrate prolonged recoveries (3 to 5 hours) from thiopental anesthesia
         f. Obesity delays drug elimination because of the high lipid solubility of barbiturates
         g. "Acute tolerance" (minimal effect with a usual dose) is rarely observed after the administration of

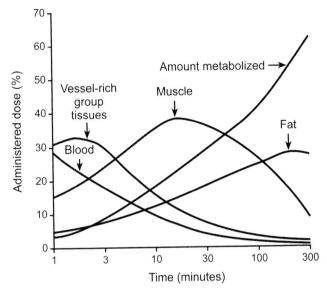

Fig. 8-2
Distribution of thiopental to various tissues. Note that the accumulation of drug in the muscle tissue corresponds to the approximate duration of thiopental anesthesia.

thiobarbiturates in horses and dogs; the mechanism is unknown but is probably related to the patient's level of excitement and the distribution of cardiac output; if this occurs, alternative anesthetic techniques should be used
  2. Barbiturates are eliminated by oxidative activity of hepatic enzymes and by renal excretion
  3. The amount of active (nonionized, nonprotein-bound) drug is increased by acidosis; alkalinization of the urine hastens drug elimination
  C. Excretion
   1. Hepatic metabolism
    a. Barbiturates are metabolized by both hepatic and extrahepatic mechanisms; metabolites are eliminated by the kidneys and appear in the urine

      b. Liver disease may prolong the duration of drug action; avoid using short-acting barbiturates in the presence of liver disease

      c. Hypothermia and depressed cardiovascular function may prolong hepatic metabolism of barbiturates

V. Dose and administration of specific barbiturate drugs

  A. Pentobarbital sodium (Nembutal)

    1. IV anesthetic dose varies from 10 to 30 mg/kg of body weight, depending on type and amount of preanesthetic medication; when administered as the only source of anesthesia, approximately half the anticipated dose should be injected rapidly; the rest should be administered in small increments until the desired effect is reached

    2. May be used in combination with other anesthetics (inhalants) to produce and maintain surgical anesthesia

    3. Preanesthetic drugs decrease the dose of barbiturates required to produce anesthesia

    4. Atropine sulfate or glycopyrrolate decreases salivary secretions, the potential for laryngospasm, and vagal activity

    5. The anesthetic duration can be prolonged by administration of 50% glucose IV; this is known as the *glucose effect*

    6. Complete recovery occurs in 8 to 24 hours

    7. The minimum lethal dose in dogs is 50 mg/kg IV

    8. Overdose is treated by cardiopulmonary support, respiratory stimulants, fluid therapy, alkalinizing solutions (Na^+ $HCO3^-$), and diuresis

    9. Oral administration is neither safe nor practical for dogs or cats

  B. Thiopental sodium (Pentothal)

    1. Administer IV in small increments to produce anesthesia (6 to 18 mg/kg)

    2. Use in 1.25% to 10% solutions

      a. Solution should be discarded after being stored for 7 days in a refrigerator at 5° to 6° C or 3 days at room temperature; precipitated solutions should not be used

   b. More concentrated solutions cause severe tissue damage (pH ≈ 13) if accidentally administered perivascularly
   c. Perivascular injection causes necrosis of tissue; tissue necrosis may be minimized by infiltrating the area with saline solution; pain can be minimized by injecting 2% lidocaine
   3. Dose for induction and intubation is 6 to 12 mg/kg; solutions of up to 10% are used in horses; repeated doses are cumulative, resulting in prolonged recovery from anesthesia
   4. Dose is based on lean body weight (body weight minus fat)
   5. Anesthesia usually occurs in 20 to 60 seconds
   6. Ventricular arrhythmias (ventricular bigeminy) may occur after induction of anesthesia (Fig. 8-3)
   7. Apnea is more common after rapid IV injections; ventilation should be supported early in anesthesia
   8. Recovery occurs in 10 to 30 minutes, but the animal may remain depressed for many hours depending on the dose; repeated doses are cumulative
   9. Overdose is best treated with O_2, controlled ventilation, fluids, alkalinizing solutions, and diuretics
C. Methohexital (Brevane)
   1. Similar to thiopental, except it is less cumulative (it is rapidly metabolized)

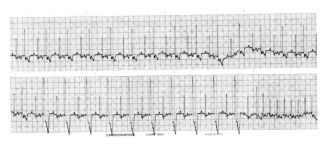

Fig. 8-3
Ventricular bigeminy (every other QRS complex is abnormal) produced by the rapid administration of thiopental to a dog.

2. 6 to 10 mg/kg provides light anesthesia in small animals; 6 mg/kg in horses and adult cattle; 3 to 5 mg/kg in calves
3. Solutions are stable at room temperature for at least 6 weeks
4. Recommended in sighthounds (e.g., greyhounds, whippets, borzois) because of its short duration of action
5. Duration is 5 to 10 minutes; less than thiobarbiturates
6. Respiratory depression and apnea are common
7. Induction and recovery may be accompanied by pronounced involuntary excitement and convulsions (delirium); CNS effects can be prevented by diazepam (0.2 mg/kg); the recovery period is characterized by muscle tremors and struggling even with preanesthetic sedation in horses
8. Not routinely used in large animals

DOSES ▪ Barbiturates			
AGENT	**ANIMAL**	**DOSE**	**DURATION**
Pentobarbital sodium	Dogs	10-33 mg/kg	30 min
	Cats	25 mg/kg	
	Horses	Not recommended	
	Cattle	15-30 mg/kg	
	Pigs	10-30 mg/kg	
Thiopental sodium	Small animals	8-20 mg/kg	10-30 min
	Horses	8.8-15.4 mg/kg	
	Cattle	7-13 mg/kg	
	Calves	15-22 mg/kg	
	Pigs	5.5-11 mg/kg	
Methohexital	Small animals	6-10 mg/kg	5-10 min
	Horses	6 mg/kg	
	Cattle	6 mg/kg	
	Calves	3-5 mg/kg	

> **CAUTIONS ▪ Barbiturates**
>
> - Respiratory depressant
> - Cardiovascular depressant (transient hypotension)
> - Tissue toxicity with a greater than 2.5% concentration; intraarterial injection may cause severe pain, vasoconstriction, and tissue necrosis
> - Liver damage, tolerance
> - Methohexital may cause excitement in recovery period

NONBARBITURATE ANESTHETIC DRUGS

  I. Etomidate (Amidate)

    A. A rapid-acting, ultrashort, nonbarbiturate, noncumulative IV anesthetic

    B. General anesthetic actions

      1. Produces hypnosis (sleep), minimal analgesia at subhypnotic doses; as with barbiturates, interacts with CNS $GABA_A$ receptors

      2. Produces depression of the reticular formation of the brain stem

      3. Enhances monosynaptic reflex activity, which may result in myoclonal activity

      4. Decreases CBF and $CMRO_2$; increases ratio of CBF to $CMRO_2$

      5. Not a good analgesic

> **USEFUL FACTS ▪ Etomidate**
>
> - Rapid onset and recovery
> - Noncumulative
> - Minimal cardiovascular effects
> - Minimal respiratory effects
> - No histamine release

    C. Organ system effects

      1. Respiratory system

        a. Brief periods of apnea may occur immediately after IV injection

       b. Tidal volume and respiratory rate are minimally affected during anesthetic maintenance; respiratory rate may increase

  2. Cardiovascular system

       a. Produces little change in heart rate, arterial BP, and cardiac output when administered at induction doses

       b. Cardiac contractility is mildly depressed

       c. Does not sensitize the myocardium to catecholamine-induced cardiac arrhythmias

       d. Does not produce histamine release

  3. GI system

       a. Nausea and vomiting are occasionally observed during induction and after anesthesia; these effects can be inhibited by proper preanesthetic medication

       b. GI motility is minimally affected

  4. Endocrine system

       a. An antiglucocorticoid and mineralocorticoid effect is produced; adrenocorticotropic hormone stimulation tests and glucose tolerance tests may be invalid

       b. Adrenocorticoid function is suppressed for 2 to 3 hours in dogs after a single IV administration of etomidate

  5. Crosses the placenta, but effects are minimal because of the rapid clearance

D. Fate and elimination

  1. Rapidly distributed to the brain, heart, spleen, lungs, liver, and intestines

  2. Anesthetic duration of action depends on drug redistribution and capacity; limited ester hydrolysis by the liver

  3. Noncumulative

E. Other

  1. Produces good muscle relaxation during anesthesia; involuntary muscle movements and myoclonic reactions occur during induction and recovery

  2. Does not trigger malignant hyperthermia in susceptible pigs but predisposes them to a more rapid onset of malignant hyperthermia if triggered by other drugs

  3. Pain may occur during IV injection

4. Decreases intraocular pressure
5. Can cause acute hemolysis
6. Nausea and vomiting can occur in recovery after the use of multiple doses

F. Clinical uses
   1. Induction agent for general anesthesia
   2. Short-term (5 to 10 minutes) anesthesia in dogs and cats; produces excessive muscle rigidity and seizures in horses and cattle

G. Doses
   1. 1.5 to 3 mg/kg IV in dogs and cats
   2. The best results are obtained after sedating the animal with diazepam, xylazine, or acepromazine

---

CAUTIONS ▪ Etomidate

- An antiglucocorticoid and mineralocorticoid effect
- Depression in adrenal function for up to 3 hours in dogs
- May cause hemolysis, nausea, or vomiting

II. Propofol
   A. A rapid-acting, ultrashort, nonbarbiturate, and relatively noncumulative IV anesthetic
   B. General anesthetic actions
      1. Produces sedation-hypnosis similar to that induced by thiopental and methohexital. Like barbiturates interact with CNS $GABA_A$ receptors
      2. Produces dose-dependent depression of the cerebral cortex and CNS polysynaptic reflexes; may enhance the effects of nondepolarizing neuromuscular blocking drugs
      3. Produces minimal analgesia at subhypnotic doses
      4. Anesthetic doses decrease CBF and $CMRO_2$; the CBF/$CMRO_2$ ratio is unchanged or minimally increased
      5. Possesses anticonvulsant properties similar to barbiturates

---

USEFUL FACTS ▪ Propofol

- Rapid onset and recovery
- Relatively noncumulative

C. Chemistry
   1. An alkylphenol poorly soluble in water
   2. Solubilized in a lecithin-containing emulsion (10% soybean oil and 1.2% egg lecithin) called *Intralipid*
D. Organ system effects
   1. Respiratory system
      a. Similar to thiopental
      b. Dose-dependent respiratory depression and initial periods of apnea
   2. Cardiovascular system
      a. Produces little change in heart rate
      b. Dose-dependent decreases in arterial BP transiently caused by decreases in cardiac output and systemic vascular resistance
      c. Minimal but dose-dependent negative inotropic effect at anesthetic doses
   3. Other organ systems: effects of propofol on the liver, kidney, and GI system are the result of changes in arterial BP and organ blood flow
   4. Crosses the placenta and can induce fetal depression, which is dose-dependent
E. Fate and elimination
   1. Termination of anesthetic effects and short duration of action are due to redistribution from well-perfused (vessel-rich) tissues such as the brain to muscle and fat
   2. Relatively rapid biotransformation by the liver compared with thiobarbiturates
   3. Rapid clearing from the body by hepatic and extrahepatic metabolism compared with thiobarbiturates
   4. Relatively noncumulative
F. Other
   1. Produces good to excellent muscle relaxation
   2. May elicit pain on induction to anesthesia
   3. Rapid recovery; little or no "hangover" effect
   4. Capable of supporting microbial growth and endotoxin production
   5. May induce oxidative injury to feline red blood cells when used repeatedly
   6. Expensive
G. Clinical uses
   1. From induction to general anesthesia

2. Maintenance of general anesthesia when combined with opioid analgesics or other sedative-analgesic drugs
3. Can be used for cesarean section surgery with generally good results

DOSES ■ Propofol		
ANIMAL	**DOSE**	**DURATION**
Small animals	4-8 mg/kg	20 min 30 min in cats
Horses (not recommended as a sole anesthetic)	2-8 mg/kg	16-49 min

CAUTIONS ■ Propofol
• Respiratory depression; transient
• Cardiovascular depression; transient
• Can support microbial growth or cause infection

H. Doses
1. 4 to 8 mg/kg IV in dogs and cats for induction
2. 0.3 to 0.8 mg/kg/min IV infusion in dogs and cats for anesthetic maintenance; usually used with diazepam and oxymorphone or fentanyl for added muscle relaxation and analgesia; medetomidine is an excellent adjunct to propofol anesthesia

III. Chloral hydrate
A. Chloral hydrate is no longer sold as an anesthetic for veterinary use but is occasionally purchased as crystals and solubilized in water for IV administration as a sedative, hypnotic, or for euthanasia in horses; administered IV or orally to cattle
B. General anesthetic actions
1. Drug is sedative-hypnotic, depressing the cerebral cortex, resulting in hyporeflexia
2. Subanesthetic doses depress motor and sensory nerves and produce mild sedation

3. The amount needed to produce anesthesia approaches the minimal lethal dose; death caused by progressive depression of the respiratory center
4. Anesthetic doses produce deep sleep lasting for several hours; recovery is prolonged (6 to 24 hours)
5. Drug is a poor analgesic at subhypnotic doses; excitement or delirium is precipitated by painful stimulation

---

USEFUL FACTS ▪ Chloral hydrate

- Excellent hypnotic, anxiolytic
- Can be administered in many routes (orally, rectally, IV, intraperitoneally, by stomach tube)

C. Chemistry
  1. Physical properties: colorless, translucent crystals that volatilize when exposed to air
  2. Chemical properties
    a. Readily soluble in both water and oil
    b. Bitter, caustic taste; irritating to the skin and mucous membranes
D. Organ system effects
  1. Respiratory system
    a. Sedative doses minimally depress both respiratory rate and tidal volume
    b. Anesthetic doses markedly affect ventilation by depression of the respiratory centers; death is usually caused by progressive respiratory center depression
  2. Cardiovascular system
    a. Anesthetic doses decrease contractility
    b. Potentiates vagal (parasympathetic) activity; bradycardia, P-R interval prolongation, and sinus arrest or atrioventricular block
    c. Supraventricular arrhythmias and atrial fibrillation have been observed
  3. GI system
    a. GI secretions and motility are increased, diarrhea may occur after anesthesia

        b. Nausea and vomiting, salivation, and defecation may occur

    4. Uterus and fetus: chloral hydrate readily crosses the placenta

  E. Absorption, fate, and excretion

    1. May be administered orally, rectally, IV, or by stomach tube; very irritating if given perivascularly, IM, or intraperitoneally

    2. A small amount is excreted unchanged in the urine; the majority is reduced to trichloroethanol

  F. Clinical uses

    1. Not used for small animal anesthesia

    2. Has lost most of its popularity as a general anesthetic in large animals but can be used as a sedative; the dose for anesthesia is variable (220 to 660 mg/kg)

    3. Casting harnesses or hobbles are generally necessary

    4. Obtained from chemical companies (Sigma-Aldrich)

  G. Dose

    1. Sedation: 2 to 3 g/45 kg IV

    2. Anesthesia: up to 10 g/45 kg IV

DOSES ■ Chloral hydrate		
ANIMAL	**DOSE**	**DURATION**
Horse	2-3 g/45 kg IV (sedation) Up to 10 g/45 kg IV (anesthesia)	1-4 hr

CAUTIONS ■ Chloral hydrate
• Narrow margin of safety • Cardiorespiratory depression

IV. Guaifenesin (glyceryl guaiacolate)

  A. Chemistry

    1. Physical properties: a white, finely granular powder that is soluble in water

    2. Chemical properties

        a. A decongestant and antitussive also noted for its centrally acting muscle relaxant properties

  b. Very similar to mephenesin chemically; mephenesin is an aromatic glycerol ether
B. General anesthetic actions
  1. Blocks impulse transmission at the internuncial neurons of the spinal cord and brain stem; guaifenesin is a centrally acting muscle relaxant
  2. Produces relaxation of skeletal muscles but produces minimal effects on the function of the diaphragm at relaxant doses
  3. Relaxes laryngeal and pharyngeal muscles, thus facilitating intubation of the trachea
  4. Compatible with preanesthetic and anesthetic agents
  5. Produces excitement-free induction and recovery from anesthesia
  6. In excessive doses, produces paradoxic increases in muscle rigidity

---

USEFUL FACTS ■ **Guaifenesin**

- Good relaxation of skeletal muscles
- The laryngeal and pharyngeal muscles are relaxed, facilitating intubation
- Good recovery

C. Organ system effects
  1. Respiratory system
    a. Little, if any, effect at relaxant doses
    b. Ventilatory rate may increase initially; tidal volume decreases
    c. Excessive doses produce an apneustic pattern of breathing
  2. Cardiovascular system
    a. Initial mild decrease in BP, which returns to normal
    b. Myocardial contractile force and cardiac rate are relatively unchanged
  3. GI system: increases GI motility
  4. Uterus and fetus: guaifenesin crosses the placental barrier but has minimal effects on the fetus
D. Absorption, fate, and excretion: excreted in the urine after conjugation in the liver to a glucuronide

E. Clinical uses
1. Used for restraint and muscle relaxation in horses and cattle
2. Used for short anesthetic procedures of up to 30 to 60 minutes
3. Used as a 5% to 10% solution; high concentrations (> 6%) may cause hemolysis and hemoglobinuria in cattle; solutions greater than 15% cause hives and hemolysis
4. Often made by mixing 50 g guaifenesin with 50 g dextrose and 1 L warm sterile water (5% solution)
5. Compatible with other IV and inhalation anesthetic drugs

CAUTIONS ▪ **Guaifenesin**

- High concentration (>6%) may cause hemolysis and hemoglobinuria in cattle; greater than 15% cause hives and hemolysis

---

F. Dose
1. The dose varies from 50 to 100 mg/kg
2. Guaifenesin may be administered to effect with the following agents:
   a. 2 g thiopental
   b. 2.5 g pentobarbital
   c. 500 mg ketamine; 500 ml of 5% guaifenesin; 20 to 50 mg xylazine for ruminants and up to 500 mg xylazine for horses has been administered to effect to produce total IV anesthesia
3. The margin of safety (guaifenesin alone) is three times the therapeutic dose (approximately 300 mg/kg IV)
4. Excessive doses cause muscle rigidity and an apneustic pattern of breathing

DISSOCIOGENIC ANESTHETIC DRUGS

Dissociative anesthetics include the arylcyclohexylamines: ketamine, tiletamine, and phencyclidine
 I. Anesthesia is characterized by profound amnesia, analgesia, and catalepsy

    A. Oral, ocular, and swallowing reflexes remain intact, and muscle tone generally increases

    B. Large doses can produce convulsions, which can be controlled with small doses of pentobarbital, thiopental, propofol, diazepam, or midazolam

II. Psychosomatic effects such as hallucinations, confusion, agitation, and fear have occurred in humans and seem to occur in animals when large doses are administered

III. Muscle rigidity is minimized by the previous administration of tranquilizers, sedatives, or benzodiazepines (diazepam, midazolam)

IV. Effects are partially reversed by adrenergic and cholinergic blockade

V. Specific drugs

    A. Ketamine HCl is the most commonly used dissociative anesthetic in veterinary practice

        1. Used for restraint, anesthetic induction, and minor surgical procedures

        2. Palpebral, conjunctival, corneal, and swallowing reflexes persist; nystagmus is common

    B. Telazol®, a 1:1 drug combination of zolazepam (a benzodiazepine) and tiletamine, is a dissociogenic drug combination for use in all species; it is very useful in aggressive dogs or cats and exotic animals

VI. Salivation and lacrimation are common and may become copious

VII. Tremors, oculogyria, tonic spasticity, and convulsions occur when excessive doses are administered

VIII. Muscle relaxation is poor; for best results, ketamine and other arylcyclohexylamines should be used with drugs that produce muscle relaxation (e.g., benzodiazepines)

IX. Animals are hyperresponsive and ataxic during recovery (a result of emergence delirium)

X. Analgesia is selective, with the best results obtained in superficial pain models; visceral pain is not abolished

XI. System effects and responses

    A. CNS

        1. Produces dissociative anesthesia characterized by poor muscle relaxation and catalepsy; inhibits N-methyl-D-aspartate, resulting in analgesia

2. Ketamine increases CBF and causes no change or an increase in $CMRO_2$; the $CBF/CMRO_2$ ratio increases; arterial BP and intracranial pressure increase; cerebral perfusion pressure decreases

B. Respiratory system
   1. Apneustic pattern of breathing (breath holding); respiratory rate may be increased; arterial Po_2 generally falls after IV administration
   2. Possible increases in Pco_2 and decreases in arterial pH caused by the irregular pattern of breathing

C. Cardiovascular system
   1. Increased heart rate
   2. Increased BP
   3. Increase in heart rate and decrease in cardiac contractility, may induce pulmonary edema or acute heart failure in animals with preexisting cardiac disease
   4. Ketamine and other cyclohexamines minimally sensitize the heart to catecholamine-induced arrhythmias

D. Kidney and liver
   1. Ketamine HCl is metabolized by the liver and excreted by the kidneys
   2. Ketamine should be used with caution in animals with hepatic or renal disease; ketamine can be used in cats with urethral obstruction, provided renal disease is absent or not severe and the obstruction has been eliminated

---

USEFUL FACTS ▪ Ketamine

- Somatic analgesia
- Activate cardiorespiratory system

XII. Dose
   A. Ketamine
      1. Cat: 6 to 10 mg/kg IM or subcutaneously; 2 to 6 mg/kg IV; doses as small as 1 to 3 mg *total* are administered IV to sick animals and cats with urethral obstruction

2. Dog: xylazine 0.1 to 1 mg/kg IV and ketamine 10 mg/kg IV; diazepam or midazolam 0.2 mg/kg IV and ketamine 5.5 mg/kg IV; 1 ml diazepam plus 1 ml ketamine administered 1 ml/10 kg IV
3. Pigs: 6 to 8 mg/kg ketamine plus 1 to 2 mg/kg xylazine administered IM produces short-term anesthesia in pigs

B. Telazol®
1. Dogs, cats, cattle, sheep, goats: 1 to 8 mg/kg IM
2. Horses: xylazine 1 mg/kg followed by 1 to 1.5 mg/kg Telazol®, IV
3. Pigs: 500 mg of Telazol® powder with 2.5 ml of xylazine (100 mg/ml) and 2.5 ml of ketamine (100 mg/ml); administer 1 to 2 ml per 50 kg IM

CAUTIONS ■ Ketamine

- Poor muscle relaxation
- Tremor

CHAPTER NINE

Inhalation Anesthesia

"O sleep! O gentle sleep! Nature's soft nurse, how have I
frightened thee, That thou no more will weigh my eyelids
down and steep my senses in forgetfulness?"

WILLIAM SHAKESPEARE

OVERVIEW

Inhalant anesthetic drugs are used to produce general anesthesia.
They are suitable for use in all species including reptiles, birds, and
zoo animals. Their safe use requires knowledge of their pharmacologic effects and physical and chemical properties. Anesthetic
doses produce unconsciousness (hypnosis), hyporeflexia, and
analgesia. Inhalant anesthetic drugs provide optimal control of
anesthesia, rapid induction and recovery from anesthesia, and
relatively few adverse side effects. This chapter outlines the basic
principles of inhalation anesthesia and its use.

GENERAL CONSIDERATIONS

   I. Inhalant anesthetic drugs are vapors or gases that are breathed
directly into the respiratory system

  II. To produce anesthesia, they must be absorbed from the
alveoli into the bloodstream and carried by the blood to
the brain

 III. Inhalant anesthetic drugs are primarily eliminated by the
lungs

 IV. Because the uptake and elimination of inhalant anesthetic
drugs are relatively rapid, the depth of anesthesia can be
controlled effectively, but constant patient monitoring is
required

PROPERTIES OF DESIRABLE INHALANT ANESTHETIC DRUGS

    I. Nonirritating and free from disagreeable odors

   II. Easily controlled, producing rapid induction and recovery from anesthesia

  III. Adequate muscular relaxation

  IV. Adequate analgesia

   V. Should not promote bleeding

  VI. Minimal to no side effects

 VII. Nontoxic to the patient or the environment

VIII. Not flammable or explosive (stable during storage)

  IX. Compatible with other drugs

   X. Easy to deliver

  XI. Inexpensive

FACTORS CONTROLLING THE BRAIN CONCENTRATIONS OF INHALANT ANESTHETIC DRUGS (Table 9-1)

  I. Factors governing the delivery of a suitable concentration of inhalant anesthetic drugs

    A. Physical and chemical properties of the agent

      1. Vapor pressure of the agent governs the volatility of inhalant anesthetic drugs

      2. Boiling points (other than nitrous oxide and desflurane) are higher than room temperature ($70°$ F or $27°$ C)

    B. Anesthetic system

      1. The concentration of inhalant anesthetic drugs delivered to the patient is primarily determined by the type of anesthetic circuit, fresh gas flow rate, type of vaporizer, and vaporizer temperature

      2. Frequent inspection and maintenance of inhalation anesthetic equipment is necessary to prevent malfunctions caused by factors such as leaks and sticky one-way valves

 II. Ventilation and uptake: The partial pressure of inhalant anesthetic drugs in the brain depends on the alveolar partial

TABLE 9-1

BOILING POINTS, VAPOR PRESSURES, AND VAPORIZATION OF INHALANT ANESHTETIC DRUGS

DRUG	BOILING POINT (°C)	VAPOR PRESSURE AT 20° C (MM HG)	MAXIMUM CONCENTRATION OF VAPOR DELIVERED BY SATURATION VAPORIZER AT 20° C (%)	USEFUL RANGES OF CONCENTRATION (AGENT USED ALONE)	
				INDUCTION (%)	MAINTENANCE (%)
Volatile anesthetic drugs					
Desflurane	23.5	664	87.4	8-15	5-9
Sevoflurane	59	160	22	4-5	2-3.5
Isoflurane	48	252	33	2-6	1-3
Halothane	50	243	32	1-4*	0.5-2
Anesthetic gas					
Nitrous oxide[†]	−89	39,500 (50 atm)			

*Up to 10% may be used in induction of large animals.
†Nitrous oxide is a gas at room temperature.

pressure; the alveolar partial pressure of the inhalant anesthetic drugs is the result of the inspired concentration, the alveolar ventilation, and uptake from the lungs. Uptake of inhalant anesthetic drugs is determined by blood/gas partition coefficient, cardiac output or lung blood flow, and the alveolar-to-venous partial pressure difference.

A. Inspired concentration
  1. Concentration effect: the greater the inspired concentration administered (vaporizer setting), the more rapid the rate of rise of alveolar concentration
  2. Second gas effect
     a. Theoretically suggests that a 50% to 80% inspired concentration of nitrous oxide initially augments the inflow and rate of uptake of the second gas (e.g., halothane, isoflurane) in the inspired mixture; it is not a clinically valid concept

B. Alveolar ventilation
  1. Generally, the greater the ventilation (tidal volume), the more rapid the approach of the alveolar gas concentration of any gas or vapor to the inspired gas concentration*
  2. Limited by lung volume; the larger the functional residual capacity, the longer it takes to wash in a new inhalant anesthetic drug
  3. Factors affecting ventilation
     a. Respiratory rate
     b. Tidal volume
     c. Increased dead space (anatomic and physiologic) during anesthesia decreases effective alveolar ventilation; tidal volume (V_T) = dead space volume (V_D) + alveolar ventilation (V_A): $V_T = V_D + V_A$
     d. Effective alveolar ventilation requires a patent airway

C. Uptake of anesthetic from the lungs
  1. Solubility: describes how much of a substance can be dissolved in a gas, liquid, or solid (e.g., fat); the solu-

---

*Excessive hyperventilation may slow induction by reducing cerebral blood flow.

bility of inhalant anesthetic drugs is usually expressed as a partition coefficient; how an inhalant anesthetic drug is distributed between two phases (e.g., between blood and gas, between tissue and blood); Ostwald's partition coefficient expresses the solubility of an inhalant anesthetic drug between blood and gas

BLOOD-GAS PARTITIONING	
AGENT	**BLOOD-GAS PARTITION COEFFICIENT (OSTWALD'S COEFFICIENT)**
Halothane	2.36
Isoflurane	1.41
Sevoflurane	0.69
Nitrous oxide	0.49
Desflurane	0.42

A gas with a blood-gas partition coefficient of 2 has *one* volume in the alveoli per *two* volumes in the blood at equilibrium (Fig. 9-1)

a. Anesthetic blood-gas partition coefficient and drug potency determine the rapidity of onset of anesthetic effect

b. The greater the blood-gas partition coefficient, the greater the solubility of anesthetic in the blood; therefore the tension of anesthetic in arterial blood rises slowly for drugs that are highly soluble in blood (high blood-gas coefficients); onset of the clinical effect is contingent on the tension of anesthetic developed in the blood; more soluble drugs produce longer induction and recovery periods because large amounts of anesthetic must be taken into the blood before the tension or partial pressure of the anesthetic rises sufficiently to produce anesthesia; clinically, slow induction may be overcome by raising the inspired concentration to values exceeding those necessary to maintain anesthesia

c. The lower the blood-gas partition coefficient, the less soluble the inhalant anesthetic drug is in the

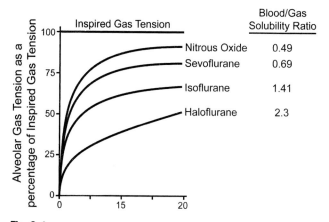

Fig. 9-1

The blood:gas solubility coefficient is a determinant of the rate of rise (rate of increase) of the alveolar anesthetic concentration. The lower the blood gas solubility coefficient, the faster the increase in alveolar anesthetic concentration and the faster induction and recovery from anesthesia (sevoflurane faster than isoflurane).

blood (only small quantities are carried in the blood; thus both alveolar concentration and tension will rise rapidly) and the more rapidly the tension or partial pressure of the drug increases in the blood; less soluble drugs such as nitrous oxide, isoflurane, and sevoflurane have relatively short induction and short recovery periods

d. Generally, inhalant anesthetic drugs with high blood-gas partition coefficients exhibit long induction and recovery times; inhalant anesthetic drugs with low blood-gas partition coefficients exhibit short induction and recovery times

2. Cardiac output: blood carries anesthetic drug away from the lungs; the greater the cardiac output, the slower the rate of rise of alveolar concentration and tension in the lung; excited, stressed animals have a slower rate of induction; animals with depressed cardiac output may be induced to anesthesia very rapidly

3. Alveolar-venous anesthetic tension difference: during induction, tissues remove nearly all the anesthetic brought to them because of the high tissue solubility of most inhalant anesthetic drugs; venous blood returning to the lungs contains little anesthetic; as time passes, increasing tissue saturation raises the venous blood concentration; less anesthetic is taken up in the lungs; anesthetic uptake by the lung is a changing but continuous process

4. Other
   a. Right-to-left intracardiac or intrapulmonary shunts (e.g., Fallot's tetralogy) delay induction; this effect is more important for poorly soluble agents (nitrous oxide)
   b. Left-to-right shunts may speed the rate of induction, particularly if cardiac output is low
   c. Pathologic changes in alveoli: if the alveolar membranes are affected by disease resulting in exudate, transudate, emphysema, or pulmonary fibrosis, diffusion may be impaired, and the uptake of the inhalant anesthetic drug is thus reduced

III. Factors governing brain and tissue uptake of anesthetic
   A. Same as those determining uptake from the lungs
      1. Solubility (blood vs tissue)
      2. Tissue blood flow
      3. Arterial blood to tissue anesthetic tension difference
   B. The uptake by tissue is dependent on anesthetic concentration, blood flow, and tissue capillary density; tissues can be divided into four groups according to blood supply (Fig. 9-2)
      1. Vessel-rich group (VRG): 75% of cardiac output (e.g., brain, heart, intestines, liver, kidneys, spleen)
      2. Vessel-moderate group, or muscle group (MG): 15% to 20% of cardiac output (e.g., muscle, skin)
      3. Neutral fat group (FG): 5% of cardiac output (e.g., adipose tissue)
      4. Vessel-poor group: 1% to 2% of cardiac output (e.g., bone, tendons, cartilage)
   C. Tissue-blood partition coefficients vary far less than blood-gas coefficients (except for fat)

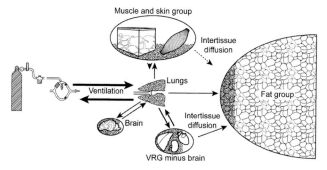

Muscle and skin group

Intertissue diffusion

Ventilation

Lungs

Fat group

Brain

Intertissue diffusion

VRG minus brain

Fig. 9-2

Anesthetic delivery to tissues is dependent on their blood flow. Tissues including lungs, brain, heart, and major organs (liver, kidney) have a relatively high blood flow (vessel-rich group) compared with other tissues of the body (muscle group, fat) and are susceptible to anesthetic drug-related effects.

    1. Lowest is approximately 1 (nitrous oxide in lung tissue)
    2. Highest is approximately 4 (halothane in muscle tissue)
  D. Important considerations
    1. Equilibration of an inhalant anesthetic drug in the VRG is complete in 5 to 20 minutes; this is approximately how long it will take for anesthesia to become deep enough to do surgery, providing the anesthetic concentration (vaporizer setting) is appropriate
    2. Equilibration in the MG may take $1\frac{1}{2}$ to 4 hours
    3. Because of a higher blood flow, arterial-tissue partial-pressure difference, and therefore uptake, decrease far more rapidly in VRG than in MG
    4. Solubility of an inhalant anesthetic drug in VRG and MG may affect recovery time
    5. The fat group occupies 10% to 30% body mass and receives approximately 5% of the cardiac output; the FG has a higher tissue solubility for inhalant anesthetic drugs than most other tissues and thus has a greater and more prolonged capacity to absorb anesthetic; because of its low blood flow, the FG has little effect on induction of anesthesia; the FG may affect recovery time after prolonged anesthetic periods (3 hours or longer)

FAT-BLOOD PARTITIONING	
AGENTS	**FAT-BLOOD PARTITION COEFFICIENT**
Halothane	65
Isoflurane	48
Sevoflurane	65
Nitrous oxide	2.3
Desflurane	27.2

6. Vessel-poor group tissues have very little effect on short-duration anesthesia
7. Rubber solubility: methoxyflurane is freely absorbed into rubber components of the anesthetic system; during recovery, they equilibrate back into the anesthetic circuitry
8. Halothane, isoflurane, and desflurane are stable in moist soda lime; sevoflurane produces a potentially toxic substance called *Compound A* when it comes in contact with dry soda lime; the concentrations of Compound A measured in circle-systems are 5 to 10 times lower than those reported to produce toxic effects

BLOOD FLOW GROUPS		
GROUP	**EXAMPLES**	**PRINCIPAL POINTS**
VRG: vessel-rich group	Brain, heart, liver	Equilibration of an inhalant anesthetic drug is complete in 5 to 20 minutes
MG: vessel-moderate group/muscle group	Muscle, skin	Equilibration of an inhalant anesthetic drug is complete in $1\frac{1}{2}$ to 4 hours
FG: neutral fat group	Adipose tissue	May affect recovery time after prolonged anesthetic periods
VPG: vessel-poor group	Bone, tendons	Have very little effect on short duration anesthesia

ELIMINATION OF INHALANT AESHTETIC DRUGS

I. By the lung
  A. Inhalation anesthetics are excreted largely unchanged by the lungs
  B. The same factors that affect the rate of anesthetic uptake are important in anesthetic elimination
    1. Pulmonary ventilation
    2. Blood flow
    3. Solubility of inhalant anesthetic in blood and tissue
  C. As anesthetic gas washes out of the lungs, the arterial blood tension falls, followed by the tension in tissues; because of the high blood flow to the brain, the anesthetic tension falls rapidly and accounts for the rapid awakening from anesthesia with insoluble agents such as sevoflurane and desflurane; decreases in anesthetic drug concentration from other tissues are progressively slower and dependent on blood flow
II. Other routes through which small quantities of inhalant anesthetic drugs may be excreted are skin, milk, mucous membrane, and urine
III. Biotransformation—Anesthetic gases are metabolized in the body to variable degrees

BIOTRANSFORMATION OF INHALANT ANESTHETIC DRUGS TO METABOLITES	
AGENT	**% RECOVERED AS METABOLITE**
Halothane	20.0
Isoflurane	0.25
Sevoflurane	3.0-5.0
Nitrous oxide	0.004
Desflurane	0.02

  A. Metabolism is generally by hepatic microsomal enzyme systems; various intermediate metabolites are formed; these may be responsible for certain toxic effects or aftereffects (Table 9-2)
    1. Approximately 20% of inspired halothane is metabolized compared with 50% of methoxyflurane;

TABLE 9-2

DEGREES OF METABOLISM AND PRINCIPLE METABOLITES OF INHALANT ANESTHETIC DRUGS IN HUMANS

	DEGREE OF METABOLISM* (%)	MECHANISM OF METABOLISM	PRINCIPAL METABOLITES
Halothane	20-45	Hepatic cytochrome P450 (2A6, 2E1, 3A4)	-Trifluoroacetic acid -Cl -Br
Isoflurane	0.2	Hepatic cytochrome P450 (2E1, 3A)	-Trifluoroacetic acid -Trifluoroacetaldehyde -Trifluoroacetylchloride
Sevoflurane	5	Hepatic cytochrome P450 (2E1)	-Hexafluoroisopropanol -F
Desflurane	0.02	Hepatic cytochrome P450 (2E1, 3A)	-Trifluoroacetic acid -F -CO_2 -Water
Nitrous oxide	0.004	Intestinal bacteria (E. coli)	-N_2 -Inactivated methionine synthase -Reduced cobalamin (vitamin B12)
Xenon	0	—	—

*Degree of metabolism includes estimates from recovery of metabolites and estimates from recovery of the unchanged drug.
†Reductive metabolism.

approximately 0.25% isoflurane is metabolized; approximately 0.02% of desflurane is metabolized
2. Toxic metabolites are primarily inorganic fluoride and bromide ions

IV. Diffusion hypoxia may occur at the end of anesthesia and is discussed in the nitrous oxide section in Chapter 10; briefly, the rapid elimination of N_2O from the blood into the alveoli results in the dilution of alveolar O_2 by N_2O and hypoxemia if ventilation is not maintained

POTENCY OF INHALANT ANESTHETIC DRUGS

I. The potency of inhalant anesthetics can be expressed in several ways; one method is to measure the minimum alveolar concentration (MAC) of the inhalant anesthetic drug at surgical anesthesia (Table 9-3); MAC is generally defined as the minimum alveolar concentration of an anesthetic (1 atm) that produces no response in 50% of patients exposed to a painful stimulus
   A. MAC is generally measured as the end-tidal concentration of an inhalant anesthetic drug
   B. MAC values are not vaporizer settings
   C. MAC values are used to compare the potency of anesthetics

II. MAC values vary among species and are affected by the following factors:
   A. Age: older patients require less inhalant anesthetic drugs
   B. Body weight: smaller patients may require more inhalant anesthetic drugs

TABLE 9-3
MINIMUM ALVEOLAR CONCENTRATIONS (MAC) OF INHALANT ANESTHETIC DRUGS IN VARIOUS SPECIES

	HUMAN	DOG	CAT	HORSE
Halothane	0.76	0.87	1.19	0.88
Isoflurane	1.2	1.3	1.63	1.31
Sevoflurane	1.93	2.34	2.58	2.34
Desflurane	6.99	7.20	9.80	7.23
Nitrous oxide	101.1	188-297	255	190

    C. Temperature: hypothermia reduces MAC
    D. Administration of other central nervous system depressant drugs
    E. Disease:
       1. Hyperthyroidism or hypothyroidism
       2. Hypovolemia, anemia
       3. Septicemia
       4. Extreme acid-base imbalances
       5. Pregnancy

III. Studies using dogs suggest the following:
    A. 1 MAC produces light anesthesia
    B. 1.5 MAC produces moderate surgical anesthesia
    C. 2 MAC produces deep anesthesia

INCREASING OR DECREASING INHALANT ANESTHETIC CONCENTRATIONS

Increasing

Turn up O_2 flow
Turn up vaporizer
DO NOT activate O_2 flush valve

Decreasing

Turn up O_2 flow or activate flush valve
Turn vaporizer down or off

Ventilate the patient

CHAPTER TEN

Pharmacology of Inhalation Anesthetic Drugs

"Sleep is pain's easiest salve, and doth fulfill all offices of death, except to kill."

JOHN DONNE

OVERVIEW

Inhalant anesthetic drugs are pharmacologically active chemicals that cause unconsciousness, various degrees of muscle relaxation and analgesia, and changes in organ system function. Their administration requires familiarity with a variety of equipment (e.g., vaporizers, flow meters, pressure valves) needed to vaporize the anesthetic liquid and the anesthetic circuits used to accurately deliver the anesthetic to the patient. Theoretically, the depth of inhalation anesthesia is easily controlled compared with that of injectable anesthesia. This chapter outlines the pharmacologic properties and the interactions of inhalant anesthetic drugs.

GENERAL CONSIDERATIONS

I. The factors that influence the ability of an inhalant anesthetic drug to produce general anesthesia are discussed in Chapter 9 and include tissue membrane effects and physiochemical properties (Table 10-1)

A. Factors that influence anesthetic uptake and delivery to the brain include:

1. Physical and chemical properties of the agent
2. Anesthetic system
3. Inspired concentration
4. Alveolar ventilation

TABLE 10-1

SUMMARY OF PHYSIOCHEMICAL PROPERTIES OF INHALATION AGENTS

PROPERTIES	ETHER	NITROUS OXIDE	HALOTHANE	ISOFLURANE	SEVOFLURANE	DESFLURANE
Chemical formula	$(C_2H_5)_2O$	N_2O				
Molecular weight	74	44	197.4	185	200	168
Specific gravity (g/ml)	0.72	1.53	1.87	1.52	1.52	1.47
Odor	Pungent, unpleasant	Pleasant	Sweet, pleasant	Pungent	Pleasant	Pungent
Preservative	Necessary	None	Necessary (thymol)	None	None	None
Stability						
To metal	May react	Nonreactive	Attacks aluminum, brass, lead with moisture	Nonreactive	Stable	Nonreactive
To alkali	Stable (traces of aldehydes)	Stable	Slight decomposition	Stable	Decomposes	Stable
To ultraviolet light	Ignitable	Stable	Decomposes	Stable	Stable	Stable
To other	Avoid halogens	Does not react with other anesthetics	Attacks rubber (softens and swells)	—	—	More stable in rubber than other volatile anesthetics

Reaction with CO₂ absorbents						
Carbon monoxide	Greatest occurrence	Least occurrence	Occurs	Least occurrence	—	—
Compound A	Occurs	Occurs	None	Occurs with a closed-circle breathing system	—	—
Heat	Occurs	Occurs	Occurs	Occurs	—	—
Explosiveness	None	None	None	None	None	Explosive (in air or oxygen)
Presentation at room temperature	Colorless liquid	Colorless liquid	Colorless liquid	Colorless liquid	Colorless gas (liquid under pressure)	Colorless liquid

5. Uptake of an anesthetic from the lungs
6. Blood-gas partition coefficient
7. Cardiac output (brain blood flow)
8. Alveolar to mixed, venous anesthetic, partial pressure difference

II. Ventilation-perfusion abnormalities and hypoventilation hinder the rate of anesthetic uptake and the rate of induction to anesthesia

III. Right-to-left intracardiac shunts may slow the rate of induction

IV. Additional drugs (sedatives, analgesics), hypothermia, older age, and some diseases decrease the dose needed for anesthesia

V. Every volatile inhalant anesthetic drug produces dose-dependent cardiopulmonary depression

VI. The metabolites of inhalation anesthetics can be toxic (e.g., fluoride)

VII. Some inhalant anesthetic drugs may produce toxic substances (e.g., compound A)

VIII. Familiarity with an anesthetic drug is the key to its safe and effective use

NITROUS OXIDE

I. General anesthetic properties (Table 10-1)
A. A gas at room temperature, but readily compressible at 30 to 50 atm (750 psi) to a colorless liquid; returns to gaseous state when released from the cylinder into atmospheric pressure
B. Nonflammable, but supports combustion by decomposing into nitrogen and oxygen

II. Effect on systems
A. Nervous system
1. Mild analgesic and anesthetic action produced by cerebrocortical depression
2. Dangerous in excessive concentrations (more than 70% total gas flow) because it interferes with patient oxygenation
B. Respiratory system
1. Nonirritating to the respiratory tract

       2. Does not depress cough reflex

       3. Causes only minimal respiratory depression; respiratory rate may increase

  C. Cardiovascular system

       1. Few side effects occur except in the presence of hypoxia

       2. Heart rate, cardiac output, and arterial blood pressure remain relatively unchanged

       3. Tachycardia may develop

       4. N_2O does not sensitize the myocardium to catecholamines

  D. Other organ systems

       1. Ileus may occur as a result of gas accumulation within the gastrointestinal tract

       2. The kidney and liver are not significantly affected

  E. Muscular system

       1. Does not cause muscle relaxation

       2. Does not potentiate muscle relaxants

  F. Uterus and fetus

       1. Passes placental barrier

       2. May cause fetal hypoxemia

III. Absorption, fate, and excretion

  A. Readily crosses alveolar membranes because of the low blood-gas partition coefficient (0.49) and relatively large inspired concentrations (40% to 75%)

  B. May accelerate the uptake of inhalant anesthetic drugs (second gas) into the blood (second-gas effect); the enhanced uptake of the second gas (e.g., isoflurane) is caused by an N_2O-dependent increase in alveolar ventilation

  C. Diffuses into closed air cavities (Fig. 10-1): N_2O is 30 times more soluble in blood than nitrogen; it diffuses into air-containing cavities faster than nitrogen diffuses out; if the cavity is closed (e.g., pneumothorax, obstructed bowel, air embolism, blocked paranasal sinuses) and N_2O administered, then either the volume or pressure inside the cavity increases

  D. Has no value as an O_2 source, nor does it form any chemical combinations in the body; carried in simple solution

Effect of anesthetic agents on
air and gases in closed body cavities

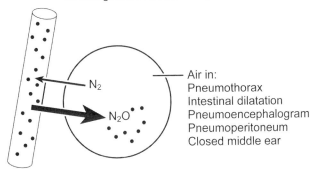

Air in:
Pneumothorax
Intestinal dilatation
Pneumoencephalogram
Pneumoperitoneum
Closed middle ear

Fig. 10-1
Distribution of N_2O from blood to air-containing cavities.

E. Eliminated through the lungs rapidly and completely in minutes
F. Diffusion hypoxia is a result of the low blood-gas partition coefficient; rapid diffusion of nitrous oxide into the alveoli at the end of anesthesia dilutes the oxygen in the alveoli; alveolar oxygen tension may be drastically reduced, especially if the patient is breathing room air; hypoxia is prevented by administering high oxygen flow rates for 5 to 10 minutes after discontinuing N_2O
G. Recovery is fast and devoid of unpleasant sequelae
H. Circumstantial evidence suggests some biotransformation; bone marrow depression may occur after prolonged exposure; N_2O may be teratogenic, especially in females after prolonged exposure in the first trimester of pregnancy

---

USEFUL FACTS ▪ Nitrous oxide

- Used to improve analgesia
- Minimal cardiorespiratory effects
- Second-gas effect

IV. Clinical use
  A. Used as an analgesic adjunct in veterinary anesthesia
  B. Adds to the effect of other inhalant anesthetic drugs; less inhalant anesthetic is needed to produce general anesthesia; cannot be used alone because of the very high minimum alveolar concentration (MAC)
  C. Often used to supplement narcotic or inhalant anesthesia drugs
  D. A minimum of 30% O_2 must be used to prevent hypoxia
  E. The ratio of N_2O to O_2 delivered by the anesthetic machine must be continually monitored; no more than 70% N_2O should be used
  F. The administration of N_2O is contraindicated during low flow or closed system anesthesia

---

CAUTIONS ▪ Nitrous oxide

- Diffusion hypoxia may occur: do NOT use more than 70% N_2O and administer 100% oxygen for 5 minutes after discontinuing N_2O
- Diffusion into closed air cavities (e.g., pneumothorax, obstructed bowel, air embolism, blocked paranasal sinuses)

V. Doses
  A. Up to 70% N_2O
  B. Maintenance concentrations are usually 50% or 66% ($N_2O: O_2$ = 1:1 or 2:1)
  C. If the patient becomes cyanotic or the cardiopulmonary status deteriorates while receiving nitrous oxide, it should be discontinued immediately
  D. N_2O is not potent enough in most animal species to make administration of less than 40% worthwhile

DIETHYL ETHER (ETHER)

  I. Ether was once a frequently used inhalation anesthetic; it is now occasionally used in laboratory animals and to make tape sticky
  II. Ether is highly flammable and explosive
  III. Ether is an ideal anesthetic in some respects because it maintains respiration and minimally depresses cardiac output

IV. Ether may cause salivation, nausea, and vomiting during induction and recovery

V. The signs and stages of ether anesthesia (Fig. 10-2), as developed by Guedel, can be loosely applied to most inhalant anesthetics

    A. Stage I: analgesia (from the beginning of induction to the loss of consciousness)

        1. Disorientation, with normal reflexes or hyperreflexia, is the most common feature

        2. Fear and subsequent release of epinephrine with increased heart rate and rapid respirations may occur

        3. Excessive salivation may occur

    B. Stage II: delirium or excitement, which represents the period of early loss of consciousness

        1. Potential hazards of stage II include struggling, physical injury, and the consequences of increased sympathetic tone

        2. Voluntary centers in the brain become depressed; the patient becomes unaware of its surroundings and its actions

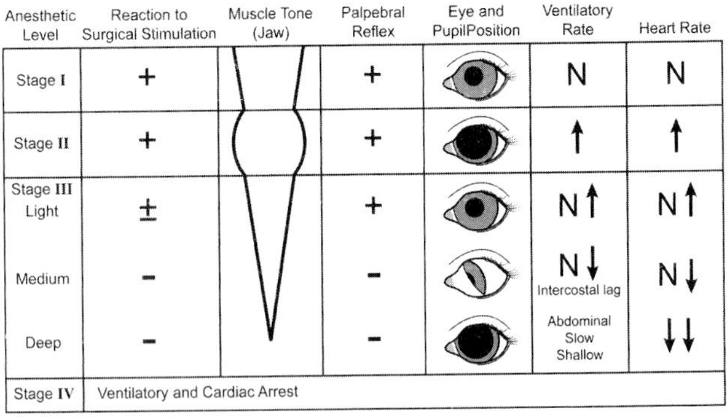

Anesthetic Level	Reaction to Surgical Stimulation	Muscle Tone (Jaw)	Palpebral Reflex	Eye and Pupil Position	Ventilatory Rate	Heart Rate
Stage I	+		+		N	N
Stage II	+		+		↑	↑
Stage III Light	±		+		N↑	N↑
Medium	−		−		N↓ Intercostal lag	N↓
Deep	−		−		Abdominal Slow Shallow	↓↓
Stage IV	Ventilatory and Cardiac Arrest					

Fig. 10-2
Increasing "depth" of anesthesia produces characteristic changes in ocular, motor reflex, respiratory, and cardiovascular responses. Medium levels of stage III anesthesia are ideal for most invasive surgical procedures. Light levels of stage III anesthesia can be used if analgesia is supplemented by local anesthetics or opioids.

3. During light anesthesia, the patient reacts to any sort of external stimuli with exaggerated reflex struggling

4. Respirations are generally irregular in depth and rate, and breath holding may occur

5. The eyelids are widely open, and the pupil is dilated because of sympathetic stimulation

6. Reflex vomiting may occur unless food has been withheld for 6 or more hours before anesthesia; defecation and urination may occur

7. The duration of stage II can be decreased by temporarily administering higher inhalant anesthetic concentrations and inhalant drugs that have a low blood-gas solubility coefficient (e.g., isoflurane versus methoxyflurane)

C. Stage III

1. Plane I: marked by the appearance of more regular respiration

   a. CO_2 retention during the preceding stages may double tidal volume for the first few minutes

   b. Preanesthetic medication directly affects the rate and volume of respiration throughout anesthesia

   c. Responses to pain, although depressed, are still present

   d. Cardiovascular function is only minimally affected

2. Plane II: respiratory rate may be increased or decreased and respiratory volume (tidal volume) is decreased; cardiovascular function is mildly depressed

3. Plane III: loss of intercostal muscle activity

   a. Respiratory depression is significant

   b. Cardiovascular function is noticeably depressed, dependent on the specific characteristics of the anesthetic drug used

   c. The level of anesthesia is potentially dangerous

4. Plane IV: complete paralysis of intercostal muscles

   a. Cessation of all respiratory effort and dilation of the pupils

   b. Cardiovascular function is generally impaired, producing decreased cardiac contractility and vasodilation leading to hypotension

D. Stage IV: respiratory arrest followed by circulatory collapse; death ensues within 1 to 5 minutes

HALOTHANE

I. General anesthetic properties (Table 10-1)
  A. Nervous system
    1. Depresses the central nervous system (CNS)
    2. Depresses body temperature-regulating centers, resulting in hypothermia
    3. Rarely causes hyperpyrexia and malignant hyperthermia in humans, pigs, horses, dogs, and cats; this has been linked to a genetic defect in humans, pigs, and dogs
    4. The stages of anesthesia: pupils may be constricted at all stages, respiration may be shallow but rapid, and the abdominal muscles are relaxed only at deeper planes of anesthesia; the arterial blood pressure may provide the best information about the depth of halothane anesthesia
    5. Increases cerebral blood flow
II. Effects on organ systems
  A. Respiratory system
    1. Respirations are depressed at all levels of halothane anesthesia
    2. Tidal volume is decreased
    3. Minute volume is smaller than in the conscious state, but breathing is usually adequate
    4. Increased breathing in response to hypercarbia does not occur during deeper anesthesia, and ventilation becomes inadequate
    5. Respiratory depression is pronounced in ruminants
    6. Tachypnea may occur; the mechanism is uncertain
  B. Cardiovascular system
    1. Hypotension is related to the depth of anesthesia
    2. Directly depresses vascular smooth muscle causing vasodilation (e.g., in cerebral, skeletal muscle, and peripheral tissues) and decreasing total peripheral resistance
    3. Directly depresses the myocardium, decreasing cardiac output, stroke volume, and cardiac contractility
    4. Decreases efferent sympathetic nervous system activity
    5. Cardiac rate is less affected but is usually decreased at deeper planes of anesthesia

      6. May cause sinus bradycardia

      7. Sensitizes the heart to catecholamines, occasionally producing ventricular arrhythmias

  C. Gastrointestinal system

      1. Decreases intestinal tract motility, tone, and peristaltic activity

      2. Liver: a number of studies on humans have related halothane to jaundice and fatal postanesthetic liver necrosis; biotransformation of halothane to hepatotoxic metabolites may produce hypersensitivity in a small number of individuals; the effect is believed to be related to halothane administration in conjunction with tissue hypoxia

  D. Renal system: no nephrotoxic effects have been reported other than those resulting from hypotension

  E. Muscular system

      1. Relaxation is only moderate during light anesthesia

      2. Skeletal muscle relaxants may be needed if pronounced muscle relaxation is required

      3. Halothane potentiates the action of nondepolarizing muscle relaxants

      4. Malignant hyperthermia can occur (especially in pigs)

  F. Uterus and fetus

      1. Decreases uterine tone; may decrease uterine involution postpartum

      2. Readily crosses the placental barrier

III. Absorption, fate, and excretion

  A. Absorption takes place rapidly in the lungs

  B. As much as 20% to 40% inspired halothane is metabolized by liver microsomes; trifluoroacetic acid, bromide, and chloride radicals are produced and excreted in the urine for many hours to days

  C. Metabolites may persist for many days in the liver

  D. The major portion of administered halothane is excreted unchanged by the lungs

IV. Clinical uses

  A. Halothane is one of the most useful anesthetics, because it is nonflammable, potent, nonirritating, controllable, and relatively nontoxic

  B. Can be used in all species

C. Accurate concentrations of halothane can be delivered from precision, thermostable or thermocompensated, calibrated vaporizers; draw-over, in-the-circle vaporizers have been used once the wick is removed

D. Decomposes slowly when exposed to light; stored in dark bottles with thymol added as a preservative; thymol is potentially tissue toxic

E. Can be used in rebreathing and nonrebreathing techniques

F. Used in in-the-circle, draw-over vaporizers during "low-flow" techniques (Chapter 14)

USEFUL FACTS ■ Halothane

- Potent anesthetic
- Relatively nontoxic
- Comparatively minimal respiratory depression at surgical anesthesia

---

V. Dose

A. 2% to 4% at induction; careful monitoring is important to avoid overdose

B. Because of the second-gas effect, induction time may be decreased if nitrous oxide is given simultaneously

C. Concurrent use of nitrous oxide reduces the amount of halothane required

D. Maintenance: 0.5% to 1.5% in small animals; 1% to 2% in large animals

---

CAUTIONS ■ Halothane

- Sensitizes the heart to catecholamines
- Significant myocardial depressant
- Liver dysfunction can occur or become worse
- Can trigger malignant hyperthermia (especially in pigs)
- Greater than 20% metabolized

ISOFLURANE (FORANE, AERRANE, ISOFLO, ISOVET)

I. General anesthetic properties (Table 10-1)

A. An isomer of enflurane and exceptionally stable

B. Produces comparatively rapid induction and recovery from anesthesia

C. Can be used in all species

II. Effects on organ systems

A. Nervous system
 1. Generalized CNS depression
 2. Cerebral blood flow is not increased if ventilation is maintained
 3. Burst suppression on the electroencephalogram is observed in moderate to deep surgical anesthesia

B. Respiratory system
 1. Produces more respiratory depression than halothane
 2. Tidal volume increases initially with depth of anesthesia; respiratory rate decreases
 3. $PaCO_2$ concentration increases with time, although surgical stimulation increases respiration and thus prevents a large rise in $PaCO_2$
 4. Ventilation may need to be assisted to prevent hypercarbia

C. Cardiovascular system
 1. Cardiac depression is less than with halothane
 2. Cardiac contractility is depressed less than with halothane at concentrations producing surgical anesthesia, and cardiac output is maintained
 3. Progressive vasodilation occurs with increasing depth of anesthesia, increasing muscle and skin blood flow
 4. Hypotensive: mean arterial blood pressure and peripheral vascular resistance decrease with depth of anesthesia
 5. Isoflurane does not sensitize the heart to catecholamine-induced arrhythmias

D. Gastrointestinal system
 1. Smooth muscle tone and motility are decreased
 2. No hepatotoxicity reported (metabolism is very low)

E. Renal system: no changes in renal function reported; very little metabolism to trifluoroacetic acid

F. Muscular system
 1. Produces excellent muscle relaxation
 2. Potentiates nondepolarizing muscle relaxants
 3. Can cause malignant hyperthermia in swine

    G. Uterus and fetus
       1. Rapidly crosses the placenta
       2. Reduces uterine tone
       3. Safety in pregnancy not evaluated

III. Absorption, fate, and excretion
    A. Absorbed and eliminated by the alveoli
    B. Primarily excreted unchanged by the lungs
    C. Very little biodegradation; approximately 0.25% is metabolized to inorganic fluoride (trifluoroacetic acid)

IV. Clinical use
    A. Produces fast, smooth induction and recovery in all species tested
    B. Rapid recovery may predispose some animals to emergence delirium
    C. Calibrated vaporizer is used to deliver accurate concentrations
    D. Can be used in in-the-circle, draw-over vaporizers during "low-flow" (closed system) techniques (Chapter 13)
    E. Can be used with nitrous oxide
    F. Can be used for mask induction
    G. Is classified as a respiratory depressant

USEFUL FACTS ▪ Isoflurane

- Potent anesthetic
- Fast and smooth induction and recovery
- Easy to control
- Less cardiac depression than halothane
- Very low metabolism
- Cheaper than sevoflurane or desflurane

    V. Doses
       A. Induction: 2.5% to 4.5% is usually necessary
       B. Induction is facilitated by the use of intravenous anesthesia or nitrous oxide
       C. Maintenance: 1% to 3%

CAUTIONS ■ Isoflurane

- More respiratory depression than halothane
- Produces carbon monoxide when exposed to dessicated CO_2 absorbent material

---

SEVOFLURANE (ULTANE®, SEVORANE®, SEVOFLO®)

I. General anesthetic properties (Table 10-1)
    A. Low blood-gas partition coefficient (0.5 to 0.7)
        1. Rapid, smooth induction; rapid recovery
        2. MAC of approximately 2.4
    B. Nonpungent
    C. Relatively stable in moist soda lime but can produce compound A, which can cause renal toxicity

II. Effects on organ systems
    A. Similar to isoflurane
    B. Nervous system
        1. Similar to isoflurane
        2. Dose-dependent CNS depression; no convulsive activity
        3. Produces good muscle relaxation and analgesia
    C. Dose-dependent cardiorespiratory depression
        1. Respiratory depression similar to isoflurane
    D. Does not sensitize the heart to catecholamine-induced cardiac arrhythmias
    E. Gastrointestinal system: decreases smooth muscle tone and motility
    F. Renal system: degradation products of sevoflurane by CO_2 absorbents, compound A, may produce renal failure (rare)
    G. Muscular system
        1. Produces good muscle relaxation
    H. Uterus and fetus
        1. Rapidly crosses the placenta, producing fetal depression

III. Absorption, fate, excretion
   A. Absorbed and eliminated by the lung
   B. Resists degradation by the liver (3%); produces inorganic fluoride similar to isoflurane
IV. Clinical use
   A. Induction and recovery from anesthesia is faster than isoflurane because of lower blood-gas partition coefficient
   B. Produces good muscle relaxation and anesthesia
   C. Can be used for mask induction
   D. Recovery may be rapid and smooth

USEFUL FACTS ■ Sevoflurane

- Similar to isoflurane
- More rapid induction and recovery than isoflurane

V. Doses
   A. Mask induction: 5% to 7% concentrations
   B. Anesthetic maintenance: 3% to 4% concentrations

CAUTIONS ■ Sevoflurane

- More respiratory depression than halothane
- Degradation produced by dessicated CO_2 absorbents could cause renal failure

---

DESFLURANE (SUPRANE)

I. General anesthetic properties (Table 10-1)
   A. Identical in structure to isoflurane, except that fluorine is substituted for chlorine
   B. Extremely low blood-gas partition coefficient (0.42); extremely rapid induction and recovery
   C. Less potent than other halogenated agents; MAC is approximately 7.2%
   D. Pungent; produces airway irritation, provoking coughing or breath holding

    E. Requires a special, electrically heated vaporizer

    F. Stable in moist soda lime

    G. Expensive

II. Effects on organ systems

    A. Similar to isoflurane

    B. Nervous system

        1. Similar to isoflurane

        2. Dose-dependent CNS depression

        3. Good muscle relaxation; enhances nondepolarizing neuromuscular blocking drugs

    C. Respiratory system

        1. Causes dose-dependent respiratory depression; decreases the breathing response to increases in $PaCO_2$

        2. Pungent odor irritates the airway; induction to anesthesia may be difficult unless preceded by a preanesthetic drug

        3. The inspired O_2 is notably less than with the other contemporary inhalant anesthetic drugs

    D. Cardiovascular system

        1. Qualitatively and quantitatively similar to isoflurane

        2. Can cause sympathetic activation "storm" in some patients

    E. Gastrointestinal system: decreases smooth muscle tone and motility

    F. Renal system: does not affect renal function

    G. Muscular system

        1. Produces good muscle relaxation

        2. Can cause malignant hyperthermia in swine

    H. Uterus and fetus

        1. Crosses the placental barrier; causes fetal depression

        2. Allows rapid recovery (fetus) from anesthesia because of low blood-gas partition coefficient (0.42)

III. Absorption, fate, excretion

    A. Absorbed and eliminated by the lung

    B. Resists degradation by the liver; produces even less inorganic fluoride than isoflurane

    C. Has shown no hepatotoxicity or nephrotoxicity

IV. Clinical use

    A. Induction and recovery from anesthesia is approximately twice as fast as with isoflurane because of the extremely

low blood-gas partition coefficient (0.42), despite comparatively low potency (MAC $\approx$ 7.2%)
B. Produces good muscle relaxation and analgesia
C. Pungent odor makes mask induction difficult unless appropriate preanesthetics are used
D. Recovery may be so rapid that resedation is needed to avoid emergence delirium

V. Doses
A. Mask induction: 10% to 15% concentrations
B. Anesthetic maintenance: 6% to 9% concentrations
C. Preanesthetic use, N_2O, and adjuncts to anesthesia (fentanyl) can reduce MAC

CHAPTER ELEVEN

Neuromuscular Blocking Drugs

"Don't fight forces; use them."
R. BUCKMINSTER FULLER

OVERVIEW

Neuromuscular blocking drugs (NMBDs), commonly referred to as *"peripheral muscle relaxants,"* as opposed to centrally acting muscle relaxants, interfere with or block neuromuscular transmission and are useful adjuncts to general anesthesia. NMBDs do *not* provide analgesia, sedation, amnesia, or hypnosis. Breathing ceases, which necessitates controlled ventilation and constant patient monitoring.

GENERAL CONSIDERATIONS

I. The primary pharmacologic effect of peripheral NMBDs is to produce skeletal muscle (SM) relaxation

II. NMBDs are potentiated by many intravenous and inhalant anesthetic drugs

III. Other clinically useful drugs (aminoglycoside antibiotics) may cause SM weakness or paralysis

IV. Potential mechanisms of SM relaxation
   A. NMBDs interfere with cholinergic (nicotinic) neuromuscular transmission in the peripheral somatic nervous system
   B. Some NMBDs enhance the activity of endogenous inhibitory mechanisms in the central nervous system, which normally modulate SM tone

V. NMBDs are used adjunctively during anesthesia to produce controlled, transient muscle weakness

195

VI. NMBDs produce muscle relaxation but do not produce analgesia or a hypnotic effect

VII. NMBDs can produce respiratory paralysis, which necessitates mechanical or manual support of ventilation

VIII. Hypothermia is an important secondary effect of prolonged SM relaxation in small animals

IX. NMBDs are positively charged (ionized) and therefore do not pass the blood-brain barrier or cross the placenta in significant amounts

X. Various electrical stimulators and stimulation protocols can be used to determine the degree of neuromuscular blockade (Figs. 11-1 and 11-2)

NORMAL NEUROMUSCULAR FUNCTION

I. Acetylcholine (ACh) is released in small amounts, even in resting muscles

    A. Random ACh release causes mini-endplate potentials at the postsynaptic muscle membrane, which are insufficient to evoke muscle contraction

II. Action potential-dependent ACh release

    A. Action potentials cause large depolarization in nerve terminals of α-motor neurons

    B. Depolarization in the presence of extracellular Ca^{++} causes simultaneous fusion of many ACh-containing vesicles with the terminal nerve membrane (Fig. 11-3)

    C. Release of ACh packets evokes a large endplate potential, leading to muscle contraction

III. Combination of ACh with postjunctional nicotine receptors (Nm receptors)

    A. Receptors on the muscle endplates are nicotinic, type IV cholinergic (Nm) receptors

    B. Strength of muscle contraction is proportional to the number of receptors activated by ACh

IV. Hydrolysis of ACh, reuptake of choline, synthesis and packing of ACh

    A. The duration of ACh activity at any cholinergic synapse is limited by the action of acetylcholinesterase (ACh esterase); ACh is metabolized to acetic acid plus choline at the synaptic cleft

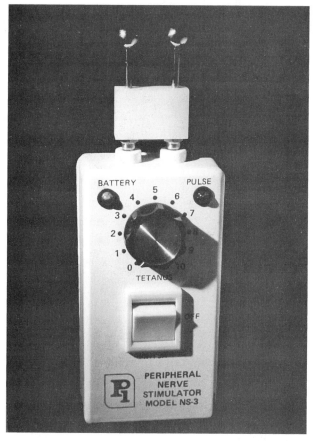

Fig. 11-1
One of a variety of peripheral nerve stimulators available to test the adequacy of neuromuscular blockade.

    B. Choline produced by hydrolysis of ACh is taken up by the nerve terminals and resynthesized into ACh at the nerve terminal membrane

    C. ACh is packaged into vesicles or stored freely in the cytoplasm of the nerve terminals

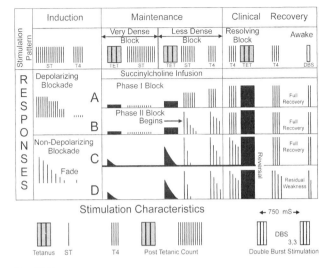

Fig. 11-2

Assessing neuromuscular function. Diagram simulates the clinical responses observed after neuromuscular stimulation. Stimulation patterns are depicted in the upper panel. (*ST*, Single twitch; *T4*, train of four; *TET*, tetanus; *DBS*, double burst-stimulation). The following four situations are demonstrated by the letters: *A*, The normal use of a succinylcholine infusion; *B*, the development of a phase II block; *C*, a nondepolarizing blockade that is reversed with full recovery; and *D*, a nondepolarizing blockade that demonstrates residual weakness.

From Barash PG, Cullen BK, Stoelting RK: *Clinical anesthesia*, ed 2, Philadelphia, 1992, JB Lippincott, p. 763.

MECHANISMS OF SKELETAL MUSCLE RELAXATION EVOKED BY INTERFERENCE WITH NORMAL PERIPHERAL NEUROMUSCULAR FUNCTION

I. At presynaptic sites
  A. Inhibition of ACh synthesis (e.g., hemicholinium blocks choline uptake)
  B. Inhibition of ACh release
    1. Ca^{++} deficiency, Mg^{++} increases
    2. Procaine
    3. Tetracyclines and aminoglycoside antibiotics

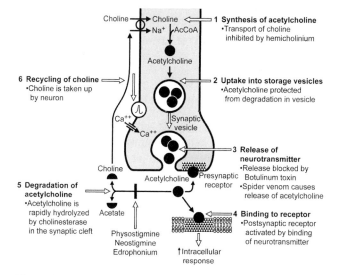

Fig. 11-3
Release of acetylcholine from neurons at the neuromuscular junction.

    4. Some β-blockers
    5. Botulinum toxin
II. At postsynaptic sites
    A. Persistent depolarization with an agonist that has a longer duration of action than ACh (e.g., succinylcholine chloride)
    B. Competitive block of ACh receptors causing *nondepolarizing* blockade (e.g., curare, pancuronium)

TYPES OF NEUROMUSCULAR BLOCKS

  I. Phase I block: depolarizing block (succinylcholine)
 II. Phase II block: nondepolarizing block (pancuronium)
III. Mixed block: any combination of I and II
IV. Dual block: excessive amounts of depolarizing agents producing phase II block
 V. Nonacetylcholine block (procaine, botulinum, decreased Ca^{++}, increased Mg^{++}, increased K^+, decreased K^+)

SEQUENCE OF MUSCLE RELAXATION

I. Oculomotor m. → palpebral m. → facial m. → tongue and pharynx → jaw and tail → limbs → pelvic m. → caudal abdominal m. → cranial abdominal m. → intercostal m. → larynx → diaphragm

    A. The sequence of motor blockade is highly variable in clinical patients

    B. Motor activity to the limbs may appear to return (twitching, jerking) before the diaphragm is fully functional

II. Intercostal and diaphragmatic muscles are thought to be affected last

III. Recovery is generally in the reverse order of paralysis

IV. It is possible but difficult to titrate the specific NMBD to paralyze the muscles of the eye while maintaining diaphragmatic function

SPECIFIC NMBDS (Tables 11-1, 11-2)

I. Depolarizing drugs act like ACh

    A. Succinylcholine chloride (Sucostrin, Anectine, Quillicine, Suxamethonium)

II. Nondepolarizing drugs; competitive blocking drugs

    A. D-Tubocurarine chloride (curare, Metubine)

    B. Gallamine triethiodide (Flaxedil)

    C. Pancuronium bromide (Pavulon)

    D. Vecuronium bromide (Norcuron)

    E. Atracurium besylate (Tracrium)

    F. Mivacurium chloride (Mivacron)

    G. Doxacurium chloride (Nuromax)

    H. Pipecuronium (Arduran)

CLINICAL DIFFERENTIATION BETWEEN DEPOLARIZING AND NONDEPOLARIZING DRUGS

I. Depolarizing

    A. First: transient muscle fasciculations caused by asynchronous depolarization

    B. Second: paralysis caused by prolonged depolarization of the motor endplate

TABLE 11-1
DOSE OF NEUROMUSCULAR BLOCKING DRUGS WITH SIDE EFFECTS AND CONTRAINDICATIONS

AGENT	SPECIES	DOSE IV (MG/KG)	DURATION OF ACTION (MIN)	SIDE EFFECTS	CONTRAINDICATIONS
Succinylcholine chloride	Dog	0.3-0.4	1-38	Little cardiovascular effect; muscarinic effect-bradycardia: nicotinic effect-hypertension, increased intraocular pressure; hyperpyrexia	Organophosphate anthelmintics, chronic liver disease, malnutrition, high-K^+, glaucoma, penetrating eye injury
	Cat	3-5 (total)	2-6		
	Pig	0.75-2	1-3		
	Horse	0.1-0.33	1-10		
Pancuronium bromide	Dog	0.02-0.06	15-108	Negligible	Liver or kidney disease
	Cat	0.02	14-15		
	Pig	0.07-0.12	7-30		
	Horse	0.08-0.14	16-35		
	Cattle	0.1	30-40		
	Calf	0.04	26		
	Sheep	5 µg/kg	21		

Continued

TABLE 11-1

DOSE OF NEUROMUSCULAR BLOCKING DRUGS WITH SIDE EFFECTS AND CONTRAINDICATIONS—cont'd

AGENT	SPECIES	DOSE IV (MG/KG)	DURATION OF ACTION (MIN)	SIDE EFFECTS	CONTRAINDICATIONS
Vecuronium	Dog	0.01-0.2	10-42	Negligible	
	Cat	0.02-0.04	5-9		
	Pig	0.1-0.2	5-20		
	Horse	0.11	20-40		
	Sheep	4.6 µg/kg	14		
Atracurium	Dog	0.1-0.4			
	Cat	0.1-0.25	10-15	Negligible	
	Pig	0.5-2.5	10-60		
	Horse	0.07-0.09	8-24	Negligible	
	Sheep	6 µg/kg/hr			
	Llama	0.15	6		
Doxacurium	Dog	8 µg/kg	16-81		
Pipecuronium	Dog	4-50 µg/kg	17-24		
	Cat	2-3 µg/kg			

TABLE 11-2
AUTONOMIC EFFECTS OF NEUROMUSCULAR BLOCKING DRUGS

DRUG	AUTONOMIC GANGLIA	CARDIAC MUSCARINIC RECEPTORS	HISTAMINE RELEASE
Succinylcholine	Stimulated	Stimulated	Slight
Pancuronium	None	Blocked weakly	None
Atracurium	None	None	Slight
Vecuronium	None	None	None
Mivacurium	None	None	Slight
Doxacurium	None	None	None
Pipecuronium	None	None	None

    C. Paralysis is not reversed by anticholinesterase drugs

    D. Paralysis is terminated by metabolism of the NMBD by pseudocholinesterase

  II. Nondepolarizing

    A. No muscle fasciculation occurs before muscle paralysis, and there is no depolarization of motor endplate; the animal gradually relaxes or "fades"

    B. Effects can be partially reversed by anticholinesterase drugs (Fig. 11-3)

      1. Neostigmine

      2. Pyridostigmine

      3. Edrophonium

 III. Onset of effect

    A. Rapid (less than 1 minute): succinylcholine

    B. Medium (1 to 2 minutes): mivacurium, atracurium, vecuronium

    C. Slow (3 to 5 minutes): doxacurium, pancuronium

 IV. Duration of effect

    A. Ultrashort (1 to 3 minutes): succinylcholine

    B. Short (5 to 10 minutes): mivacurium, atracurium

    C. Intermediate (10 to 20 minutes): vecuronium

    D. Long (20 to 40 minutes): doxacurium, pancuronium, pipecuronium

  V. Speed of antagonism by anticholinesterases

    A. Rapid (less than 1 minute): mivacurium

    B. Medium (1 to 2 minutes): atracurium, vecuronium

    C. Slow (3 to 5 minutes): doxacurium, pancuronium

VI. Metabolism
   A. Hoffmann elimination: atracurium
   B. Plasma cholinesterase: succinylcholine, mivacurium
   C. Liver: vecuronium, pancuronium, pipecuronium, atracurium

DEPOLARIZING BLOCKING DRUGS

I. Mechanism of action
   A. Persistent depolarization alone may result in neuromuscular block because of Na^{++} inactivation, which prevents electrical impulse generation
   B. Dual block: prolonged exposure of ACh membrane receptors to large doses of depolarizing drugs (ACh, succinylcholine, C-10) reduces the ability of these drugs to cause conductance changes; the reason for this is uncertain

II. Indications
   A. Diagnostic or surgical procedures requiring a short duration of muscle relaxation
   B. Facilitation of endotracheal intubation in humans and primates
   C. Cesarean sections
   D. Fracture reductions

III. Contraindications with depolarizing drugs
   A. Disease states causing prolonged NMBD activity
      1. Liver disease: pseudocholinesterase is produced in the liver
      2. Chronic anemia: acetylcholinesterase is associated with red blood cell membranes
      3. Chronic malnutrition
      4. Organophosphates (anthelmintics): enzyme activity is inhibited
   B. Other conditions
      1. High serum K^+ levels
         a. Burns, muscle trauma, renal failure
         b. Depolarizing blockade can cause potassium release from muscles
      2. Ophthalmologic conditions
         a. Glaucoma, penetrating eye wounds

       b. Depolarizing blockade can transiently increase intraocular pressure

IV. Specific depolarizing drugs: succinylcholine (Table 11-2)

    A. Succinylcholine: adverse effects

       1. Muscle soreness: reason unknown; probably related to muscle fasciculations and K^+ release before paralysis

       2. Histamine release

       3. Cardiovascular effects

          a. Potential for bradycardia

          b. The more common response is tachycardia and hypertension caused by sympathetic stimulation

       4. Hyperkalemia: caused by increased efflux of K^+ from endplate region of skeletal muscle

       5. Some patients have a deficiency of plasma cholinesterase; in these patients, neuromuscular block may be prolonged

       6. Genetic anomaly in which plasma cholinesterase is replaced by an atypical cholinesterase may prolong drug effects; differentiation is possible with dibucaine, which inhibits normal plasma cholinesterase 80% and atypical cholinesterase, only 20%

       7. Malignant hyperpyrexia: manifested by a severe, rapid rise in temperature, which may be accompanied by significant muscle rigidity

          a. Usually occurs when using succinylcholine and halothane together

          b. Treat with 100% O_2, rapid cooling, sodium bicarbonate to control acidosis, and dantrolene sodium (2 mg/kg)

          c. A genetic disease of pigs and humans

NONDEPOLARIZING BLOCKING DRUGS

   I. Mechanism of action

     A. Competitive blocking drugs: compete with ACh for postsynaptic receptors, thereby reducing the depolarization caused by ACh

   II. Indications

     A. Same as depolarizing drugs

    B. High-risk cases as part of a balanced anesthetic technique with narcotics, inhalation, or other analgesic drugs

    C. Ocular surgery

    D. Control of ventilation at any time

III. Specific nondepolarizing drugs (Table 11-2)

    A. Pancuronium (Pavulon)

        1. No histamine release or ganglionic block; no catecholamine release or inhibition

        2. Effects are enhanced by inhalation anesthetics

        3. Major portion is excreted unchanged in urine

        4. Tachycardia is occasionally seen after administration

    B. Atracurium (Tracrium)

        1. Developed as a rapid-onset and duration-competitive NMBD; can be administered by infusion

        2. pH and temperature-dependent degradation (Hoffman elimination); a potential benefit is that biologically mediated metabolism and elimination by the liver and kidneys are not needed

        3. Some histamine release at high doses

        4. Occasionally decreases heart rate and arterial blood pressure

    C. Vecuronium (Norcuron)

        1. Developed in an attempt to produce a competitive NMBD with short onset and duration and to eliminate the tachycardia seen occasionally with pancuronium

        2. Eliminated in bile (40%) and through the kidneys (15%) — a potential advantage in patients with compromised renal function

        3. Minimal cardiovascular effects; no histamine release; no ganglionic block

    D. Mivacurium

        1. Slight histamine release

        2. Rapid clearance by plasma cholinesterase

        3. Occasional decrease in arterial blood pressure

    E. Doxacurium

        1. No histamine release

        2. Low clearance eliminated by the kidney

        3. Minimal cardiovascular effects

    F. Pipecuronium

        1. No histamine release

2. Low clearance eliminated by the kidney
3. Minimal cardiovascular effects
G. Tubocurarine
1. Infrequently used in veterinary medicine
2. Used to poison the tips of arrows
H. Gallamine
1. Infrequently used
2. Causes tachycardia and occasionally hypertension

FACTORS THAT MAY INFLUENCE NEUROMUSCULAR BLOCKADE (Table 11-3)

I. Temperature
   A. Hyperthermia antagonizes competitive blockade but enhances and prolongs depolarizing blockade
   B. Hypothermia prolongs nondepolarizing NMBDs
II. Acid-base balance
   A. Respiratory acidosis augments nondepolarizing neuromuscular blockade
   B. Inadequate reversal of nondepolarizing drugs causes depressed ventilation and respiratory acidosis, which enhances the blockade (a vicious cycle)

TABLE 11-3
FACTORS ALTERING INTENSITY OF DEGREE AND DURATION OF MUSCLE RELAXATION

FACTOR	DEPOLARIZING AGENT	NONDEPOLARIZING AGENT
Tranquilizers	↑	↑
Volatile anesthetic agents	↑	↑
Decreased body temperature	↑	↑
Decreased cardiac output/kg body weight	↓	↓ (Gallamine)
Increased age	↑	↑
Antibiotics		
Streptomycin	↑	↑
Neomycin	↑	↑
Kanamycin	↑	↑
Organophosphates	↑	—

↑, Increase; ↓, decrease; —, no effect.

III. Fluid and electrolyte imbalance
   A. Hypokalemia and hypocalcemia potentiate nondepolarizing drugs
   B. Dehydration increases the plasma concentration of a normal dose of a nondepolarizing drug, augmenting its effect
   C. High Mg^{++} blood levels enhance both depolarizing and nondepolarizing NMBDs
IV. Other drugs
   A. The following antibiotics potentiate nondepolarizing drugs: neomycin, streptomycin, gentamicin, kanamycin, paromomycin, viomycin, polymyxin A and B, colistin, tetracycline, lincomycin, and clindamycin

ANTICHOLINESTERASE DRUGS

I. Reversal of neuromuscular block
   A. Anticholinesterase drugs such as edrophonium, physostigmine, pyridostigmine, and neostigmine can be used with or without anticholinergic drugs
      1. Atropine is used to block the undesirable muscarinic effects of anticholinesterase drugs; muscarinic effects include bradycardia and increased bronchial and salivary secretions, increased intestinal motility, and bradycardia
      2. This regimen is ineffective against depolarization block; in fact, it exacerbates the block because of additional depolarization by excess ACh
      3. This regimen may be effective when a depolarizing, blocking drug is producing a phase II block
   B. Reverse with 0.02 to 0.04 mg/kg neostigmine combined with 0.01 to 0.02 mg/kg atropine (average dose); do not repeat the neostigmine dose more than three times
   C. Edrophonium dose is 0.5 mg/kg IV; it may be repeated up to five times
   D. Complete reversal takes 5 to 45 minutes

CENTRALLY ACTING SKELETAL MUSCLE RELAXANTS

I. Guaifenesin (see Chapter 8)
   A. The mechanism of action is poorly understood but probably relates to depression of transmission through spinal polysynaptic pathways, which normally maintain SM tone
   B. No effect on cerebral arousal
      1. Mild sedation
      2. Variable, mild analgesia
   C. Clinical use: significantly reduces the dose of induction drug required to produce recumbency
   D. Doses and route of administration
      1. 50 to 100 mg/kg or to ataxic effect by intravenous infusion; 100 mg/kg for recumbency by intravenous infusion
      2. Typically administered as a 5% solution
II. Benzodiazepines (see Chapter 3)
   A. Mechanism of skeletal muscle relaxant activity is probably related to the ability to activate benzodiazepine receptors, activate chloride channels, and potentiate γ-aminobutyric acid, a central nervous system inhibitory neurotransmitter

CHAPTER TWELVE

Anesthetic Toxicity, Oxygen Toxicity, and Drug Interactions

"Can we ever have too much of a good thing?"
DON QUIXOTE DE LA MANCHA

OVERVIEW

All drugs that produce chemical restraint and anesthesia have the potential to produce toxic effects. These toxic effects, if allowed to continue or if sufficiently severe, can jeopardize the patient's life. Toxicity occurs when drugs are administered by individuals who are either unfamiliar with the pharmacologic properties of a drug or who have insufficient knowledge about how to counteract the toxic effects of the drug. Intravenous drug toxicity is usually due to the administration of too much drug too fast. Inhalation anesthetic drug toxicity is a major concern for operating room personnel. All inhalation anesthetics are central nervous system (CNS) depressants. When these agents are used, waste anesthetic vapors should be scavenged to minimize personnel exposure. Oxygen can be both beneficial and detrimental, depending on the tension of the oxygen and the duration of exposure. Drug interactions underscore the importance of obtaining a comprehensive history and preliminary physical examination.

GENERAL CONSIDERATIONS

I. All drugs used to produce chemical restraint and anesthesia are potentially toxic; toxicity is caused by the following:
   A. Inhibition of nervous system activity

    B. Alteration of normal physiology and depression of cardiopulmonary function

    C. Inhibition of enzyme systems

    D. Direct cytotoxic effects

    E. Differences in species' sensitivity to drugs

    F. Idiosyncratic reactions

II. The toxic manifestations of drugs used to produce chemical restraint and anesthesia are generally reversible

III. Many drugs used to produce chemical restraint and anesthesia can be antagonized

    A. Opioids by narcotic antagonists such as naloxone

    B. α_2-Antagonists by α_2-antagonists such as yohimbine, tolazoline, and atipamezole

    C. Nondepolarizing muscle relaxants by acetylcholinesterase inhibitors such as neostigmine and edrophonium

    D. Benzodiazepines by the antagonist flumazenil

    E. General anesthetic-induced depression can be antagonized partially by analeptics such as doxapram, yohimbine, tolazoline, and atipemazole

IV. Waste gas scavenging minimizes the potential danger of drug-induced toxicity

V. Drug interactions may significantly potentiate or inhibit the actions of drugs used for chemical restraint and anesthesia

VOLATILE ANESTHETICS

I. The anesthetic molecule is nontoxic; however, volatile anesthetics are not completely inert and are metabolized to varying degrees (except for nitrous oxide)

    A. Metabolites are believed to be responsible for drug toxicity

    B. Chloride, bromide, and fluoride metabolites have been reported

    C. Inhalation anesthetics interact with CO_2 absorbents (barium hydroxide lime, soda lime) to produce potentially toxic metabolites and heat

        1. Isoflurane—CO

            a. Volatile agents containing a difluoromethoxy moiety (CHF_2) may react with the absorber to form carbon monoxide (CO); the magnitude of

CO production is greatest with desflurane and enflurane, intermediate with isoflurane, and least with halothane and sevoflurane

   b. To reduce the accumulation of CO in circle and to-and-fro systems, inhalant anesthetics should not be used with dry carbon dioxide (CO_2) absorbent

2. Sevoflurane—compound A and heat

   a. Sevoflurane may react with carbon dioxide absorbents (especially barium hydroxide lime) and be degraded to haloalkenes and compound A, which are nephrotoxic

   b. The interaction of desiccated absorbents with inhalant anesthetics can produce absorbent temperatures of several hundred degrees centigrade (Fig. 12-1)

     (1) Desflurane and isoflurane can increase the temperature up to approximately $100°$ C ($212°$ F) with barium hydroxide lime

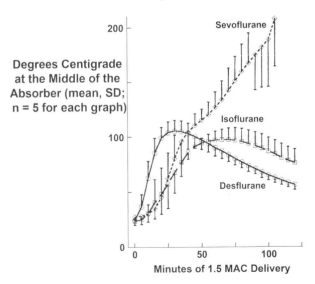

Fig. 12-1

Temperatures recorded within the CO_2 absorbent canister during inhalation anesthesia.

(2) Sevoflurane can increase the temperature up to 350° to 400° C (662° to 752° F) with barium hydroxide lime; melting of plastic components, smoldering, fire, explosion have been reported

D. Low-flow anesthesia increases the possibility of interactions between volatile anesthetics and CO_2 absorbents; barium hydroxide lime should not be used for low-flow anesthesia with isoflurane and sevoflurane

II. Metabolism of inhalation anesthetics occurs primarily in the liver; metabolites are excreted predominantly by the kidneys

III. Volatile anesthetics are amazingly uniform in distribution, except in areas high in fat, in the thymus, and in the adrenal gland

IV. Three general mechanisms of tissue injury are associated with inhaled anesthetics

A. Toxic intracellular accumulation of metabolites

B. Initiation of immune responses caused by hapten formation

C. Destructive free-radical chain reactions initiated by reactive intermediate products of metabolism

V. Normal metabolic functions are affected as long as anesthetic is present; at normal metabolic rates, no toxic side effects may occur; however, some individual animals may have metabolic rates far below normal, which may augment toxic effects

A. Animals in shock

B. Hypothermic animals

C. Animals with liver disease

D. Animals with kidney disease

VI. Metabolism of all inhalant anesthetics may be increased after the administration of enzyme-inducing agents (i.e., phenobarbital)

VII. Several inhalant anesthetic agents have demonstrated teratogenicity in mice when administered chronically or at high concentrations; further investigations are needed to clarify the importance of these findings and their relationship to other animals and humans

VIII. Materials that are properly prepared, stored, and used have not led to any known catastrophes attributable to

contaminants; toxic impurities can be and have been caused by human error
A. Cylinders of nitrous oxide (N_2O) have been mislabeled as nitrogen dioxide (NO_2)
B. Improper storage can lead to decomposition of initially pure anesthetics
C. Halogenated compounds are unstable in light
D. Unsuitable handling of CO_2 absorbents, hotness or dryness of CO_2 absorbents make the risk higher

TOXICOLOGY OF ANESTHETIC DRUGS

I. Halothane toxicity
  A. Halothane sensitizes the myocardium to catecholamine-induced dysrhythmias
  B. Halothane predisposes some animals to hyperpyrexia and malignant hyperthermia
  C. Halothane is extensively metabolized
    1. Major metabolites
      a. Trifluoroacetic acid
      b. Fluoride ion
      c. Chloride ion
      d. Bromide ion
    2. Prolonged exposure to subanesthetic concentrations increases metabolism
  D. Hepatotoxicity
    1. Many halogenated hydrocarbons are hepatotoxic
    2. Degree of halogenation increases the incidence of toxicity
    3. Hepatic necrosis is believed to be caused by toxic effects of the fluoride or bromide molecules released after halothane metabolism by the liver
    4. Toxic effects are potentiated by halothane-induced decreases in liver perfusion
    5. The National Study of Hepatic Necrosis was unable to identify any unique or consistent lesion resulting from halothane administration
  E. Toxicity to halothane
    1. Dose-related
    2. Increases with multiple uses

3. Thymol preservative in commercially prepared halothane is potentially toxic to both the liver and the kidney; however, it is present in minute quantities

II. Isoflurane, sevoflurane, and desflurane toxicity

A. Metabolism

1. Defluoridation of isoflurane and desflurane does not result in clinically significant concentrations of serum fluoride ions

2. Metabolism of sevoflurane may result in higher fluoride concentrations, but they seldom reach the threshold for nephrotoxicity

B. All agents predispose some animals to malignant hyperthermia

C. Future clinical and laboratory evaluation of these agents may reveal additional concerns

IV. Nitrous oxide toxicity

A. Nitrous oxide is not metabolized in vivo

B. It undergoes a physiochemical reaction with vitamin B_{12}

1. This reaction results in megaloblastic bone marrow changes and neurologic disease

2. Indirectly inhibits deoxyribonucleic acid synthesis, resulting in reproductive disorders

C. Toxic effects appear after relatively long-term exposure (more than 10 hours)

D. Clinical use is not associated with any direct toxic effects

V. Barbiturate toxicity

A. In general, clinical use of barbiturates does not manifest any direct cellular toxicities

1. Barbiturates stimulate liver microsomal enzymes and may alter the metabolism of other drugs

2. Some seemingly normal animals appear to be sensitive to the cardiorespiratory depressant effects of barbiturate anesthetics; this clinical observation is probably a result of inadvertent overdose, but it may result from idiosyncrasy (although unlikely)

3. Thiobarbiturates increase the susceptibility to the development of ventricular arrhythmias

4. Thiobarbiturates are metabolized slowly and accumulate, especially in sight hounds or animals with poor

liver function, resulting in prolonged recovery from anesthesia

VI. Propofol toxicity
  A. Administration on consecutive days results in significant Heinz body production, lethargy, anorexia, and diarrhea in normal cats
  B. Prolonged administration (>3 hours) will lead to drug accumulation and longer recovery from anesthesia

VII. Local anesthetic toxicity
  A. In general, the proper administration of local anesthetics has little or no deleterious effects on tissues
  B. Toxic reactions primarily affect the CNS and the cardiovascular system
    1. Acidosis and hypoxia potentiate toxicity
    2. Sensitivity is increased by rapidity of injection
  C. CNS toxicity
    1. Dose necessary to produce CNS toxicity is usually less than the dose that causes cardiovascular collapse
    2. Excessive levels of agents such as lidocaine can cause hypotension, anxiety, tremors, convulsions, paralysis, or coma
  D. Cardiotoxicity
    1. Rapid intravenous injection of more potent local anesthetics (e.g., bupivacaine) may cause cardiovascular collapse
    2. Ventricular dysrhythmias and fatal ventricular fibrillation result
    3. Resuscitation is more difficult after bupivacaine
    4. Pregnant animals may be more sensitive

VIII. Narcotic, ataractic, and cyclohexamine toxicity
  A. These drugs have little or no toxic effect on the different organ tissues when administered in anesthetic doses
  B. Deleterious side effects
    1. Narcotics
      a. The most common are hyperexcitability, respiratory depression, and bradycardia
      b. Anaphylactic reactions
      c. Blood dyscrasias, thrombocytopenia
    2. Ataractics
      a. Phenothiazine tranquilizers

(1) Noted for their sympatholytic and hypotensive effects
(2) Rarely cause extrapyramidal behavioral changes and bradycardia
(3) Paraphimosis in horses and cattle
b. Butyrophenone tranquilizers can cause aggressive behavior and, rarely, excitement
c. Benzodiazepines; propylene glycol, a preservative and diluent for diazepam, may cause respiratory depression, bradycardia, and cardiac arrest
d. α_2-Agonists cause significant respiratory depression and bradycardia
3. Cyclohexamines
a. Produce an apneustic pattern of ventilation and increased arterial PCO_2, resulting in respiratory acidosis
b. Prolonged recovery from anesthesia may occur after the administration of Telazol® to cats and pigs

WASTE ANESTHETIC GAS POLLUTION

I. Waste anesthetic gases are anesthetic vapors that escape the patient and/or the anesthetic system and enter the environment
II. Pollution and staff exposure occur when anesthetic waste gases leak into the environment
III. Health concerns
A. Adverse effects associated with chronic exposure to trace levels of waste gases include increased incidence of spontaneous abortion, birth defects, neoplasia, hepatic and renal disease, neurologic disturbances, hematopoietic changes, infertility, and pruritus
1. Individuals at highest risk
a. Persons with preexisting hepatic or renal disease
b. Persons with immune system compromise
c. Women in the first trimester of pregnancy
B. Anesthetics incriminated
1. Nitrous oxide
2. Halothane

3. Methoxyflurane
4. Enflurane
5. Isoflurane

C. Epidemiologic studies, animal studies, and human volunteer studies reveal conflicting evidence
   1. To date, there is no definitive cause-and-effect relationship between exposure to waste gases and disease
   2. Overall evidence implies a potential hazard

IV. Environmental concern
   A. Nitrous oxide
      1. A greenhouse gas (implicated in global warming)
   B. Halogenated hydrocarbons
      1. Ozone layer depletion

V. Regulations regarding waste anesthetic gas levels
   A. Standards for maximum allowable concentrations have been established by the National Institute for Occupational Safety and Health (http://www.cdc.gov/niosh/homepage.html)
   B. Recommended acceptable levels
      1. Volatile agents used alone: less than 2 ppm
      2. Volatile agents combined with nitrous oxide: less than 0.5 ppm
      3. Nitrous oxide: less than 25 ppm
      4. Levels are time-weighted averages over the span of surgical procedure(s)
   C. These standards are used by the Occupational Safety and Health Administration when inspecting veterinary hospitals

V. Monitoring for waste gas levels
   A. Continuous sampling
      1. Instantaneous point sampling in many areas
      2. Immediate results
      3. Expensive equipment
   B. Instantaneous (grab) sampling
      1. Room air aspirated into a container and sent to a laboratory for evaluation
      2. Delayed results
      3. Results may not reflect overall exposure
      4. Inexpensive and easy to perform

      C. Time-weighted average sampling
         1. Samples absorbed by a collection device over a period of time
         2. Delayed results
         3. Best indication of overall exposure
         4. Inexpensive and easy to collect

VI. Collection and removal of waste gases
      A. Scavenging is the collection and removal of waste gases from the anesthetic system and the workplace (Fig. 12-2)
      B. Scavenging systems are made up of the following major components:
         1. Pressure relief valve (pop-off)
            a. Collects excess gases for conduction to removal system
            b. May need to be modified or replaced for leak-free connection to transfer tubing
            c. In nonrebreathing circuits, waste gases are collected from the reservoir bag

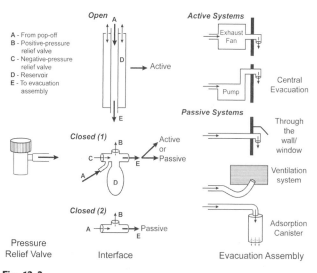

Fig. 12-2
Different methods of scavenging waste anesthetic gases.

2. Interface
   a. Protects breathing circuit and patient from excessive positive or negative pressures
   b. Located between the pop-off valve and the disposal system
   c. Open interfaces contain no valves and are open to the atmosphere
      (1) Best suited for use with high-flow active evacuation systems
      (2) Must have reservoir to buffer pressure differences
      (3) Safety depends on the number of vents
      (4) Economical and easily made
   d. Closed interfaces contain mechanical pressure relief valves
      (1) Best suited for use with low-flow active or passive evacuation systems
      (2) Positive-pressure relief valve protects system from pressure buildup if the line is occluded
      (3) Negative-pressure relief valve required for use with active evacuation system
      (4) Does not require a reservoir, except when active evacuation is used
      (5) More costly, but safer and more versatile
3. Evacuation systems
   a. The evacuation system moves the collected waste gases to a remote area for release
   b. Passive evacuation systems
      (1) The flow of gases is controlled by ventilation
      (2) Gases are exhausted into a nonrecirculating ventilation system, directly out into the atmosphere
      (3) Inexpensive and easy to install
      (4) Inefficient and a potential hazard to the patient because of potential resistance to exhalation
   c. Active evacuation systems
      (1) Mechanical flow-inducing devices
      (2) Consist of a central vacuum system or a dedicated fan or pump
      (3) Negative pressure produced requires an interface with a negative pressure relief valve

(4) More costly and complex than passive systems

(5) More effective than passive systems

d. Activated charcoal absorption canisters

(1) Remove hydrocarbons

(2) Do not remove nitrous oxide

(3) Require frequent replacement

4. Transfer tubing

a. Connects the different components of the system

b. Tubing should be resistant to kinking, easily differentiated from the breathing circuit, and able to transfer high flows

c. Tubing for passive systems should be as short and wide as practical

VII. Additional control methods

A. Pressure check all breathing circuits and machines for leaks (see Chapter 14)

B. Use agent-specific bottle cap adaptors when filling vaporizers to avoid spillage, and fill at the end of the workday when fewer people are present

C. Use low-flow or closed-system techniques whenever possible

D. Check endotracheal tube cuff before use and be sure it is adequately inflated during use

E. Avoid chamber and mask inductions; when they cannot be avoided, use tight-fitting mask and attach scavenger tubing to chamber

F. Ventilate areas where inhalation anesthesia is commonly used and areas where animals are recovering; remain at least 1 m from the recovering patient's head

G. Do not turn on vaporizer until patient is connected to the circuit

H. When disconnecting the patient from the breathing circuit, turn off flowmeter and vaporizer, occlude Y piece, and evacuate remaining gas in the system into the scavenger

I. Wear a half-mask respirator if waste gases cannot be avoided

J. Inform all employees of potential risks associated with waste gas exposure and emphasize measures to reduce exposure

OXYGEN TOXICITY (HYPEROXIA)

I. Tolerance to oxygen
   A. Exposure of animals to increased oxygen tensions at atmospheric pressures for prolonged periods (100% for 12 hours, more than 46% for more than 24 hours) causes metabolic derangements resulting in pulmonary dysfunction; changes include decreases in vital capacity, lung compliance, minute ventilation, respiratory rate, pH, arterial oxygen partial pressure, total lung volume, carbon dioxide-diffusing capacity, dizziness, and convulsions
   B. Animals show considerable variation in the susceptibility to oxygen toxicity
   C. The rate of onset of the disease process is proportional to the inspired tension of oxygen and the duration of exposure
   D. Reductions in vital capacity and pulmonary compliance are the best criteria for identifying the onset of toxicity
   E. Safety range is 18% to 25%
II. Mechanisms of pulmonary oxygen toxicity
   A. Although oxygen is necessary for the production of energy and survival of all aerobic cells, it is also a cellular poison
      1. Cellular injury results from the metabolic processing of oxygen itself
      2. Most oxygen entering the body is metabolized to create adenosine triphosphate and enzymatically reduced to form water
      3. Free radicals are active products of this process: superoxide anion (O_2^-), the hydroxyl radical (OH^-), and hydrogen peroxide (H_2O_2)
      4. Elevated levels of oxygen-free radicals are thought to be the cause of biologic membrane damage related to oxygen toxicity
      5. Interaction of free radicals with side chains of membrane lipids results in the formation of lipid peroxides, which inhibit many enzyme activities and further byproducts that can create holes in cell membranes

6. Damaged membranes leak fluids into extracellular spaces
7. Inflammation and phagocytosis occur, producing additional free radicals

III. Lesions
  A. Pulmonary responses to increased oxygen tension
      1. Low doses of oxygen (25% to 60%) are associated with proliferative changes in endothelium and epithelium and permanent widening of the interstitium caused by increased collagen and elastin fiber deposition
      2. Exposure to high concentrations (more than 60%) of oxygen for more than 12 hours results in the following:
          a. Pulmonary capillary endothelial congestion and hyaline accumulation, type 1 epithelial cell death
          b. Enhanced alveolar epithelial permeability
          c. Interstitial and alveolar edema
          d. Atelectasis; increased shunting
          e. Intraalveolar hemorrhage
      3. Bronchiolar epithelium is also damaged to a lesser degree
  B. Hemolysis
  C. Multiorgan damage (retinal, hepatic, renal, and myocardial)

IV. Signs of toxicity
  A. Early signs
      1. Restlessness
      2. Coughing
      3. Anorexia and lethargy
      4. Dyspnea
  B. Late signs
      1. Respiratory insufficiency
      2. Cyanosis
      3. Frothy or bloody fluid from mouth
      4. Asphyxia

V. Conditions contributing to toxicity
  A. General rate of metabolism affects the response to oxygen toxicity
  B. Hyperthyroidism and elevations of adrenocortical hormones hasten toxicity

    C. The depression of cellular activity by anesthesia decreases susceptibility to oxygen toxicity

    D. Preexisting pulmonary disease and hypoxia may help protect against rapid onset

    E. Increased susceptibility may result from extremes in humidity, hypercapnia, acidosis, hyperthermia, and pulmonary edema

  VI. Recommendations

    A. Do not overreact to the use of oxygen

      1. Hypoxia is commonly associated with anesthesia and hypoventilation, and the damage it causes occurs rapidly

      2. Pulmonary injury from oxygen is uncommon, and onset is slow

      3. Early symptoms are fully reversible on termination of oxygen administration

    B. There are no known contraindications to the use of pure oxygen for brief periods or in emergencies; in the normal lung, no significant toxicity develops if pure oxygen is given for 12 hours or less

ANESTHETIC DRUG INTERACTIONS

  I. Pharmacologic drug interactions: combinations of two or more drugs may be additive, supraadditive (synergistic), or antagonistic, thereby enhancing or negating expected effects and side effects; experience with tested drug combinations is the best way to avoid problems; for example, the combination of opioids (morphine) and α_2-agonists (medetomidine) can produce bradycardia and apnea

    A. Blood or blood products with calcium-containing solutions other than saline solution

    B. Acidic drug with basic drug

      1. Thiobarbiturate plus lidocaine

      2. Sodium bicarbonate with calcium-containing solutions

      3. Diazepam with oxymorphone or butorphanol

  II. Pharmacokinetic interactions: interactions affecting absorption, distribution, metabolism, or elimination of a drug

    A. Protein-binding effects

      1. Phenylbutazone displaces thiobarbiturates from binding sites, resulting in relative barbiturate overdose

      2. Decreased protein binding is caused by hemodilution of intravenous fluid administration

  B. Alterations in biotransformation

      1. Barbiturates enhance liver microsomal enzyme activity (enzyme induction)

      2. Organophosphates inhibit plasma cholinesterase, prolonging the duration of action of ester-linked local anesthetics and depolarizing muscle relaxants

      3. Cimetidine and chloramphenicol reduce hepatic microsomal enzyme activity, thus prolonging the duration of action of some drugs

      4. Epinephrine prolongs local anesthetic duration of action, and hyaluronidase increases the area of local anesthetic spread

III. Chemical interactions: combining two or more drugs in solution may result in a chemical incompatibility; unless you are certain there is not incompatibility, do not combine drugs

IV. Pharmacodynamic interactions: the actions of a drug on a particular organ system or on the body as a whole can be altered by concurrently administered drugs

  A. Agonist-antagonist interactions

      1. Narcotic agonists-antagonists: butorphanol

      2. α_2-Agonists: yohimbine/tolazoline/atipamezole

      3. Nondepolarizing muscle relaxants-cholinesterase inhibitors

      4. Benzodiazepines: flumazenil

      5. Autonomic receptor agonists-antagonists

  B. Other alterations in pharmacodynamics

      1. Arrhythmogenicity of halothane in presence of catecholamines

      2. Enhancement of halothane-catecholamine arrhythmias by certain drugs such as barbiturates, xylazine, or ketamine

      3. Decrease in digitalis-induced arrhythmias by halothane

      4. Epinephrine can induce hypotension after acepromazine administration

      5. Aminoglycoside antibiotics prolong effects of muscle relaxants

      6. Tetracyclines enhance nephrotoxicity

      7. The development of acute (thiobarbiturates) and delayed tolerance (opioids) to drugs

CHAPTER THIRTEEN

Anesthetic Machines and Breathing Systems

"Give the tools to him that can handle them."
NAPOLEON BONAPARTE

OVERVIEW

A variety of equipment is used to deliver inhalant anesthetic drugs. Volatilizing the liquid anesthetic and safely delivering it to the patient, while minimizing environmental pollution, requires relatively sophisticated, expensive, and, at times, cumbersome devices. Regardless of their apparent complexity, most inhalant anesthetic drug delivery systems use similar, simple designs for the delivery of oxygen, safe anesthetic concentrations, and the removal of carbon dioxide and waste gases. This chapter describes the anesthetic machine, breathing circuits, and ancillary equipment for delivering inhalant anesthetic drugs to animals.

GENERAL CONSIDERATIONS

Most anesthetic delivery systems contain the same components. They reduce the pressure of stored oxygen and nitrous oxide and precisely mix these gases with potent inhalant anesthetic drugs for delivery through a breathing system.

ANESTHETIC EQUIPMENT

I. Compressed gases: oxygen, nitrous oxide, and other select gases come in color-coded cylinders of varying size (Tables 13-1 and 13-2). They are used as carrier gases for delivering inhaled anesthetics

TABLE 13-1
COMPRESSED GASES

CYLINDER SPECIFICATION (LITERS, STP)

AGENT	E (8.8 cm × 66 cm)	G (17.6 cm × 121 cm)	H (19.8 cm × 121 cm)	FILLING PRESSURE (PSI)
Oxygen	655	5290	6910	2200
Nitrous oxide	1590	12,110	14,520	750
Carbon dioxide	1590	4160		800
Helium	500	4350	5930	1650

STP, Standard temperature and pressure; *psi,* pounds per square inch.

TABLE 13-2
UNITED STATES AND IOS (INTERNATIONAL ORGANIZATION FOR STANDARDIZATION) GAS COLOR CODES

	US	ISO
Oxygen	Green	White
Nitrous oxide	Light blue	Light blue
Medical air	Yellow	Black and white
Suction	White	Yellow
Nitrogen	Black	Black
Carbon dioxide	Grey	Grey
Helium	Brown	Brown

A. Cylinders should be handled carefully
   1. Never leave an unsupported or unsecured cylinder sitting upright
      a. Store E cylinders in a rack
      b. Secure H cylinders anchored to a wall or a transport cart with a chain
   2. If dropped, a cylinder may explode because it is under high pressure
   3. Open cylinder valves slowly and completely
   4. Crack the cylinder valve (open and shut quickly) before attaching it to the machine to remove dust from the connecting port (dirt or dust plus rapid compression at the connecting port can cause a fire)

    5. Install a new gasket supplied with each full cylinder to the connecting port

B. Most machines have a hanger yoke for attaching one or more E cylinders; hanger yokes and E cylinders are keyed (coded) with a pin index safety system that prevents inadvertent connection of the wrong cylinder to the wrong gas yoke on the machine (Fig. 13-1)

C. Centralized oxygen sources usually use G or H cylinders

    1. H cylinders require an individualized pressure regulator (thread size and connection are coded for different types of gas)

    2. These cylinders are attached to the machine by a length of high-pressure hose connected to the Diameter Index and Safety System fitting of the machine

    3. In other systems, the high-pressure hose is connected to a special yoke-block connector that attaches to the pin index system in the hanger yoke

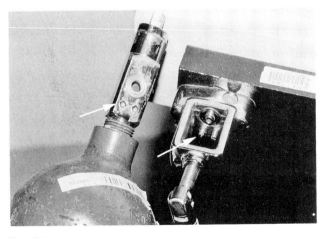

Fig. 13-1

The pin index system ensures that the appropriate tank is properly secured to the anesthetic machine.

D. Oxygen and nitrous oxide
   1. Oxygen is present within the cylinder only as a gas, and its pressure is proportional to gas volume
   2. Nitrous oxide is present within the cylinder as a liquid and a gas; pressure within the tank remains constant at 750 psi until all the liquid is gone. The pressure then falls
E. Oxygen generators can be installed for central gas supply; they extract oxygen from room air to 90% to 95% O_2
   1. Various sizes are available according to projected volume used

II. Hanger yoke site of E cylinder attachment (Fig. 13-1)
   A. Pin index system configuration avoids improper cylinder connection
   B. A brass filter prevents particulate contamination of the anesthetic machine's gas lines
   C. Pressure gauges located on the anesthetic machine or attached directly to the cylinder measure cylinder pressure
   D. One-way (check) valves prevent transfilling of cylinders or cylinder into pipeline supply

III. Pressure-reducing valves (pressure regulators) are built into some anesthetic machines or they attach directly to the cylinder
   A. Reduces the pressure of the gas within the cylinder to a constant pressure of approximately 50 psi
   B. Provides constant pressure to the flowmeter
   C. Allows a wide range of flowmeter settings
   D. Ensures that the flowmeter does not have to operate at high pressures
   E. Hospital supply cylinders (G and H) require individualized regulators

IV. Oxygen "fail-safe" system
   A. If the oxygen supply is interrupted, nitrous oxide and any other gas flow is automatically interrupted
   B. An audible oxygen supply failure alarm is also activated on some machines

    C. Not all machines are so equipped, which means if the oxygen supply is interrupted, then N_2O may be delivered without oxygen

V. Flowmeters

    A. A flowmeter controls the rate at which a specific gas is delivered (milliliters per minute; liters per minute). The most common gas flowmeter is the rotameter. It contains a ball or bobbin that rises within a glass tube to a height proportional to the flow of gas through the tube. The gas flow rate is read at the widest diameter of the ball or bobbin

    B. Ideally, the oxygen flowmeter should be the last in a series of flowmeters (a hypoxic gas mixture is less likely to develop if a flowmeter tube is cracked)

    C. Avoid excessive torque when closing flowmeters, because the knobs can be twisted off

    D. Flowmeter tubes are gas-specific; an N_2O flow tube cannot be substituted for an O_2 tube

    E. Individual gas flows are combined downstream from the flowmeters; from here, gases move to an out-of-circuit vaporizer or directly to the anesthetic circuit

    F. Some machines are equipped with two oxygen flowmeters

        1. They are typically connected in series; the flow from both is additive

            a. One flowmeter is used for low flows (up to 1 L/min)

            b. The other is used for flows greater than 1 L/min

VI. Oxygen flush valve

    A. Bypasses the vaporizer and delivers oxygen directly to the common gas outlet or anesthetic circle

    B. Delivers oxygen to the circle at 35 to 75 L/min

    C. Dilutes the anesthetic gases in the system

VII. Common gas outlet: the point-of-gas-exit from the machine for oxygen, nitrous oxide, and vaporized (out-of-circuit) gas anesthetic. It has a 15-mm connector

VIII. Anesthetic vaporizers

    A. Vaporizers are designed to volatilize liquid inhalant anesthetic drugs and to deliver clinically useful concentrations of anesthetic vapor

B. Vaporizers are located near the flowmeters out of the anesthetic breathing circuit (vaporizer out-of-circle [VOC], non-rebreathing system) or within the anesthetic circle (vaporizer in-the-circle [VIC])

C. VOCs
   1. These vaporizers deliver precise anesthetic concentrations (%) of anesthetic vapor that are relatively independent of temperature and flow rate; the manufacturer specifies limits of temperature and flow
   2. Gas flow within the vaporizer is split between the bypass and vaporization chamber. The splitting ratio is determined by the desired output (%) of anesthetic vapor, and the specific anesthetic can change anesthetic concentration relatively rapidly
   3. VOCs are agent-specific
      a. Isoflurane vaporizers
         (1) Ohio Calibrated Vaporizer for Isoflurane (Ohmeda)
         (2) Vapor 19.1 (Dräger)
         (3) Isotec (Ohmeda)
      b. Halothane vaporizers
         (1) Fluotec Mark II, III, IV, V (Cyprane, Matrix)
         (2) Vapomatic (old Foregger Fluomatic; A.M. Bickford)
         (3) Vapor and Vapor 19.1 Halothane (Dräger)
         (4) Ohio Calibrated Vaporizer for Halothane (Ohmeda)
      c. Sevoflurane vaporizers
         (1) Tec III (converted enflurane vaporizers); Sevotec (Tec 5) (Ohmeda)
         (2) Sevomatic (A.M. Bickford)
         (3) Sigma Delta (InterMed Penlon)
      d. Desflurane vaporizer
         (1) Tec 6 vaporizer (Ohmeda): electronically heated vaporizer; unique construction because of the physical-chemical properties of desflurane
      e. Nonagent-specific vaporizers can be used for various inhalant drugs except desflurane
         (1) Copper Kettle (Foregger)

(2) A separate flowmeter controls carrier gas flow through vaporizer

(3) Slide rule or calculator needed to determine vaporizer flowmeter setting

    (a) Vapor pressure (depends on inhalant anesthetic drugs chosen and temperature)

    (b) Desired total gas flow

    (c) Desired anesthetic percent

(4) A slide rule is provided by most manufacturers for calculating flow rate through the vaporizer; an exception is the Metomatic 980; it is a Vernitrol with specific calibration marks for methoxyflurane that should not be used for other inhalant anesthetic drugs

  f. Maintenance

    (1) Vaporizers should be sent to the manufacturer yearly for cleaning and recalibration

    (2) They should also be serviced whenever the dial setting (%) does not match clinical perception of anesthetic depth

D. VICs (also called draw-over vaporizers); the animal's breathing moves the gas through the vaporizer and volatizes the inhalant anesthetic drugs

  1. Draw-over vaporizers are not agent-specific

  2. Output depends on the following:

    a. The inhalant anesthetic's volatility

      (1) Less volatile agents (e.g., ether) require a wick; current inhalant anesthetic drugs (isoflurane, sevoflurane) need no wick

    b. Temperature

      (1) Vapor pressure and therefore vaporizer output increases or decreases with ambient temperature

      (2) Overdose can occur at high ambient temperatures

      (3) Animals may be difficult to keep anesthetized at low ambient temperatures

    c. Flow-through vaporizer

      (1) Controlled by animal's minute ventilation; increases in depth and rate of ventilation

(spontaneous or assisted) increase the vaporizer output
   d. Vaporizer construction
      (1) Wick versus no wick; adjustable sleeves; distance between the surface of the liquid and the gas flow
   e. Location of vaporizer in the breathing circuit
      (1) The vaporizer should be mounted on the inspiratory side to reduce the condensation of water in the vaporizer
3. Calibration marks on top of the vaporizer are not synonymous with the percentage output of VIC vaporizers
4. Types
   a. Ohio No. 8 Vaporizer (Pitman-Moore); wick must be removed when using with isoflurane or sevoflurane
   b. Stephens (Henry Schein); wick must be removed when using with isoflurane or sevoflurane
5. Maintenance: wick should be allowed to dry weekly to rid system of excess water vapor
E. General comments
   1. Vaporizers ideally should be filled with anesthetic in a well-ventilated area at the beginning or end of the day to minimize exposure of personnel to vapor
   2. Vaporizers must be in the off position when filling or draining
   3. Special filling devices are available to minimize spills and escape of vapors into the environment
   4. Vaporizers should not be tilted or laid on their sides unless completely drained; dangerously high concentrations can result during subsequent use

ANESTHETIC BREATHING SYSTEMS

I. Purpose
   A. The safe delivery of inhaled anesthetics and oxygen
   B. Removal of carbon dioxide and excess anesthetic gases by one of three methods
      1. Dilution (e.g., T piece systems)

2. One-way valve systems: rarely used because disadvantages outweigh advantages (currently used in manual resuscitators)
3. Carbon dioxide absorbents (Baralyme, Sodasorb, Amsorb)

II. Types of systems
  A. Open drop or cone system (Fig. 13-2)
    1. Features
      a. No reservoir
      b. Minimal or no rebreathing of expired gases
      c. Carbon dioxide removal by dilution
    2. Advantages
      a. Low cost of equipment

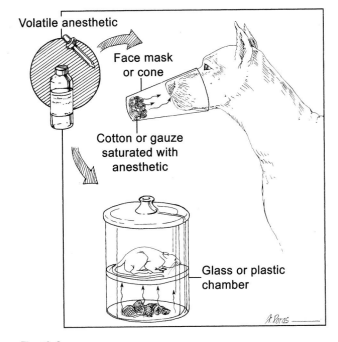

Fig. 13-2

Open system. Gauze or cotton is saturated with anesthetic and placed in a cone or chamber from which the animal breathes.

b. Minimal or no rebreathing of expired gases

c. Minimal resistance to breathing (especially open drop)

3. Disadvantages

a. Wasteful because so much anesthetic is vaporized

b. Difficult to control anesthetic concentration delivery

c. No method of assisting ventilation

d. Difficult or impossible to scavenge waste gas

e. Vaporization of anesthetic depends on room temperature (open drop and cone)

B. Non-rebreathing valveless systems (Mapleson classification) rely on relatively high, fresh gas flow rates (Table 13-3) to remove carbon dioxide. The following classifications are based on the location of fresh gas inlet and opening (or valve) for exit of exhaled gas. The relative location of the fresh gas inlet and the valve opening determine the efficiency of the circuit

1. Types

a. Rees modification of Ayre's T piece (Fig. 13-3) (Mapleson F: fresh gas enters near the patient and exits from the reservoir bag)

TABLE 13-3
RECOMMENDED OXYGEN FLOW RATES FOR ANESTHETIC SYSTEMS

Non-rebreathing systems	
Mapleson systems*	
Magill system	100 ml/kg/min
Lack system	150 ml/kg/min
Ayre's T piece	150 ml/kg/min
Bain circuit	150 ml/kg/min
Insufflation	200-300 ml/kg/min
Rebreathing or circle systems	
Closed	3-5 ml/kg/min†
Semi-closed low flow	5-10 ml/kg/min‡
Semi-closed high flow	20-30 ml/kg/min‡

* Do not use during controlled or assisted ventilation.
† Do not use nitrous oxide in a closed circle unless in-circuit oxygen analyzer is used.
‡ If using nitrous oxide, add to the O_2 flow.

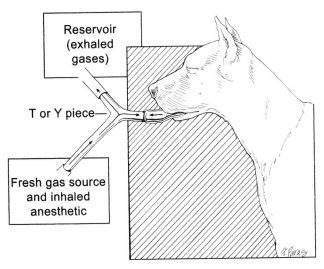

Fig. 13-3
Mapleson F (Ayres T piece). Low-resistance method of delivering anesthetic and oxygen. High fresh gas flow rates are used to minimize or eliminate the rebreathing of exhaled gas. Exhaled gas flows through corrugated tubing into a rebreathing bag. Excess gas is vented through an opening in the bag.

    b. Bain circuit (modified Mapleson D): fresh gas enters circuit near the bag, but in the coaxial (tube in a tube) design, it delivers anesthetic near the patient; exhaled gas passes around the fresh gas line to exit near the bag (Figs. 13-4 and 13-5)

    c. Lack system (modified Mapleson A): fresh gas is delivered via a large-bore corrugated tube surrounding a smaller inner tube that carries exhaled gas to a pressure relief valve at the distal end of the circuit (opposite of the Bain; Fig. 13-4)

      (1) Above three systems are relatively efficient during both spontaneous and controlled ventilation. Fresh gas flow rate during spontaneous and controlled ventilation should be set to equal 150 ml/kg/min

Bain (modified Mapleson D)

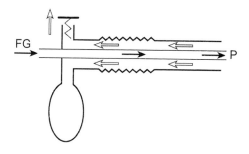

Lack (modified Mapleson A)

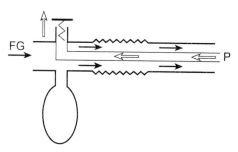

Fig. 13-4
Examples of non-rebreathing systems. *FG,* Fresh gas; *P,* patient.

      d. Magill system (Fig. 13-6) (modified Mapleson A): fresh gas enters near bag and exhaled gas exits through a pressure relief valve located near the patient
        (1) Very efficient during spontaneous ventilation (fresh gas flow only needs to match minute alveolar ventilation)
        (2) Very inefficient during controlled ventilation (fresh gas flow = 3 to 5 × minute ventilation)
  2. Advantages and disadvantages of all non-rebreathing circuits
    a. Advantages: low equipment dead space, low resistance to breathing

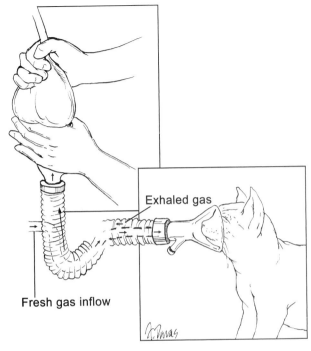

Fig. 13-5
Modified Mapleson D Bain circuit. Functions similarly to Ayres T piece system. It is designed to minimize equipment dead space and facilitate warming of the inspired gases.

      b. Disadvantages: wasteful; high gas (O_2) flow rates can rapidly decrease patient's temperature; difficult to scavenge

    C. Rebreathing systems allow rebreathing of exhaled gases minus carbon dioxide; amount of rebreathing depends on the fresh gas flow rate

      1. Circle system (Figs. 13-7 and 13-8)

        a. Components

          (1) Pressure relief ("pop-off") valve

            (a) Allows the release of excess pressure from

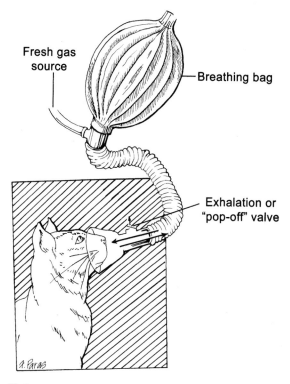

Fig. 13-6
Mapleson A Magill system. Low fresh gas flow rates can be used during spontaneous ventilation because of the presence of a pressure relief valve near the patient that preferentially exhausts alveolar gas.

the system; the volume of gas in excess of the animal's minute oxygen consumption is vented from the system

(b) Fitted with spring-loaded or variable orifice valves; when in the fully open position, modern valves usually "pop off" or open when pressure exceeds 0.5 to 1 cm H_2O; as valve is tightened down, more pressure is required to open valve

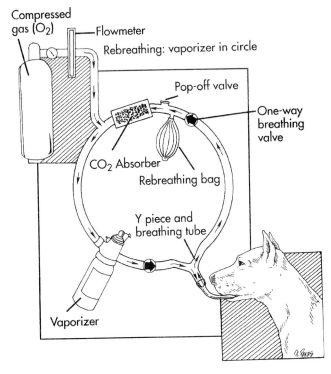

Fig. 13-7
Anesthetic circle system with the vaporizer in-circle

      (c) Fitted with orifice or hood for scavenging waste gas
  2. Carbon dioxide absorbent canister (Table 13-4)
    a. Contains the material that chemically removes carbon dioxide from the expired gases
    b. Capacity should be one to two times tidal volume ($V_T = 10$ ml/kg)
    c. Active ingredients are various proportions of K^+, Ca^{++}, and Na^+ hydroxide. These hydroxides react with exhaled CO_2 and water to form carbonate; heat is liberated, pH decreases

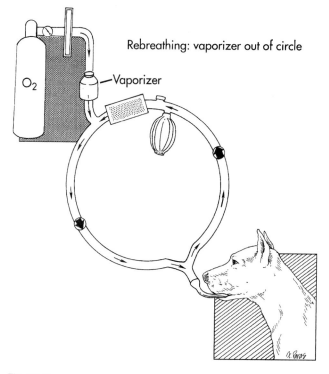

Fig. 13-8
Anesthetic circle system with the vaporizer out-of-circle.

    d. Uses 4- to 8-mesh, granule-size

    e. Absorbent has a pH color-change indicator (usually ethyl violet) that turns blue on consumption; the indicator may revert to its original color when allowed to rest; absorbent should be changed after 6 to 8 hours of use, depending on fresh gas flow rates and size of the animal (Fig. 13-9)

    f. Absorbent becomes brittle, dusty, and clumps together when no longer useful

TABLE 13-4
CHEMICAL COMPOSITION OF SOME CARBON DIOXIDE ABSORBENTS

CO_2 ABSORBENT	$BA(OH)_2$ (%)	$CA(OH)_2$ (%)	KOH (%)	NA(OH) (%)	$CACL_2$ (%)	$CASO_4$ (%)	H_2O (%)	SILICA (%)	POLYINYLPYRROLIDINE (%)
Barium hydroxide lime	16	64	4.6	—	—	—	14-18	—	—
Sodium hydroxide lime (classic)	—	80-81	2.0-2.6	1.3-3.0	—	—	14-18	0.1	—
Sodium hydroxide lime (KOH-free)	—	81.5	0.003-0.005	2.0-2.6	—	—	14-18	0.1	—
Calcium hydroxide lime	—	75-83	—	—	0.7	0.7	14.5	—	0.7

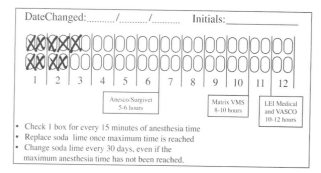

DateChanged:........./........./.......... Initials:_____

1 | 2 | 3 | 4 | 5 | 6 | 7 | 8 | 9 | 10 | 11 | 12

Anesco/Surgivet 5-6 hours

Matrix VMS 8-10 hours

LEI Medical and VASCO 10-12 hours

- Check 1 box for every 15 minutes of anesthesia time
- Replace soda lime once maximum time is reached
- Change soda lime every 30 days, even if the maximum anesthesia time has not been reached.

Fig. 13-9

The total time that the CO_2 absorbent is used should be monitored to ensure maximum CO_2 removal from the anesthetic circuit.

g. Desiccated absorbent can liberate various toxins (e.g., compound A, carbon monoxide, formaldehyde, methanol) (see Chapter 12)

h. Change absorbent at appropriate intervals to avoid accumulation of compound A from sevoflurane, desflurane, and halothane and accumulation of carbon monoxide from desflurane, isoflurane, sevoflurane, and halothane

3. Two unidirectional flow valves prevent exhaled gas from being rebreathed before it passes through the absorbent canister

4. Vaporizer (in or out of the circle; see Figs. 13-7 and 13-8)

5. Rebreathing bag (reservoir bag) is available in the following sizes:

1L: for animals less than 5 to 7 kg

2L: for animals more than 7 kg but less than 15 kg

3L: for animals more than 15 kg but less than 50 kg

5L: for animals more than 50 kg but less than 150 kg

35L (large-animal system): for animals more than 150 kg

6. Pressure manometer

a. Monitors pressure within breathing system

b. Typically calibrated from −30 to +50 cm H_2O

c. Pressure within circle increases when bag is squeezed, particularly when the "pressure relief" valve is closed

7. Corrugated breathing tubes and Y piece
   a. Generally 1 meter long and 22 mm in diameter for small animal patients
   b. Longer tubes are used when machines cannot be located near the patient's head
   c. Shorter tubes with small diameter (13 mm) are used for animals less than 5 kg
   d. Large animal tubes are 50 mm in diameter
   e. Advantages of circle system:
      (1) Relatively low gas flow rates can be used (economical and minimize pollution)
      (2) Carbon dioxide-absorbent canister is located away from patient, as opposed to to-and-fro system
      (3) Ventilation is readily observed and controlled by reservoir bag
      (4) Minimal heat loss and airway drying
      (5) Absence of abrupt fluctuations in anesthetic depth
   f. Disadvantages:
      (1) System is bulky
      (2) Parts may be inappropriately rearranged or may malfunction
      (3) Resistance to gas flow is greater than with Mapleson systems; conventional circle systems should not be used in animals less than 3 kg
      (4) Some components are difficult to clean
      (5) Cross-infection of patients is possible; bag and hoses should be disinfected after each use
      (6) Concentration within system typically does not match the vaporizer setting
      (7) System concentration changes slowly when vaporizer setting is adjusted, especially with relatively low fresh gas flow rates

8. Fresh gas flow rates for rebreathing systems (Table 13-5)
   a. Minimum flow rate equals minute oxygen consumption
      (1) Approximately 3 to 5 ml/kg/min

TABLE 13-5
GENERIC ANESTHESIA MACHINE AND BREATHING CIRCUIT CHECK

I. Inspect machine
    A. Turn off vaporizers, fill vaporizers, tighten filler caps
    B. Fill CO_2 canister, with absorbent
    C. Confirm proper function of undirectional valves in circle—with surgical mask inhale and exhale through Y piece*
II. Confirm oxygen supply and failsafe
    A. Check cylinder pressure
    B. Turn on N_2O cylinder and flowmeter; turn O_2 cylinder off; N_2O float should drop to zero; reopen O_2 cylinder*
III. Verify proper flowmeter functions—bobbin or float should move freely throughout length of tube*
IV. Check breathing circuit
    A. Proper, tight connections
    B. Occlude Y piece, close pressure relief valve, pressurize circuit to 30 cm H_2O; check for leaks; open pressure relief valve and confirm release of pressure
V. Check waste gas scavenging system (if attached)*
    A. Confirm that scavenging system is connected to pressure relief valve
    B. Turn on vacuum pump or verify patency of passive system
VI. Check ventilator function*
    A. Verify connection to breathing circuit
    B. Check for leaks according to manufacturer

*Need only be performed daily.

        (2) Because the volume of fresh gas delivered equals patient uptake, the volume of the system will not change; the pressure relief valve can, but does not have to, remain closed
        (3) Advantages of closed system
            (a) Minimal pollution
            (b) Economical
            (c) Breathing system warmth and humidity maximized
        (4) Disadvantages
            (a) Difficult to rapidly change concentration with VOC; VOC cannot be used with closed-system flow rate for the first 10 to 15 minutes because anesthetic uptake is too

great; VIC can be used with closed-system flow rates from the beginning of anesthesia
(b) System volume must be more closely monitored
(c) Increased CO_2 absorbent use
(d) N_2O cannot be used without an oxygen monitor in the system

b. Flow rates in excess of 4 to 6 ml/kg/min require an open pressure relief valve (semi-closed)

VETERINARY ANESTHETIC MACHINES

I. Machines are currently manufactured for veterinary use by the following companies:
   A. A.M. Bickford: several small animal models (Wales Center, New York, www.ambickford.com)
   B. AnescoSurgivet/Smith Medical: a variety of anesthetic machines, and ventilators for small and large animals (Waukesha, Wisconsin, www.surgivet.com)
   C. DRE: small animal machine (Louisville, Kentucky, www.dreveterinary.com)
   D. Engler Engineering Corp.: small animal combination ventilator/anesthetic machine (Hialeah, Florida, www.englerusa.com)
   E. Hallowell Engineering and Manufacturing Corp.: a variety of anesthesia ventilators and accessories (Pittsfield, Massachusetts, www.hallowell.com)
   F. Highland Medical Equipment: a variety of small animal machines (Temecula, California, www.highlandmedical.net)
   G. iM3: in-circle vaporizer for small animals (Vancouver, Washington, www.im3vet.com)
   H. J. D. Medical: several large and small animal machines with ventilators (Phoenix, Arizona, www.jdmedical.com)
   I. Mallard Medical: large and small animal machines and ventilators (Redding, California, www.mallardmedical.net)
   J. Matrx: several small animal machines and ventilators and one large animal machine (Orchard Park, New York, www.matrxmedical.com)
   K. Moduflex Anesthesia Equipment: small animal anesthe-

sia machines (San Diego, California, www.moduflex-anesthesia.com)
  L. Summit Hill: a variety of small animal machines (Tinton Falls, New Jersey, sales@summithilllaboratories.com, 732-933-0800)
  M. Vetland: small and large animal anesthesia machines (Louisville, Kentucky, www.vetland1.com)
 II. Veterinary machines no longer manufactured
  A. Dupaco compact 78: small-animal machines
  B. North American Dräger Narkovet: small and large animal machines
  C. Pitman-Moore: 970, 980, and Vetaflex-5
III. Used human anesthesia machines are available through most anesthesia equipment dealers

CLEANING AND DISINFECTION

  I. Breathing hoses and reservoir bags should be cleaned and disinfected after each use
  A. Wash with hot, soapy water and rinse
  B. Soak in a cold disinfectant solution such as Nolvasan or Cidex and thoroughly rinse
  C. Clean the external surfaces of the anesthetic machine daily with a spray cleaner
  D. Occasionally disassemble the dome valves and absorbent canister and wipe dry
 II. Gas or steam autoclaving is not necessary unless gross contamination is present
III. Anesthetic machine check (Table 13-4)
  A. Verify proper machine function before each use; some checks should be performed daily, others before each use
  B. Consult the owner's manual for manufacturer's recommendations

TROUBLESHOOTING ANESTHETIC EQUIPMENT PROBLEMS

  I. Rebreathing bag empty
  A. Flow rate is too low or the flowmeter control knob is turned off

B. System leak
  1. Gasket on carbon dioxide canister improperly installed
  2. Hole in rebreathing bag or tubing
  3. Leak in endotracheal tube cuff
  4. Waste-gas scavenging system using active suction improperly regulated
  5. Water drain near carbon dioxide absorbent canister is open

II. Rebreathing bag overly distended (positive pressure in circuit)
  A. Pressure relief valve inadvertently left closed
  B. Flow rate too high in closed system
  C. Waste-gas scavenging system improperly regulated

III. Patient seems "light"
  A. Vaporizer empty, not working properly, or on an inadequate setting
  B. Excessive carbon dioxide buildup
    1. Exhausted carbon dioxide absorbent
    2. Sticky unidirectional valve
  C. Vaporizer needs service
    1. Water buildup on wick
    2. Recalibration necessary
  D. Patient receiving hypoxic gas mixture
    1. Nitrous oxide flowmeter set too high relative to oxygen flow
    2. Oxygen cylinder(s) filled with wrong gas

IV. Patient seems "deep"
  A. Vaporizer set too high or not working properly
  B. Patient severely hypercarbic or hypoxic
  C. Patient is hypotensive

CHAPTER FOURTEEN

Ventilation and Mechanical Assist Devices

"You don't need a weatherman to know which way the wind blows."

BOB DYLAN

OVERVIEW

One of the most crucial aspects of providing safe general anesthesia is the maintenance of normal ventilation. Normal ventilation is defined as the maintenance of arterial carbon dioxide levels within normal limits (35 to 45 mm Hg). Generally, respiratory effort can be verified by observing the movements of the patient's chest and abdominal wall. Although these movements may be regular and give the appearance of satisfactory gas exchange, they do not ensure adequate movement of air in and out of the lungs. Adequate gas exchange can be provided by inflating the lungs to a predetermined pressure or predetermined volume by manually squeezing a rebreathing bag on an anesthetic machine or by using a mechanical ventilatory-assist device. Controlled ventilation helps to maintain a more stable plane of anesthesia because the lungs serve as the exchange site for inhalant anesthetic uptake and elimination. High-frequency ventilation of patients is a unique procedure based on the principle that diffusion is the primary means by which fresh gases are delivered to peripheral airways and gas exchange sites.

GENERAL CONSIDERATIONS

I. Artificial ventilation can do more harm than good if improperly used, but if properly applied can be used to maintain

249

stable inhalant anesthesia (the drug delivery system is the lung) and blood gases for prolonged durations with minimal untoward effects

II. Anyone attempting controlled ventilation should be thoroughly familiar with the equipment, procedure, and normal cardiopulmonary physiology and blood gas interpretation

III. Generally, mechanical ventilatory-assist devices do no more than compress a rebreathing bag to inflate the lungs; they are an extra pair of hands

IV. The use of controlled ventilation should be considered in patients who are not breathing adequately or are difficult to keep anesthetized

V. Blood gas determinations are the best test of ventilatory adequacy

REASONS FOR RESPIRATORY INADEQUACY

I. Depression of respiratory centers
   A. Drug-induced
      1. Anesthetic
      2. Drug toxicities
   B. Metabolic
      1. Acidosis
      2. Coma
      3. Toxic metabolites (endotoxins)
   C. Physical
      1. Head trauma (increased intracranial pressure)

II. Inability to adequately expand the thorax
   A. Pain (splinting of chest)
   B. Chest trauma
   C. Thoracic surgery
   D. Abdominal distention
   E. Muscle weakness
   F. Obesity
   G. Bony deformities of the chest wall
   H. Positioning
      1. Weight of viscera may impede expansion
      2. Abdominal compression may impede expansion
   I. Neuromuscular blocking drugs

J. Severance of nerves
K. Nerve trauma (edema)
III. Inability to adequately expand the lungs
   A. Pneumothorax (especially tension pneumothorax)
   B. Pleural fluid
   C. Diaphragmatic hernia
   D. Lung disease
   E. Neoplasia
   F. Pneumonia
   G. Atelectasis
   H. Positioning
   I. Airway obstruction
IV. Acute cardiopulmonary arrest
V. Pulmonary edema or insufficiency

MANAGEMENT OF VENTILATION IN ANESTHESIA

I. Anesthetics are respiratory depressants; therefore ventilation may need to be assisted if hypoventilation occurs
II. Special indications for controlled ventilation in anesthesia
   A. Thoracic surgery
      1. Controlled respiration minimizes extraneous chest wall movements, which aids the surgeon
      2. With the chest open, the patient cannot adequately expand the lungs (pneumothorax)
   B. Neuromuscular blockers (see Chapter 11): clinical doses of neuromuscular blocking drugs, which produce muscular relaxation, also paralyze the diaphragm and intercostal muscles
   C. Prolonged anesthesia (more than 60 minutes), especially in the horse
   D. Trauma
      1. Flail chest
      2. Diaphragmatic hernia
   E. Maintain a more stable plane of anesthesia
   F. Drug overdose
   G. Convenience: eliminate concerns about hypoventilation and poor gas exchange (low O_2; high CO_2)

PHYSIOLOGIC CONSIDERATIONS

I. Pulmonary system
   A. Normal lungs are well ventilated during spontaneous breathing as a result of the generation of different pressures, volumes, and flow rates (Fig. 14-1)
   B. During spontaneous ventilation, the portions of the lung in closest contact with moving surfaces (i.e., the peripheral lung field) undergo the greatest volume changes
   C. Increased CO_2 can cause:
      1. Respiratory acidosis
      2. Sympathetic stimulation
      3. Cardiac arrhythmias
         a. A mix of sympathetic stimulation and hypoxemic effects
      4. Variable peripheral vasoconstriction (sympathetic effect) followed by peripheral vasodilation as a direct effect on peripheral vessels
      5. Central nervous system depressant effect and eventually, narcosis
         a. $PaCO_2$ levels above 100 mm Hg have an anesthetic effect

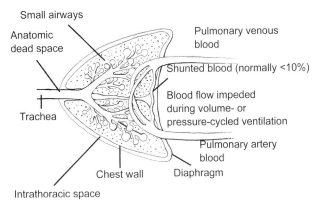

Fig. 14-1
Lung volume and airway pressure can augment or impede blood flow through the lung.

6. Increased cerebral blood flow and intracranial pressure
7. Tachypnea and an increased work of breathing, which can negatively affect a debilitated patient

D. During controlled ventilation, pressure is introduced into the trachea, which inflates the peribronchial and mediastinal areas of the lung; the peripheral segments remain relatively hypoventilated compared with normal spontaneous breathing; pressure or volume ventilation increases airway diameter and thus anatomic dead space, further reducing alveolar ventilation

E. Positive-pressure ventilation results in a significant reduction in lung compliance; the lung becomes stiffer, which can lead to atelectasis and hypoxemia

1. Small airway closure can occur
2. The distribution of ventilation is altered
3. Ventilators delivering a preset volume compensate for worsening lung mechanics to a greater degree than do those delivering a preset pressure (by ensuring delivery of a constant volume); the latter must be reset to compensate for "stiffened" lungs (periodic "sighs" are important)

II. Cardiovascular system (Table 14-1)

TABLE **14-1**
CARDIOVASCULAR SYSTEM: EFFECTS OF BREATHING AND INTERMITTENT POSITIVE-PRESSURE VENTILATION

PHASE OF CYCLE	INTRATHORACIC PRESSURE	TOTAL THORACIC BLOOD VOLUME	LEFT VENTRICLE CARDIAC OUTPUT
Normal breathing			
Inspiration active	$(-5$ cm of $H_2O)$	↑	↓
Expiration passive	↑$(-2$ cm $H_2O)$	↓	↑
IPPV			
Inspiration passive	↑ $(10\text{-}20$ cm $H_2O)$	↓	— (↓ if IPP prolonged)
Expiration generally passive	↓ To atmospheric pressure	↑	↓

IPPV, Intermittent positive-pressure ventilation; *IPP,* intermittent positive pressure.

A. During spontaneous ventilation, the subatmospheric pressure within the thorax augments venous return; this subatmospheric pressure is reduced (made more negative) during inspiration by downward movement of the diaphragm

B. During controlled ventilation, the pressure in the trachea and lung is transmitted to the thoracic cavity, thus impeding venous return and potentially decreasing cardiac output (Fig. 14-2; also see Fig. 14-1)

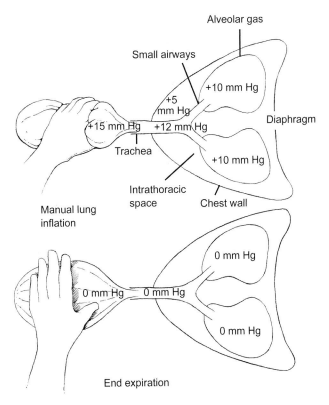

Fig. 14-2
Manual lung inflation produces a positive pressure in the lung and thoracic cavity, which impedes lung blood flow and lowers cardiac output.

C. Controlled ventilation decreases arterial blood pressure and cardiac output in any of the following instances:
  1. Average airway pressure consistently more than 10 mm Hg
  2. Low circulating blood volume caused by dehydration, anemia, and blood loss
  3. Impaired sympathetic nervous system activity caused by anesthesia, local anesthetics, and shock
D. Controlled ventilation decreases pulmonary blood flow and therefore may lead to ventilation-perfusion abnormalities
E. Circulatory changes during controlled ventilation are caused by prolonged increases in mean airway pressure and decreased CO_2

III. Important normal values to remember (Fig. 14-3)
  A. Tidal volume (V_T): the amount of gas exchanged in one respiratory cycle
    1. 10-15 ml/kg in animals weighing less than 200 kg
    2. 14-16 ml/kg in animals weighing more than 200 kg
    3. Ventilator bellows volume is usually increased by 2 to 4 ml/kg over V_T during intermittent positive-pressure breathing to compensate for the increased positive pressure-induced volume of the breathing hoses and conducting airways (wasted ventilation)

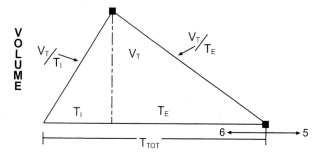

Fig. 14-3
Important components of the breathing cycle include tidal volume (V_T; ml) and inspiratory (T_I) and expiratory time (T_E). The T_E should always be longer than the T_I.

B. Minute volume (V_m): the volume of gas exchanged in 1 minute
   1. Dependent on V_T and breaths per minute (BPM): $V_T \times BPM = V_m$
C. Adequate inflation of the lungs of a normal animal requires approximately 15 to 20 cm H_2O pressure; lung compliance (volume/pressure/kg) is important in determining the pressure required to inflate the lung
D. The spontaneous ventilatory cycle
   1. Inspiration (I) is active
      a. 1 second in small animals
      b. 1.5 to 2 seconds in large animals
E. Guides to adequate mechanical controlled ventilation in the normal patient (Table 14-2, Fig. 14-4)
   1. V_T (under normal conditions)
      a. Up to 10 to 15 ml/kg in small animals
      b. Up to 14 to 16 ml/kg in large animals
   2. Pressures
      a. 10 to 20 cm H_2O in small animal species with normal lungs; 20 to 30 cm H_2O in large animal species with normal lungs

TABLE **14-2**

INITIAL SETTING FOR PULMONARY VERSUS EXTRAPULMONARY PATHOLOGY

PARAMETER	NORMAL LUNGS	ABNORMAL LUNGS
F_IO_2	100% initially	
V_T	8-15 ml/kg	
Respiratory rate	8-15 breaths/min	
Minute ventilation	150-250 ml/kg/min	
PIP	10-20 cm H_2O	12-25 cm H_2O
PEEP	0-2 cm H_2O	2-8 cm H_2O
Trigger sensitivity	−2 cm H_2O or 2 L/min	
I:E ratio	1:2	
Inspiratory time	Approximately 1 sec	

F_IO_2, Fraction of inspired O_2; *I:E ratio,* inspiratory time to expiratory time ratio; *PEEP,* positive end expiratory pressure; *PIP,* peak inspiratory pressure; V_T, tidal volume.

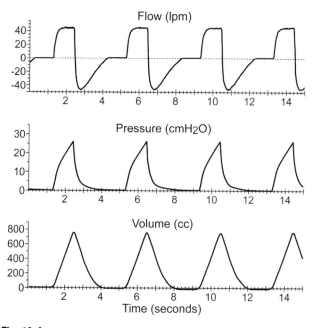

Fig. 14-4

Flow, pressure, and volume (V_T) waveforms associated with normal breathing. Note the timing and changes in flow and pressure associated with the increase or decrease in volume during a single breath.

      b. During open-chest procedures or in the presence of "stiff" or mechanically inhibited lungs, pressure must be increased

   3. I/E (inspiration/expiration) ratios; can be preset or will vary based on rate and tidal volume

      a. 1:2 to 1:3 in small animals

      b. 1:2 to 1:4.5 in large animals

   4. Inspiratory times during controlled ventilation

      a. Less than 1 second in small animals

      b. Less than 2 to 3 seconds in large animals (e.g., 2 seconds in a 450-kg horse)

      c. Observation of chest wall movements can be a useful indicator of lung inflation

CLASSIFICATION OF VENTILATORS

I. Volume preset (Fig. 14-5)

A. A gas or gas mixture is delivered to a preset volume by the ventilatory-assist device

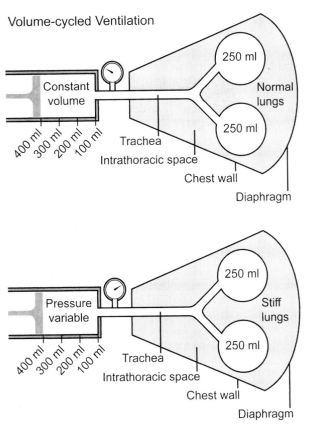

Fig. 14-5

Volume preset ventilation delivers a constant volume of gas. The pressure is variable. If the lung becomes stiffer, the pressure required to deliver a constant volume increases.

B. Advantages
  1. Delivers a known V_T regardless of the pressure imposed
    a. Most volume-cycled ventilators are equipped with a blow-off safety valve to prevent the development of extremely high pressure (more than 60 cm H_2O)
    b. Delivers a constant volume despite changes in compliance and resistance of the lungs during anesthesia
  2. Relatively simple machine
C. Disadvantages
  1. High airway pressures may develop
  2. Volume ventilators do not compensate for small leaks in the system; eliminating them requires an airtight system; a major leak prevents the patient from receiving an adequate V_T
D. Piston or bellows-type ventilator delivers a predetermined volume
E. Some are equipped with the ability to select a maximum pressure

II. Pressure preset (Fig. 14-6)
A. A gas or gas mixture is delivered by a ventilatory-assist device during the inspiratory phase until the system reaches a preset pressure
B. Advantages
  1. High safety factor; high pressure will not develop unless preset by the operator
  2. Compensates for small leaks; large leaks prolong inspiratory time
C. Disadvantages
  1. Volume delivered is variable and depends on the following:
    a. Lung compliance
    b. Airway resistance
    c. Number of functional alveoli
    d. Pressure within the thorax
  2. Measurement of tidal volume may be difficult if the ventilator is not equipped with bellows or a respirometer
  3. Pressure may need to be increased during a procedure to maintain adequate V_T

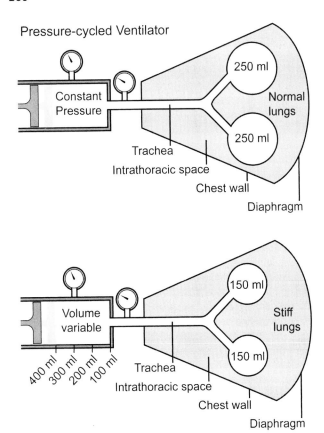

Fig. 14-6
Pressure-preset ventilators deliver a predetermined pressure regardless of the volume delivered.

III. Time cycled: most volume-preset ventilators can be adjusted to limit the volume delivered through a combination of adjustments to the I:E ratio, frequency or respiratory rate (f), and inspiratory flow rate (most modern anesthesia ventilators are this type)

IV. Anesthesia ventilators classified by bellows movement during expiration

A. Standing: preferred design because leaks are easily identified; bellows rise during expiratory phase
B. Hanging: bellows fall during expiratory phase

MODES OF OPERATION OF VENTILATORY-ASSIST DEVICES

I. Assist mode: patient triggers the ventilatory device by initiating an inspiratory effort
II. Controlled mode
   A. Operator sets the desired respiratory rate
   B. Ventilator is insensitive to the patient's inspiratory efforts
   C. If the patient resists controlled ventilation ("bucks" the ventilator), severe cardiopulmonary compromise may occur
III. Assist-controlled mode: a minimal respiratory rate is set by the operator, which the patient may override by initiating spontaneous ventilatory efforts at a faster rate
IV. Intermittent mandatory ventilation: used in intensive care unit ventilation; a predetermined number of positive breaths is set by the operator; the patient also breathes spontaneously through a parallel breathing circuit

TERMS USED FOR VARIABLE MODES OF OPERATION DURING MECHANICAL VENTILATION

I. **IPPV** (intermittent positive-pressure ventilation): positive pressure maintained only during inspiration
II. **CPPV** (continuous positive pressure ventilation): mechanical ventilation with positive pressure maintained during inspiration and at lower pressure on expiration
III. **PNPV** (positive/negative pressure ventilation): positive pressure during inspiration and negative pressure during expiration
IV. **PEEP** (positive end-expiratory pressure): used to open small airways after lung trauma or pulmonary edema
V. **ZEEP** (zero end-expiratory pressure): normal passive expiration
VI. **NEEP** (negative end-expiratory pressure): used to hasten expiration

   VII. CPAP (continuous positive airway pressure): spontaneous breathing with positive pressure during both inspiratory and expiratory cycles

VIII. IMV (intermittent mandatory ventilation): breaths supplied by ventilator, in addition to normal negative pressure breaths supplied by the patient

VENTILATORS COMMONLY USED IN VETERINARY MEDICINE

Most ventilators used during general anesthesia connect to the anesthesia breathing system where the rebreathing bag attaches; other free-standing ventilators are used without a breathing circuit

   I. Mallard medical microprocessor-controlled large animal anesthesia ventilator (Fig. 14-7)

      A. Classification: standing bellows; time cycled, microprocessor controlled

      B. Controls

         1. Inspiratory flow rate is adjustable

         2. Respiratory rate

         3. Inspiratory time

      C. Volume, I:E ratio, and pressure delivered are a function of adjustments in inspiratory flow rate, frequency, and inspiratory time

      D. Ventilator bellows connect to rebreathing bag port of large animal circle system

      E. PEEP capability

   II. Hallowell EMC 2000-time-cycle Small Animal Ventilator (also sold by Matrix, Inc. as model 3000)

      A. Standing bellows

      B. V_T adjustable from 0 to 3000 ml

      C. Volume and pressure delivered are a function of adjustments in frequency and inspiratory time

      D. Interchangeable bellows for animals weighing 1 kg to 200 kg

   III. Surgi-Vet SAV 2500-Small Animal Anesthesia Ventilator

      A. Standing bellows

      B. Time cycled with adjustments for inspiratory flow rate and inspiratory time

      C. V_T adjustable from 0 to 3000 ml

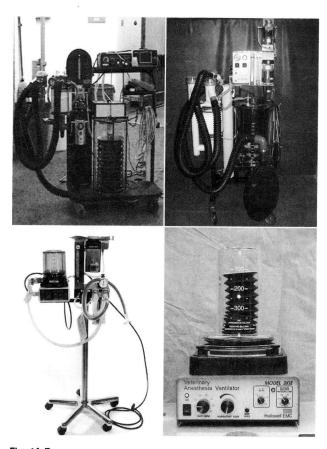

Fig. 14-7
Ventilators are used to provide intermittent positive-pressure ventilation in large (top) and small (bottom) animals. Both pressure (15 to 20 cm H_2O) and volume (12 to 15 ml/kg) should be monitored.

    IV. Surgi-Vet Large Animal Ventilator
        A. Classification: volume preset; hanging bellows; time cycled
        B. Volume delivered depends on frequency, inspiratory flow rate, and inspiratory time

V. Engler ADS 1000
   A. Microprocessor controlled
   B. Can be used with a vaporizer for anesthesia or without a vaporizer
   C. Non-rebreathing circuit principle of operation
      1. No CO_2 absorbent necessary
      2. No conventional anesthesia breathing circuit necessary
   D. Machine automatically selects ventilation parameters based on patient weight
   E. PEEP capability
VI. North American Dräger Large and Small Animal Anesthetic Ventilator
   A. Classification: volume-preset ventilator; time cycled; hanging or standing bellows
      1. Volume is adjusted by raising and lowering bellows support to appropriate level
      2. Pressure manometer indicates the pressure within the system
   B. Controls
      1. On/off switch
      2. Frequency is adjusted to breaths per minute
      3. Flow is adjustable; inspiratory flow rate determines inspiratory time
      4. I:E ratio is adjustable from 1:1 to 1:4.5
      5. Adjustment of flow rate, I:E ratio, and inspiratory time determine delivered volume
      6. Operates only in the control mode
   C. Pressure relief valve
      1. Manual pressure relief valve of breathing system must be closed during ventilator use
      2. Automatic pressure relief closes with the inspiratory cycle
VII. Bag-in-a-barrel type ventilator, generally powered by a Bird pressure-cycled ventilator (J. D. Medical anesthetic machine)
   A. Classification: pressure-preset ventilator; hanging bellows
   B. Large animal ventilator
      1. Bag or bellows in a cylinder is compressed by the flow generated by a modified Bird Mark 7 ventilator

2. Volume is indicated on the chamber encasing the bellows
3. The pressure and f can be adjusted for the desired volume

C. Mode
1. Assisted: the sensitivity can be adjusted so that the patient can trigger the machine
2. Controlled: the value of sensitivity can be decreased so that the patient cannot trigger the machine
3. Assist-controlled: the operator can control the minimum number of breaths delivered; the patient can also trigger ventilator operation

D. Controls
1. Inspiratory pressure
   a. Usually set at 20 to 30 cm H_2O
   b. Adjusted for the desired tidal volume
2. Expiratory time
   a. Controls respiratory rate by controlling time between breaths
   b. Rate usually set at 6 to 10 breaths/min for horses
3. Flow rate (adjust to an inspiratory time of 1.3 to 2 seconds for horses)
4. Air mix: pull air mix knob to "out" position
   a. Set at 50% to conserve oxygen
   b. Does not affect oxygen supply to the animal
5. Sensitivity
   a. Governs the animal's ability to trigger the ventilator
   b. Numbers are merely a rough guide to indicator of position

VIII. Bird Mark 7 and Bird Mark 9 ventilators
A. Classification: pressure preset ventilator; volume delivered is controlled by the pressure developed unless the machine is equipped with a bellows
B. Must be equipped with a bag-in-a-barrel or a bellows to be used as an anesthetic system; otherwise, it can stand alone as an intensive care ventilator
C. Controls
1. Inspiratory pressure
   a. Controls peak pressure

b. Normally set at 15 to 30 cm H_2O
2. Sensitivity
   a. Controls animal's ability to trigger the machine
   b. Low numbers; easily triggered
   c. High numbers; difficult to trigger
3. Inspiratory flow rate
   a. Controls inspiratory time
   b. Set equal to or less than expiratory time
4. Expiratory time
   a. Controls respiratory rate by controlling expiratory time
   b. Respiratory rate is normally 6 to 12 breaths/min
5. Air mix
   a. Varies percentage of inspired oxygen from 50% (knob out) to 100% (knob in)
   b. Negative pressure: (Bird Mark 9 only) allows the operator to produce NEEP

HIGH-FREQUENCY VENTILATION

I. High-frequency ventilation is a form of mechanical ventilation in which f is greater than 1 Hz (hertz), and V_T is less than anatomic dead space
II. High-frequency ventilation is used to minimize breathing effects and chest wall movement while maintaining adequate oxygenation
III. Potential uses include acute respiratory distress syndrome, hyaline membrane disease, bronchopleural fistula, and pulmonary contusion

WEANING THE PATIENT OFF THE VENTILATOR

The initiation of spontaneous respirations after controlled ventilation can be hastened by the following methods:
I. Decreasing the rate of controlled respiratory frequency
II. Decreasing anesthetic depth
III. Reversing neuromuscular blockade
IV. Antagonism of opioid-induced respiratory depression

  V. Patients undergoing long-term ventilation require a more sophisticated approach to weaning from a ventilator (e.g., use of intermittent mandatory ventilation)

  VI. Physical manipulation: rolling the patient, twisting an ear, pinching a toe

 VII. Respiratory stimulants: doxapram administration, 0.2 to 0.5 mg/kg intravenously

HAZARD PREVENTION (SEE BOX)

  I. Always be prepared to convert the anesthesia system back to the nonventilator mode in case of unforeseen ventilator problems; keep the rebreathing bag near the ventilator

 II. Verify proper ventilator function before use; follow manufacturer's recommendations

    A. Verify that all controls are operational

    B. Perform a leak test

       1. Standing bellows: fill bellows using O_2 flush valve on anesthesia machine; occlude ventilator delivery hose; bellows will remain in fully ascended position if no leaks are present

       2. Hanging bellows: fully contract bellows; occlude ventilator delivery hose; bellows will remain fully contracted if no leaks are present

---

COMPLICATIONS ASSOCIATED WITH MECHANICAL VENTILATION

Pulmonary

Ventilator-induced lung injury
Ventilator-associated pneumonia
Pneumothorax
Patient-ventilator asynchrony
Endotracheal tube occlusion and accidental disconnection
Oxygen toxicosis
Tracheal necrosis

RESPIRATORY ASSIST DEVICES

I. Manual resuscitators
   A. Several models available
   B. Self-inflating bags (e.g., Ambu) and one non-rebreathing valve
   C. Useful for rapid emergency ventilation
II. Demand valves
   A. An apparatus that can be inserted into the proximal end of an endotracheal tube and is capable of delivering oxygen on demand from a patient-initiated breath or from operator assistance
   B. Inspiration is passive or assisted
   C. Expiration is passive
   D. Adapters are available for large and small animal use

CHAPTER FIFTEEN

Patient Monitoring During Anesthesia

"You see only what you look for, you recognize only what you know."

MERRIL C. SOSMAN

"Diligence is the mother of good fortune."

MIGUEL DE CERVANTES

OVERVIEW

A variety of simple and complex monitoring equipment is available for determining patient status during anesthesia. The electrocardiogram (ECG), the electroencephalogram, and the electromyogram can be displayed and recorded. Blood pressure (arterial or central venous pressure [CVP]), heart sounds and/or peripheral blood flow, arterial and venous pH, oxygen and carbon dioxide tensions, and arterial or capillary blood oxygen saturation (pulse oximetry) can be determined. End-expired samples of respiratory gases can be analyzed for oxygen/carbon dioxide and inhalation anesthetic concentration. "Point of care" devices are available that permit patient side evaluation of the hemogram, acid-base values, blood chemistries, and serum enzyme values within minutes of collecting a peripheral blood sample. All the monitoring equipment in the world, however, cannot replace an educated, attentive anesthetist.

GENERAL CONSIDERATIONS

I. A patient's physiology and ability to compensate for cardiorespiratory changes are altered by anesthetic drugs and by the pathophysiologic processes of disease

269

II. Intraoperative patient monitoring optimizes safety during anesthesia:
   A. Frequent monitoring facilitates informed and timely responses to changes in patient status by tracking physiologic variables
   B. The completion of an anesthetic record provides a database for comparison withsubsequent anesthetic procedures
III. Prerequisites for intraoperative monitoring
   A. Applied understanding of normal physiology and pathophysiology
   B. Thorough, accurate knowledge of the patient's physiologic status
   C. Knowledge of pharmacokinetics, pharmacodynamics, and toxicity of anesthetic drugs and adjuncts
   D. Availability of a convenient system for recording observations (anesthetic record)
   E. A thorough knowledge of the monitoring devices, their operation and limitations, and the inherent assumptions associated with their use

BASIC PRINCIPLES

I. Monitor body functions (see Chapter 2 for normal values)
   A. Formulate a monitoring plan based on the following:
      1. Patient's health status and disease(s)
      2. Specific procedure and duration
      3. Available monitoring equipment
      4. Anticipated duration of anesthesia
   B. Intraoperative decisions are based on comparisons with normal values (i.e., Are observed responses qualitatively and/or quantitatively appropriate? Are measured variables within normal limits?)
II. Monitor more than one body system and more than one variable per body system, if possible
   A. Evaluating several values (e.g., heart rate, respiratory rate) rather than fragments of information increases the likelihood of correct assessment
   B. Determining trends in the individual variables facilitates an early response

III. Use monitoring techniques that are specific, accurate, and complementary
  A. Use simple, reliable techniques (e.g., visual inspection, palpation, auscultation)
  B. Check instrument calibrations frequently; instruments may provide specific data. Inaccurate information may be confusing, misleading, and dangerous
  C. Never totally depend on one piece of monitored information

NONINVASIVE (INDIRECT) MONITORING TECHNIQUES

I. Information is gathered by observing readily apparent variables (e.g., counting respiratory rate) and/or noninvasive diagnostic testing (e.g., ECG, pulse oximeter, arterial blood pressure [ABP])
  A. Advantages
    1. Techniques are simple, reliable, and informative
    2. Patient is not placed at risk for complications caused by the monitoring technique
  B. Disadvantages
    1. Not all useful physiologic variables (e.g., pH and blood gases) can be accurately monitored noninvasively
    2. Inaccurate information (highly variable) is sometimes gathered when a noninvasive technique (e.g., noninvasive ABP) is substituted for a more invasive procedure (e.g., arterial catheterization) to determine the same information

INVASIVE (DIRECT) MONITORING TECHNIQUE

I. Information is gathered by placing instruments inside the body (e.g., intravascular pressure catheters)
  A. Advantages
    1. Physiologic database is increased
    2. Many techniques are accurate, reliable, and simple to perform
    3. A direct measurement of a physiologic variable is often provided with fewer assumptions

B. Disadvantages
   1. Patient is at risk for secondary complications depending on technique; these complications include the following:
      a. Hemorrhage, infection
      b. Direct tissue damage
      c. Inflammation with subsequent tissue damage
      d. Acute perturbation of tissue function (e.g., cardiac dysrhythmias)
   2. Some monitors require advanced technical knowledge and skills

PHYSIOLOGIC CONSIDERATIONS

I. Homeostasis
   A. Monitoring compensatory responses to anesthesia and surgical stimulation (Tables 15-1 and 15-2)
      1. Responses observed
         a. Individual organ systems
         b. Integrated responses
      2. Invasive monitoring techniques may evoke additional responses
II. Monitoring key organ systems
   A. Central nervous system
      1. Observe reflex activity to monitor degree of central nervous system depression
         a. Eye reflexes
            (1) Palpebral
            (2) Corneal
            (3) Nystagmus
            (4) Lacrimation
         b. Jaw tone
         c. Anal reflex
         d. Pedal reflex
      2. Monitor skeletal muscle tone and degree of relaxation
      3. Electroencephalography
         a. Records and averages brain activity
         b. Correlates to depth of anesthesia
            (1) The bispectral index can be used to monitor depth of anesthesia

TABLE 15-1
AMERICAN COLLEGE OF VETERINARY
ANESTHESIOLOGISTS SUGGESTIONS FOR MONITORING

Circulation

Objective: to ensure that blood flow to tissues is adequate

Methods:
1. Palpation of peripheral pulse
2. Palpation of heartbeat through chest wall
3. Auscultation of heartbeat (stethoscope, esophageal stethoscope, or other audible heart monitor)
4. Electrocardiogram (continuous display)
5. Noninvasive blood flow or blood pressure monitor (e.g., Doppler ultrasonic flow detector, oscillometric flow detector)
6. Invasive blood pressure monitor (arterial catheter connected to transducer/oscilloscope or to aneroid manometer)

Oxygenation

Objective: to ensure adequate oxygen concentration in the patient's arterial blood

Methods:
1. Observation of mucous membrane color
2. Pulse oximetry (noninvasive estimation of hemoglobin saturation)
3. Oxygen analyzer in the inspiratory limb of the breathing circuit
4. Blood gas analysis (PaO_2)
5. Hemoximetry (direct measurement of hemoglobin saturation in the blood)

Ventilation

Objective: to ensure that the patient's ventilation is adequately maintained

Methods:
1. Observation of chest wall movement
2. Observation of breathing bag movement
3. Auscultation of breath sounds
4. Audible respiratory monitor
5. Respirometry (measurement of tidal volume ± minute volume)
6. Capnography (measurement of CO_2 in end-expired gas)
7. Blood gas monitoring ($PaCO_2$)

Continued

TABLE 15-1
AMERICAN COLLEGE OF VETERINARY ANESTHESIOLOGISTS SUGGESTIONS FOR MONITORING—cont'd

Anesthetic record

Objective: to maintain a legal record of significant events and to enhance recognition of trends in monitored parameters

Methods:
1. Record all drugs administered to each patient, noting the dose, time, and route of administration
2. Record monitored parameters (minimum: heart rate, respiratory rate) on a regular basis (minimum: every 5 min) during anesthesia

Personnel

Objective: to ensure that a responsible individual is aware of the patient's status at all times during anesthesia and recovery and is prepared either to intervene when indicated or to alert the veterinarian in charge about changes in the patient's condition

Methods:
1. If a veterinarian, technician, or other responsible person is unable to remain with the patient continuously, a responsible person should check the patient's status on a regular basis (at least every 5 min) during anesthesia and recovery
2. A responsible person may be present in the same room, although not necessarily solely occupied with the anesthetized patient (for instance, the surgeon may also be responsible for overseeing anesthesia)
3. In either of the above situations, audible heart and respiratory monitors are suggested
4. A responsible person, solely dedicated to managing and caring for the anesthetized patient during anesthesia, remains with the patient continuously until the end of the anesthetic period

TABLE 15-2
COMMONLY MONITORED PARAMETERS AND POTENTIAL CAUSES OF ABNORMAL RESPONSES

Respiratory rate and pattern

Tachypnea	Too "light," pain, hypoxemia, hypercarbia, hyperthermia, true or paradoxical CSF acidosis, drug effects (e.g., doxapram)
Apnea	Too "deep," hypothermia, recent hyperventilation (especially while breathing O_2-enriched gases), musculoskeletal paralysis (pathologic or pharmacologic), drug effects (e.g., ketamine, thiobarbiturates, propofol)

Heart rate

Tachycardia	Too "light," pain, hypotension, hypoxemia, hypercarbia, ischemia, acute anaphylactoid reactions, anemia, drug effects (e.g., thiobarbiturates, ketamine, catecholamines), fever, hypokalemia
Bradycardia	Too "deep," hypertension, elevated intracranial pressure, surgically induced vagal reflexes (e.g., visceral stretch responses), hypothermia, hyperkalemia, myocardial ischemia/anoxia, drug effects (e.g., xylazine, narcotics)

Arterial blood pressure

Hypertension	Too "light," pain, hypercarbia, fever, drug effects (e.g., catecholamines, ketamine)
Hypotension	Too "deep," relative or absolute hypovolemia, sepsis, shock, drug effects (e.g., thiobarbiturate boluses, inhalation anesthetics)

Corneal reflexes*

Hyperactive	Too "light," pain, hypotension, hypoxemia, hypercarbia, drug effects (e.g., ketamine)
Hypoactive	Too "deep," CNS depression (e.g., excessively deep anesthesia, acidosis, hypotension)

*Pertains to horses and ruminants only; not useful in pigs, dogs, and cats.
CSF, Cerebral spinal fluid; *CNS,* central nervous system.

> 4. End-tidal concentration of anesthetic gases can be monitored and correlated to anesthetic depth (Fig. 15-1)
>
> B. Respiratory system (Tables 15-1 and 15-2; Figs. 15-2 through 15-8)

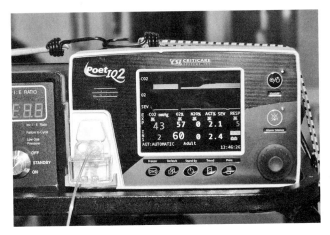

Fig. 15-1
The end-tidal concentration of CO_2 and anesthetic circuit concentrations of O_2 and inhaled anesthetic can be monitored.

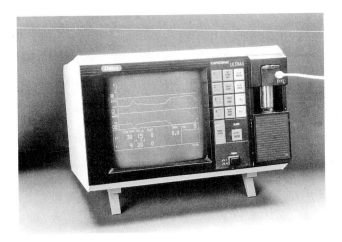

Fig. 15-2
Monitor that measures end-tidal concentration of inhalant anesthetics (halothane, isoflurane, sevoflurane) to ensure that proper anesthetic concentrations are being delivered to the patient.

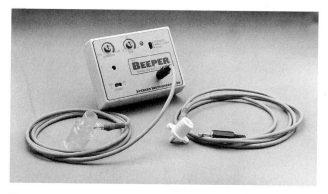

Fig. 15-3
This monitor issues a "beep" when the patient breathes.

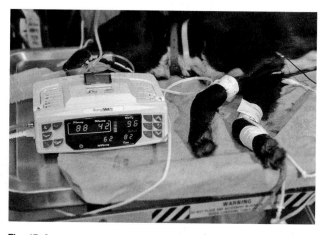

Fig. 15-4
Pulse oximeters are used to monitor the saturation of hemoglobin with oxygen. Because pulse oximeters detect a peripheral pulse, they also detect heart rate. The total amount of oxygen delivered to tissues is still dependent on the amount of hemoglobin or packed cell volume. Many pulse oximeters are part of multiparameter modules.

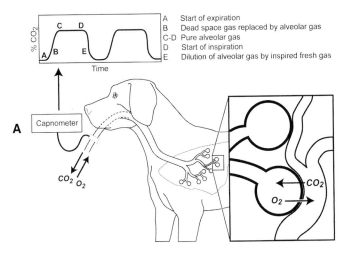

A Start of expiration
B Dead space gas replaced by alveolar gas
C-D Pure alveolar gas
D Start of inspiration
E Dilution of alveolar gas by inspired fresh gas

Fig. 15-5
End-tidal CO_2 monitoring: the amount of carbon dioxide in the expired gas increases during exhalation (**A**) and can be used to assess the adequacy of breathing (goes up during hypoventilation). The increases and decreases in the end-tidal concentration of CO_2 during expiration and inhalation, respectively, produce a characteristic capnogram *(upper inset)*. Portable handheld capnometers are available (**B**).

1. Noninvasive measurements
   a. Respiratory frequency
   b. Respiratory pattern
      (1) Irregular patterns suggest respiratory depression
   c. Changes in tidal volume, noted by observing thorax and rebreathing bag
2. Noninvasive equipment
   a. Esophageal or precordial stethoscope
   b. Breathing frequency monitors (Fig. 15-3)
      (1) Activated by changes in airway temperature or gas flow
      (2) Some emit an audible tone and digitally display respiratory rate
      (3) Some units contain alarms

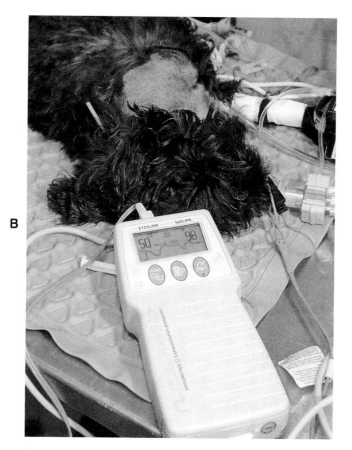

B

Fig. 15-5—cont'd

c. Pulse oximetry (Fig. 15-4)
   (1) Measures percent saturation of oxygen in arterial blood (SpO_2)
   (2) A spectrophotoelectric device applied directly to nonhaired skin over a pulsating vascular bed; light absorbance of oxygenated versus reduced hemoglobin detected and percentage of saturated hemoglobin is displayed numerically

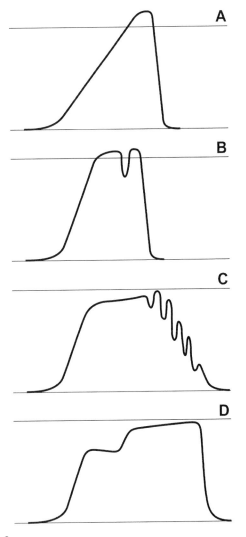

Fig. 15-6
Analysis of the capnogram can be used to identify kinked endotracheal tubes (**A**), high CO_2 and diaphragmatic twitches (**B**), cardiac oscillations (**C**), and uneven emptying of the lungs (**D**).

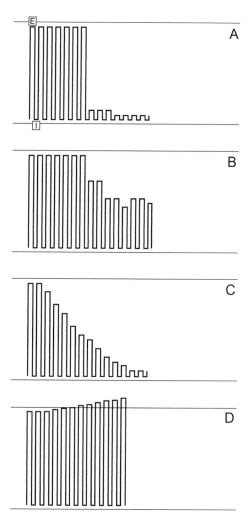

Fig. 15-7

A sudden drop in end-tidal concentration of CO_2 to zero suggests that the endotracheal tube has become dislodged (esophageal intubation), kinked, or that the CO_2 sensing circuit has been disconnected (**A**); a gradual drop in end-tidal concentration of CO_2 to a lower value could indicate a CO_2 sampling problem or hyperventilation (**B**); an exponential decrease in CO_2 is indicative of circulatory arrest, pulmonary embolism, or severe hyperventilation (**C**); a gradual increase in CO_2 is generally indicative of hypoventilation (**D**). *E,* Expiration; *I,* inspiration.

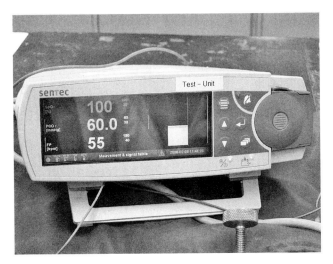

Fig. 15-8
Some capnometers monitor the end-tidal concentration of CO_2, SpO_2, and transcutaneous CO_2. Transcutaneous CO_2 increases (tissue pH decreases) when tissue blood flow is reduced.

    (a) Inaccurate in the presence of carboxyhemoglobin or methemoglobin

    (b) The pulsatile signal is reduced by hypotension, hypothermia, and altered vascular resistance, which limits SpO_2 determination

  (3) Sites for attachment of probes

    (a) Tongue

    (b) Symphysis of mandible

    (c) Gastrocnemius tendon

    (d) Digit

    (e) Esophagus

    (f) Rectum

    (g) Superficial artery

    (h) Prepuce

    (i) Vulva

    (j) Scrotum

    (k) Pinna

  d. Analysis of inspired oxygen concentration

  e. Analysis of inspired or expired carbon dioxide concentration (capnography) or transcutaneous carbon dioxide concentration (Figs. 15-6 through 15-8)

   (1) End-tidal carbon dioxide measurements estimate arteriolar concentrations of CO_2 ($PaCO_2$)

   (2) Useful when controlled ventilation is used

   (3) True alveolar concentrations are underestimated by 5 to 10 mm Hg

   (4) Measurements become more inaccurate during hypoventilation or abnormal breathing patterns

  f. Spirometry (Fig. 15-9, *B*)

 3. Invasive measurements

  a. Hematocrit (packed cell volume percentage) and/or hemoglobin concentration

  b. Arterial and/or venous blood gas, pH and lactate analysis (Fig. 15-10) (also see Chapter 16)

  c. Oximetry (arterial oxygen saturation; SaO_2)

C. Cardiovascular system (Tables 15-1 and 15-2)

 1. Heart rate

  a. Range of normal heart rates, by species (beats per minute) (see Chapter 2)

   (1) Dog: 70 to 100

   (2) Cat: 100 to 200

   (3) Horse: 30 to 45; up to 80 in foals

   (4) Cow: 60 to 80

   (5) Sheep: goat: 60 to 90

   (6) Pig: 60 to 90

   (7) Llama: 50 to 100

  b. Limits of heart rate during anesthesia in beats per minute (values outside these limits indicate that cardiovascular function may be impaired)

   (1) Dog: <50, >160

   (2) Cat: <100, >200

   (3) Horse: <28, >50

   (4) Cow: <48, >90

   (5) Sheep, goat: <60, >150

   (6) Pig: <50, >150

   (7) Llama: <50, >150

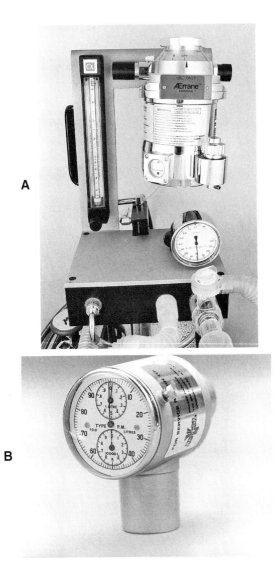

Fig. 15-9
Respiratory monitors used in anesthesia practice. **A,** P-N pressure gauge used to monitor inspiratory pressure during ventilation. **B,** Ventilometer used to measure tidal volume and minute volume.

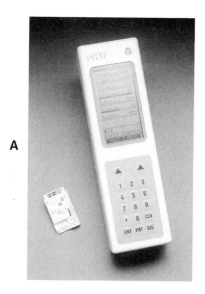

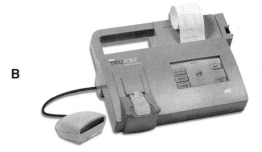

Fig. 15-10
Point of care blood chemical analyzers. **A,** i-STAT (Heska/Sensor Devices, Inc.). **B,** IRMA TRUpoint (Photo courtesy ITC, Edison, NJ).

c. Techniques for monitoring heart rate
(1) Palpation of arteries or the heart
(a) Dog: femoral, dorsal pedal, digital, and lingual arteries; precordium
(b) Cat: femoral artery, precordium
(c) Cow, sheep, and goat: auricular, digital, coccygeal, and dorsal metatarsal arteries
(d) Horse: facial, transverse facial, dorsal metatarsal, and palatine arteries
(e) Pig: femoral and auricular arteries
(f) Llama: auricular and femoral arteries
(2) Indirect method uses esophageal stethoscope (Fig. 15-11)
(a) Coupled to earpieces or to an electronic amplifier
(b) Advantages: inexpensive; can detect abnormalities in rhythm and rate; can monitor breath sounds

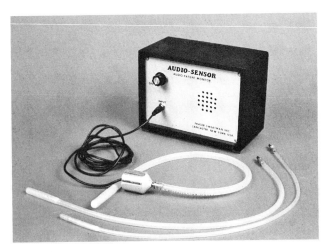

Fig. 15-11
Esophageal catheters are attached to a stethoscope or audio monitor to hear heart sounds and determine heart rate.

(c) Disadvantages: difficult when sounds are muffled or when surgery involves the mouth or throat

d. Peripheral pulse amplifiers
   (1) Applied over peripheral arteries; audible beep heard with each pulse
   (2) Advantages: can determine heart rate and rhythm
   (3) Disadvantages: prone to electrical interference; difficult to keep in place

e. Ultrasonic Doppler device
   (1) Doppler crystal applied over peripheral artery (e.g., palmar artery); sound of blood flow amplified
   (2) Advantages: detects abnormalities in rhythm and rate; can also be used to estimate systolic blood pressure (BP); reliable once signal is acquired
   (3) Disadvantages: accurate for systolic BP only if appropriate cuff size is used, rate is not displayed

f. ECG, handheld monitors are available; an example is Biolog (Fig. 15-12)
   (1) Direct visualization of ECG, or sound amplifier that beeps with each R wave
   (2) Advantages: direct visualization of ECG allows interpretation of heart rate and rhythm
   (3) Disadvantages: ECG activity can continue to look normal in the absence of a perfusing blood pressure (pulseless electrical activity)

g. Pulse oximeters
   (1) Most units indicate heart rate digitally
   (2) Signal is frequently lost after 20 to 30 minutes; probe needs to be repositioned

h. Reasons for abnormal heart rates (Table 15-2)
   (1) Bradycardia
      (a) Drugs: opioids, α_2-agonists (e.g., xylazine, medetomidine, detomidine, romifidine), anticholinesterases (e.g., neostigmine)
      (b) Excessive anesthetic depth

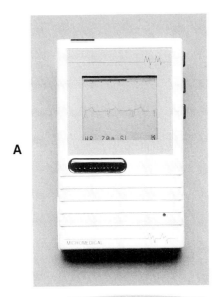

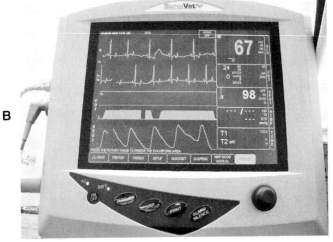

Fig. 15-12
Small handheld monitors can be used to record, store, and transmit the electrocardiogram (**A**). Larger multiparameter monitors facilitate monitoring of the ECG, SpO_2, end-tidal concentration of CO_2, and direct or indirect arterial blood pressure (**B**).

(c) Hyperkalemia

(d) Preexisting heart disease (second- or third-degree heart block)

(e) Vagal reflex (intubation, oculocardiac reflex)

(f) Terminal stages of hypoxemia

(g) Hypothermia

(2) Tachycardia

(a) Drugs: ketamine, thiobarbiturates, anticholinergics, sympathomimetics, pancuronium

(b) Hypokalemia

(c) Hyperthermia

(d) Inadequate anesthetic depth

(e) Hypercarbia and hypoxemia

(f) Anemia, hypovolemia

(g) Hyperthyroidism, pheochromocytoma

(h) Anaphylaxis

2. Peripheral perfusion

  a. A function of ABP and local vasomotor tone

  b. Assessment

    (1) Capillary refill time

      (a) Normal: less than 1 to 2 seconds

      (b) Assess on oral or vulvar mucous membranes

    (2) Peripheral pulse strength

      (a) Pulse pressure (systolic–diastolic)

      (b) May be weak or rapid and weak during hypotension or vasodilation

    (3) Urine production

      (a) Palpation of bladder

      (b) Urinary catheterization

      (c) Dog and cat: 1 to 2 ml/kg/hr

3. CVP is obtained by measuring the mean right atrial pressure; awareness of the CVP and monitoring its changes can be important in some clinical situations (Fig. 15-13)

  a. Physiologic significance

    (1) Right atrial pressure is a balance between the following:

      (a) Cardiac output: the forward flow of blood

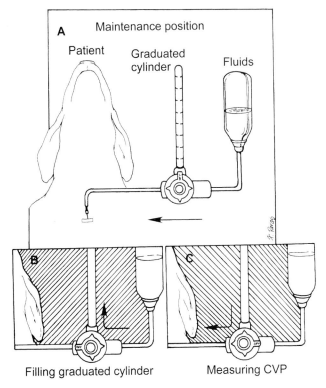

Fig. 15-13
A, CVP monitoring. **B,** A graduated cylinder at or below the level of the heart is filled with saline solution. **C,** The cylinder is then opened to the patient.

    (b) Venous return: tendency for blood to flow from the peripheral veins back into the right atrium
  b. Range of normal values
   (1) 0 to 4 cm H_2O: standing, awake animals
   (2) 2 to 7 cm H_2O: anesthetized small animals
   (3) 15 to 25 cm H_2O: anesthetized large animals

c. Indications
   (1) Monitoring fluid therapy

NOTE

CVP is not always an accurate indicator of fluid overload.

---

   (2) Assessing cardiac output
       (a) Shock (CVP$\downarrow$)
       (b) Heart failure (CVP$\uparrow$)
       (c) Anesthesia (CVP$\uparrow$)
d. Primary factors affecting CVP
   (1) Blood volume
       (a) Increase in circulating blood volume may cause an increase in CVP. Overzealous intravenous (IV) fluid administration can cause a transient increase in CVP
       (b) Decrease in effective circulating blood volume may cause a decrease in CVP, as in acute hemorrhage
   (2) Vascular tone
       (a) Venous dilation (e.g., acepromazine) may cause CVP to decrease because of peripheral pooling of blood and decreased venous return
       (b) α_2-Agonists produce venous constriction and an increase in CVP
   (3) Cardiac contractility
       (a) Decreased by most anesthetic agents
       (b) Decreases may cause CVP to increase because of the decreased contractile force of the heart
   (4) Heart rate
       (a) May decrease CVP with onset of tachycardia or increase CVP with onset of bradycardia
   (5) External cardiac factors
       (a) Intrathoracic pressure: elevations in intrathoracic pressure (positive-pressure ventilation) increase CVP; decreases in intrathoracic pressure decrease CVP

    (b) Intrapericardial pressure increases CVP
- Cardiac tamponade
- Congenital pericardial herniation
- Ventricular filling is decreased or eliminated

    (c) Body position: primarily a factor in large animal species because of hydrostatic pressure (CVP may increase 10 to 15 cm H_2O when a horse is taken from standing to lateral recumbency)

e. Clinical approach to low CVP
- (1) Increase blood volume
- (2) Patients with relative or absolute hypovolemia should receive appropriate IV fluids (crystalloids, blood, colloids) until the CVP approaches the upper limit of normal range

f. Clinical approach to elevated CVP
- (1) Generally indicates hypervolemia or myocardial depression/heart failure
  - (a) Decrease or stop IV fluid administration rate
  - (b) Administer drugs to improve cardiac function (dobutamine)

g. Hazards of CVP measurement
- (1) Air embolism
- (2) Thrombophlebitis
- (3) Hemorrhage

h. Equipment
- (1) IV catheter of sufficient length to reach the great veins in the chest (preferably the right atrium)
- (2) CVP manometer (Fig. 15-13)
  - (a) Homemade
    - Three-way stopcock
    - Graduated cylinder or pipette
    - Connecting tubes
  - (b) Commercially available
    - Baxter
    - Abbott
  - (c) Appropriate fluids and a fluid administration set
    - i. Procedure (Fig. 15-13)

(1) Thread a fluid-filled IV catheter into the jugular vein (toward the heart)
(2) Flush the catheter with saline solution
(3) Attach fluid-connecting tubes to the IV catheter
(4) Attach a three-way stopcock and graduated cylinder
(5) Attach the fluid administration line to the other port of the three-way stopcock
(6) Suspend the graduated cylinder or pipette so that the three-way stopcock is below the animal's heart base; draw an imaginary line parallel to the floor between the animal's heart base and the cylinder; this marks the point of zero pressure on the cylinder
    (a) The heart base is marked by the sternum when the animal is in lateral recumbency
    (b) The heart base is marked by the point of the shoulder when the animal is standing or in dorsal recumbency
(7) Let the fluid run through the system at the calculated flow (5 to 10 ml/kg/hr) until ready to record CVP

4. ABP
  a. Noninvasive

NOTE

Occluding cuffs should be one half the circumference of the extremity around which they are placed.

---

(1) Oscillometric method (Fig. 15-14)
    (a) An air-filled occlusion cuff is placed around a peripheral limb (small animal, foal) or at the base of the tail (small animal, large animal); air is gradually released from the cuff until arterial pulsations (oscillations) are detected and electronically displayed
    (b) Advantages: easy to use; determines heart rate and systolic, mean, and diastolic BP

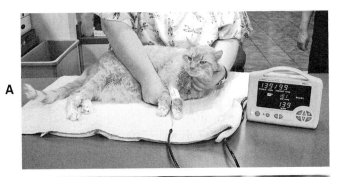

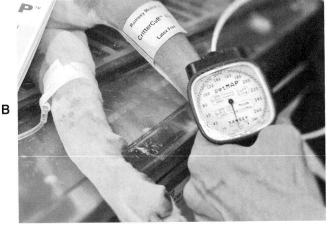

Fig. 15-14
Smaller, more portable multiparameter monitors can also be used to monitor SpO_2, end-tidal concentration of CO_2, and indirect arterial blood pressure (**A**). Handheld electronic sphygmomanometers can be used to monitor arterial blood pressure indirectly (**B**).

      (c) Disadvantages: may not be absolutely accurate but should accurately reflect trends; difficult to get accurate data in animals weighing less than 3 kg (e.g., cats); accuracy depends on occluding cuff size; inaccurate at low BPs

  (2) Ultrasonic Doppler apparatus (Fig. 15-15)

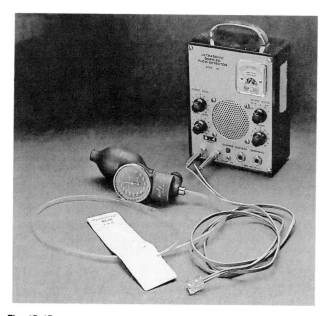

Fig. 15-15
An electronically activated Doppler crystal senses blood flow, which can be used to audibly broadcast and monitor blood pressure.

(a) Doppler crystal placed over peripheral artery (e.g., dog: digital, dorsal pedal; horse: coccygeal)

(b) Place appropriately sized inflatable cuff with pressure gauge proximal to Doppler crystal; inflate cuff until pulse sound stops, then slowly deflate until pulse is first heard; this corresponds to the systolic BP as displayed on the pressure gauge

(c) Advantages: can count pulse rate and detect abnormalities in pulse rhythm

(d) Disadvantages: accuracy related to many factors; cuff size should be one half the limb circumference; measures systolic pressure only; inaccurate at low BPs

b. Invasive
  (1) The technique of invasive arterial pressure monitoring provides an accurate quantitative value of the arterial pressure and a qualitative representation of the pulse waveform; BP is not an indicator of cardiac output (CO) (Figs. 15-16 and 15-17)
    (a) Monitoring patient's hemodynamic status
    (b) Monitoring of hemodynamic effects of anesthetic drugs
  (2) Physiologic significance
    (a) ABP is expressed clinically in millimeters of mercury (mm Hg) with the zero reference at the level of the right atrium
    (b) The mean pressure required to adequately perfuse organs is approximately 60 mm Hg; the systolic blood pressure should be >80 mm Hg

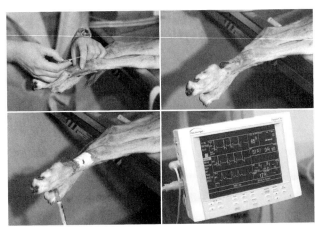

Fig. 15-16
A catheter can be placed in the dorsal pedal artery of the dog to directly record arterial blood pressure. The dorsal pedal artery of a dog is catheterized (*top figures*). The catheter is secured and is connected to a pressure transducer and then to a multiparameter monitor (*lower figures*).

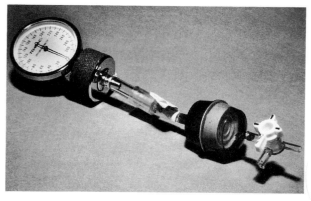

Fig. 15-17
A small blood filter attached to a three-way stopcock and then to a sphygmomanometer. This is an inexpensive method of monitoring mean arterial blood pressure.

    (c) Normal arterial pressure values
- Systolic: 110 to 160 mm Hg
- Diastolic: 50 to 70 mm Hg
- Mean: 60 to 90 mm Hg
- Systolic – diastolic = pulse pressure

    (d) Components of the pulse pressure (Fig. 15-18)

    (e) Inotropic component: the steep ascending limb of the pressure pulse

  (3) Primary factors affecting the ABP

    (a) ABP = CO × total peripheral resistance (TPR)

$$ABP = CO \times TPR$$

- Factors increasing stroke volume or cardiac output favor an increase in arterial pressure
- Factors increasing TPR favor an increase in arterial pressure

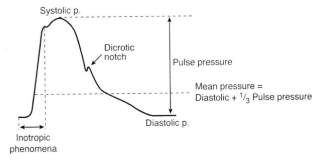

Fig. 15-18
Characteristics of the arterial pressure waveform.

(b) CO = heart rate (HR) × stroke volume (SV)
(c) Therefore:

$$ABP = HR \times SV \times TPR$$

NOTE

Decreases in HR, SV, or TPR individually or in any combination can decrease ABP.

(d) Pulse pressure curves (Fig. 15-19)
(4) Clinical value of arterial pressure monitoring
   (a) Determine the effects of anesthetic drugs on cardiac output and peripheral resistance
   (b) Determine the adequacy of fluid therapy, drug administration (e.g., dobutamine), and ventilatory assist devices (Fig. 15-20)
   (c) Prevention of tissue ischemia and subsequent metabolic acidosis relies on normal mean BPs (greater than 60 mm Hg)
(5) Treatment of hypotension
   (a) Rapid IV fluid administration
   (b) Decreased depth of anesthesia
   (c) Initiation of positive inotrope therapy (e.g., dopamine, dobutamine)

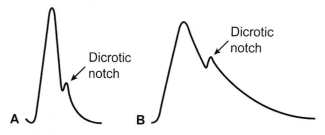

Fig. 15-19

Effects of peripheral artery vasodilation (**A**) and vasoconstriction (**B**) on the arterial blood pressure waveform.

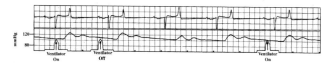

Fig. 15-20

ECG and arterial pressure waveform in an anesthetized 3-year-old horse. Note change in arterial pressure waveform during expiration.

(6) Hazards of invasive arterial pressure monitoring
  (a) Hematoma formation
  (b) Air embolization
  (c) Arterial thrombosis and occlusion (rare)
  (d) Infection (rare)
  (e) Formation of atrioventricular fistula or aneurysm (rare)
(7) Equipment
  (a) Intraarterial catheter with three-way stopcock
  (b) Pressure-sensing device (e.g., pressure transducer and oscilloscope, mercury manometer)
(8) Procedure
  (a) Cannulate a peripheral artery (e.g., dorsal pedal artery in dogs; facial artery in horses) aseptically with the arterial catheter

    (b) Flush the catheter with heparinized saline solution; always aspirate first to prevent air embolism

    (c) Attach the pressure transducer while stopcock is closed to the artery

    (d) Open the transducer to air to establish the baseline (zero) reference pressure with the transducer at the level of the right atrium

    (e) Open the arterial line to the pressure transducer; pulse-pressure curve should be displayed at this point

    (f) After removing the arterial catheter, place manual pressure on the site of cannulation for 5 minutes to prevent hematoma formation

5. CO

    a. CO can be monitored noninvasively or minimally invasively

    b. CO = SV × HR or ABP/TPR

    c. Equipment (Fig. 15-21)

       (1) CO_2 rebreathing method (NICO, Novametrix Medical Systems)

       (2) Indicator dilution method—lithium dilution (LiDCOplus, LiDCO), thermodilution

       (3) Doppler technology (USCOM, USCOM)

D. Musculoskeletal system (see Chapter 11)

  1. Skeletal muscle tone

  2. Quality of elicited reflexes

  3. Peripheral nerve stimulator; used to assess quality of skeletal muscle responses during onset and reversal of neuromuscular blocking agents

E. Thermoregulation

  1. Body temperature regulation is an integrated process involving the following body systems or organs:

    a. CNS

    b. Cardiovascular system

    c. Musculoskeletal system

    d. Respiratory system

    e. Skin

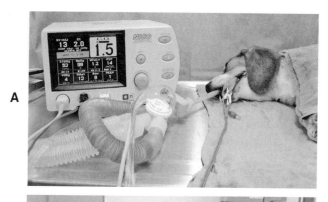

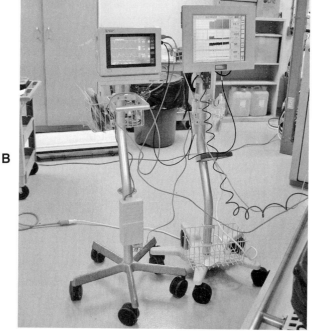

Fig. 15-21
Cardiac output (total blood flow) can be determined by monitoring exhaled gases (Fick principle) (**A**) or by using various indicators (cold saline solution, lithium) (**B**).

2. Abnormalities of thermoregulation during anesthesia
   a. Hypothermia
      (1) Heat loss in excess of production
      (2) Most often encountered in small animals because of the larger ratio of body surface area to body mass
      (3) Potential causes
          (a) CNS depression
          (b) Vasodilation
          (c) Reduced heat production by skeletal muscle
          (d) Other causes
              • Cold IV fluids
              • Open body cavities
              • Cold surgical preparation solutions
   b. Hyperthermia
      (1) Heat production exceeding loss
      (2) Iatrogenically produced in response to specific drug combinations in certain species
          (a) Drugs: isoflurane, succinylcholine, and ketamine
      (3) Malignant hyperthermia is a genetic (autosomal recessive) defect most commonly reported in pigs; on rare occasions it is observed in dogs and other species
   c. Monitoring body temperature during anesthesia and postoperative periods should be considered an integrated response involving the specific species, drugs, and each of the body systems listed (Fig. 15-22)

III. Integrated responses (Table 15-2)
   A. Observed responses represent the outcome of a series of events involving simultaneous input and output of many systems, leading to combined autonomic endocrine and somatic responses
   B. Integrated responses to diseases, surgical stress, and anesthetic-induced depression of certain functions are modulated by the autonomic nervous system and the adrenal medulla
      1. Sympathetic tone mediates "fight-or-flight" responses to any type of stress

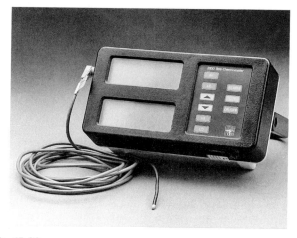

Fig. 15-22
Digital-display temperature monitoring device.

      a. Causes of increased sympathetic tone
        (1) Pain
        (2) Hypotension
        (3) Hypoxemia
        (4) Hypercarbia
        (5) Ischemia
    2. Parasympathetic tone may change as part of an integrated reflex
      a. Vasovagal
      b. Vagophrenic
      c. Vagal efferent (baroreceptor)
  C. Correct interpretation of isolated responses requires an understanding of integration and the ability to work backwards from the observation to its cause
  D. Acute intervention should be initiated and justified on the basis of the following:
    1. A set of monitored observations
    2. Rational selection of therapies to achieve desired physiologic goals
    3. The anticipated patient response

CHAPTER SIXTEEN

Acid-Base Balance and Blood Gases

"The management of a balance of power is a permanent undertaking, not an exertion that has a foreseeable end."

HENRY KISSINGER

OVERVIEW

Traditionally, the diagnosis of acid-base disorders has hinged on the interpretation of changes in blood pH, PCO_2, and HCO_3^- concentration. Changes in pH signal either an increase (acidosis) or decrease (alkalosis) in hydrogen ions. The associated changes in carbon dioxide and bicarbonate concentration help determine the precise cause for the pH change. Alternatively, the diagnosis of acid-base disorders may be determined by changes in independent variables, which include PCO_2, strong ion concentration (e.g., Na^+, K^+, Cl^-), unmeasured anions, and total protein, which are responsible for determining the values of pH, PCO_2, and HCO_3^- (dependent variables). From a clinical standpoint, both approaches work, although the latter is usually more revealing when mixed acid-base disorders exist. Evaluation of a patient's acid-base status is useful in the diagnosis of disease processes and the formulation of therapy. Electrolyte abnormalities are frequently associated with, and may be responsible for, acid-base disorders, further emphasizing the importance of a basic understanding of pH, PCO_2, and electrolyte abnormalities.

GENERAL CONSIDERATIONS

I. Definitions

Acid: A substance that can donate a hydrogen ion (H^+)

$$Ex.: H_2CO_3 \rightarrow H^+ + HCO_3^-$$

Actual bicarbonate: The amount of bicarbonate (HCO), expressed in milliequivalents per liter of plasma

Base (B): A substance that can accept a hydrogen ion (H^+)

$$Ex.: OH^- + H^+ \rightarrow H_2O$$
$$HCO_3^- + H^+ \rightarrow H_2CO_3$$

Base excess (BE): The amount of base above or below the normal buffer base, expressed in milliequivalents per liter, in blood attributed to the metabolic component; positive values (+) reflect excess of base (or deficit of acid), metabolic alkalosis; negative values (−) reflect a deficit of base (or excess of acid), metabolic acidosis; decrease or increase of 0.1 in pH is equal to decrease or increase of 7 in BE when $PaCO_2$ is 40 mm Hg

Buffer: A mixture of substances in a solution that resists or reduces changes in hydrogen ion concentration (changes in pH); important buffers in the body include hemoglobin and bicarbonate

COMPONENTS OF BUFFERING IN BLOOD	
BUFFERS IN WHOLE BLOOD	**% BUFFERING**
Hemoglobin and oxyhemoglobin	35
Organic phosphate	3
Inorganic phosphate	2
Plasma proteins	7
Plasma bicarbonate	35
RBC bicarbonate	18
Total	100

Free water: Water without electrolytes (pure H_2O); increases in free water can cause dilution acidosis; decreases in free water can cause contraction alkalosis

Partial pressure: The pressure an individual gas exerts on a column of mercury; expressed in millimeters of mercury; see the following example of gaseous components of air

COMPOSITION OF AIR		
GAS (MM HG)	FRACTIONAL CONTENT (%)	PARTIAL PRESSURE
Nitrogen (N_2)	78.084*	593.44
Oxygen (O_2)	20.948*	159.2
Argon (Ar)	0.934	7.1
Carbon dioxide (CO_2)	0.031	0.24
Others	0.003	0.02
Total	100	760
		(atmospheric pressure)

*PH_2O varies according to humidity and has a proportionate effect on PO_2 and PN_2.

pH: The negative log of the hydrogen ion (H^+) concentration; the pH is inversely proportional to the log of the H^+ concentration (Fig. 16-1)

$$Ex.: \ (H^+) = 0.000001 = 1 \times 10^{-6} \ pH = 6.0$$
$$(H^+) = 1 \times 10^{-7} \ pH = 7.0$$
$$(H^+) = 1 \times 10^{-8} \ pH = 8.0$$

P_{tot}: Total protein; increases in P_{tot} (weak acids) can cause metabolic (nonrespiratory) acidosis; decreases in P_{tot} cause metabolic alkalosis

Strong ions: Salts that are completely dissociated in water (e.g., Na^+, K^+, Cl^-)

Strong ion difference (SID): The difference between the sums of the positive and negative strong ions; normally (Na^+, K^+, Cl^-); increases in SID usually cause metabolic (nonrespiratory) alkalosis; decreases in SID usually cause metabolic (nonrespiratory) acidosis

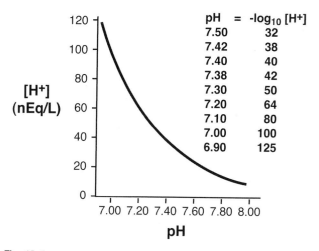

pH	=	$-\log_{10}$ [H+]
7.50		32
7.42		38
7.40		40
7.38		42
7.30		50
7.20		64
7.10		80
7.00		100
6.90		125

Fig. 16-1
The hydrogen ion-pH relationship.

Total CO_2 content: The amount of carbon dioxide gas extractable from plasma; total CO_2 consists of:
Bicarbonate (85% of the total CO_2 is HCO_3^-)
Carbonic acid (10% of the total CO_2 is H_2CO_3)
Carbon dioxide
Unmeasured anions: Strong ions (anions) that are not routinely measured (e.g., lactate; PO_4^{+2}, SO_4^{+2})

II. Many factors influence a patient's acid-base balance
  A. Species
  B. Diet (carnivorous versus herbivorous)
  C. Physical status
  D. Temperature
  E. Concentration of "strong" ions or salts that completely dissociate in water (e.g., Na^+, K^+, Cl^-, lactic acid)
  F. Total protein
III. Normal cellular metabolism continuously produces excess hydrogen ions, the concentration of which is regulated and eliminated by the lungs, kidneys, and gastrointestinal system to maintain an extracellular pH of approximately 7.4

A. The kidneys eliminate hydrogen ions by excreting fixed acids and reabsorption of HCO_3^-

B. The lungs reduce plasma hydrogen ion concentration by eliminating carbon dioxide

C. The gut participates in regulating pH by modulation of acid (HCl), base (Na^+, HCO_3^-), and water excretion

IV. Substances within the body known as *buffers* help minimize changes in pH (e.g., hemoglobin, HCO_3^-. HPO_4^-, $Prot^-$)

V. Determination of pH and blood gases is useful in determining patient acid-base status during anesthesia

VI. When interpreting the absolute values of a patient's pH and blood gases, the patient's clinical history and physical status should be considered

FORMATION AND ELIMINATION OF ACIDS AND BASES IN ANIMALS

I. The waste products of oral intake or metabolism are mostly acidic substances that release hydrogen ions

A. Volatile acid: an acid that produces a gas

$$H_2CO_3 \rightarrow H_2O + CO_2$$

B. Nonvolatile or fixed acids: acids that cannot be converted to gas

1. Lactate + H^+
2. Sulfate + H^+
3. Phosphate + H^+

II. The pathways for acid removal include the kidney, lung, and gastrointestinal tract

$$\text{Input} \rightarrow \text{Oral intake} \quad \underset{\downarrow}{\overset{\text{Metabolism and}}{\text{oral intake}}} \quad \underset{\downarrow}{\overset{\text{Aerobic}}{\text{metabolism}}}$$

$$\underset{\downarrow}{HCO_3^-} \quad + \quad \underset{\downarrow}{H^+} \leftrightarrow \underset{\downarrow}{H_2CO_3} \leftrightarrow \underset{\downarrow}{H_2O + CO_2}$$

$$\text{Output} \leftarrow \text{Kidney} \quad \underset{\text{Gastrointestinal tract}}{\text{Kidney}} \quad \text{Lung}$$

This is the carbonic acid equation or CO_2 hydration equation and is the basis for explaining acid-base kinetics in the body

A. High-protein diets (cats, dogs, pigs, humans)

1. H^+ excess is derived from oxidation of neutral sulfur in these amino acids
   a. Methionine
   b. Cystine
   c. Cysteine
B. Diets high in plant material and grain have HCO_3^- excess from salts in:
   1. Fatty acids (acetate, propionate)
   2. Citrate (fruits)
   3. Gluconates

Ex.:

$$\underset{\text{(sodium acetate)}}{H - \overset{\overset{H}{|}}{\underset{|}{C}} - \overset{\overset{O}{\|}}{C} - O - Na^+} + 2O_2 + H^+ \rightarrow 2\underset{\downarrow}{CO_2} + 2H_2O + Na^+ \quad \overset{H_2CO_3 \; H^+ + HCO_3^-}{\frown}$$

Lung

Metabolizable salts of fatty acids yield HCO_3^- after metabolism

C. Based on primary dietary intake
   1. Carnivores have acid urine or excess acid to excrete (pH: 5.5 to 7.5)
   2. Herbivores have alkaline urine or excess base to excrete (pH: 6 to 9)
D. Dietary and metabolic intake of acid or base equals the urinary and respiratory output, thereby maintaining the pH of the body fluids near 7.4
E. Many approaches to the diagnosis and treatment of acid-base disorders are based on the following (Henderson-Hasselbalch equation):
   1. $CO_2 + H_2O \overset{CA}{\leftrightarrow} H^+ + HCO_3^-$ (carbonic anhydrase [CA])
   2. $K_1 = \dfrac{[CO_2] + [H_2O]}{[H_2CO_3]}$ (K; the dissociation constant for the each acid)

   $\dfrac{K_2}{K_1} = \dfrac{[H^+] + [HCO_3^-]}{[H_2CO_3]}$

   3. $\dfrac{K_2}{K_1} = \dfrac{[H^+] + [HCO_3^-]}{[CO_2] + [H_2O]} = K_3$

   4. Given: $[CO_2] = \alpha \times PCO_2$ ($\alpha = 0.0301$ – solubility coefficient)

5. $\dfrac{K_3 \times \alpha PCO_2}{[HCO_3^-]} = (H^+)$

$-\log (H^+) = pH; -\log K_3 = pK$

pK is that pH at which 50% of an acid or a base is in the ionized state; the pK of the acid $(pK_3 = pK_a)$ H_2CO_3 is 6.1

6. $-\log K_3 -\log \alpha PCO_2 + \log [HCO_3^-] = -\log [H^+]$

$pH = pK_3 + \log \dfrac{[HCO_3^-]}{[\alpha PCO_2]}$ (Henderson-Hasselbalch eq)

F. In the body: $pH = 7.4$, $pK_3 = 6.1$, $PCO_2 = 40$ mm Hg

1. $pH = pK_a + \log \dfrac{[HCO_3^-]}{[\alpha PCO_2]}$

2. $7.4 = 6.1 + \log [HCO_3^-] - \log \alpha PCO_2$

3. $1.3 = \log [HCO_3^-] - \log \alpha PCO_2$

4. Antilog $1.3 = \dfrac{[HCO_3^-]}{0.0301 \times 40}$ antilog $1.3 = 20$

$(HCO_3^-) = 20 \times 0.0301 \times 40 = 24$ mEq/L

ARTERIAL OXYGENATION

I. Normal gas partial pressures (expressed in millimeters of mercury) during inspiration in ambient air, conducting airways, terminal alveoli, and arterial and mixed venous blood[*]

PARTIAL PRESSURE OF INHALED GASES				
	AMBIENT AIR	**CONDUCTING AIRWAYS**	**TERMINAL ALVEOLI**	**ARTERIAL BLOOD**	**MIXED VENOUS BLOOD**
P_{O_2}	156	149	100	95	40
P_{CO_2}	0	0	40	40	46
P_{H_2O}	15†	47	47	47	47
P_{N_2}	589	564	573	573	573
P total	760	760	760	755	706

P_{H_2O} varies according to humidity and has a proportionate effect on P_{O_2} and P_{N_2}.

* From Murray JF: *The normal lung,* ed 2, Philadelphia, WB Saunders, 1986.

II. The inspired oxygen-arterial tension (FIO_2) relationship
   A. Relationship between FIO_2 and PaO_2

THE EFFECT OF INSPIRED OXYGEN FRACTION ON PARTIAL PRESSURE OF OXYGEN

FIO_2 (%)	PREDICTED IDEAL PaO_2	
	(mm Hg)	(kPa)
20	95-100	12.6-13.3
30	150	20.0
40	200	26.6
50	250	33.3
80	400	53.2
100	500	66.5

   B. The alveolar gas equation

$$PAO_2 = PIO_2 - \frac{PaCO_2}{0.8}$$

III. Causes of arterial hypoxia (a reduction in PaO_2) and their effect on alveolar-arterial $P(A\text{-}a)O_2$ differences ($[A\text{-}a]O_2D$)

CAUSES OF ARTERIAL HYPOXEMIA

CAUSE	EFFECT ON ARTERIAL PO_2	EFFECT ON $(A\text{-}a)O_2D$
Hypoventilation	Decreased	No change
Diffusion abnormality	No change or decreased*	No change or decreased*
Ventilation perfusion imbalance	Decreased	Increased
Right-to-left shunt	Decreased	Increased
Reduction in inspired PO_2	Decreased	No change

*Effects of diffusion abnormalities are infrequently encountered at rest and are most likely to be evident during exercise.

IV. Oxygenation
  A. Efficiency of oxygenation
    1. $P_{(A-a)}O_2$ Difference
    2. PaO_2/PAO_2
    3. Right-to-left shunt (when breathing 100% O_2)

$$Qs \text{ (shunt blood flow)} = \frac{(P_{A}O_2 - PaO_2)\,(0.003)}{4 + (P_{A}O_2 - PaO_2)\,(0.003)}$$

  B. Adequacy of tissue oxygenation PvO_2

DELIVERY OF OXYGEN TO TISSUE

I. Dissolved
  A. Henry's law: amount of O_2 dissolved is proportional to Po_2; for each 1 mm Hg of PO_2, there is 0.003 ml $O_2/100$ ml of plasma; content = solubility partial pressure
  B. Dissolved O_2 is not adequate to meet the animal's oxygen needs
II. Hemoglobin
  A. Conjugated protein of iron and porphyrin joined to the protein globin; globin has two alpha and two beta chains made of differing amino acid sequences
    1. Hemoglobin A: adult
    2. Hemoglobin F: fetal
    3. Hemoglobin S: sickle (valine-glutamic acid); poor oxygen-carrying capability
  B. Hemoglobin A is transferred from a ferrous to a ferric ion by oxidation (methemoglobin), which is not useful in O_2 carriage
    1. Nitrites
    2. Sulfonamides
    3. Benzocaine

O_2 DISSOCIATION CURVE (Fig. 16-2)

I. $O_2 + Hb = HbO_2$ (oxyhemoglobin); O_2 capacity is the amount of O_2 that can be combined with Hb; 1 g Hb can combine with 1.39 ml of O_2; for example, if there are 15 g Hb, then $1.39 \times 15 = 20.8$ ml $O_2/100$ ml at 100% saturation

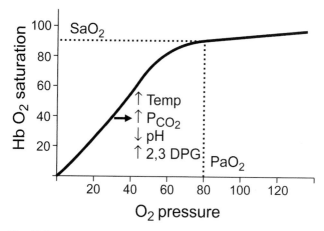

Fig. 16-2

The oxyhemoglobin dissociation curve. The effects of pH, PCO_2, temperature, and 2, 3-diphosphoglycerate on hemoglobin saturation with O_2 are noteworthy, as is the effect of anemia (low Hb) on O_2 content.

II. O_2 saturation

$$\frac{O_2 \text{ combined with Hb} \times 100}{O_2 \text{ capacity}} \; (\%)$$

III. O_2 content is the amount of O_2 present as dissolved O_2 and combined with Hb. Example: What is the O_2 content of blood if the hemoglobin concentration is 12 g/dl and the hemoglobin saturation is 96% when the PaO_2 is 100 mm Hg?

1.39 ml $O_2 \times$ 12 g (Hb) $\times$ 96% = 16 ml O_2 (with Hb)

+) 100 mm Hg (PaO_2) $\times$ 0.003 ml O_2/mm Hg = 0.3 ml O_2 (in plasma)

16.3 ml O_2/100 ml (O_2 in blood)

IV. O_2 dissociation curve shape (Fig. 16-2)
   A. Upper portion: PO_2 (partial pressure of oxygen) can fall slightly without affecting O_2 loading of Hb
   B. Lower portion: peripheral tissues can withdraw large amounts of O_2 with only small changes in PO_2; more than 5 g/dl of deoxygenated (unsaturated) Hb can cause

cyanosis (blue or purple discoloration of the mucous membranes)
V. Shifts in the O_2 dissociation curve are most commonly caused by changes in pH, PCO_2, and temperature
   A. Increasing temperature and PO_2 and decreasing pH shifts the O_2 dissociation curve to the right; reverse changes have the opposite effect
   B. 2,3-diphosphoglycerate increases within red blood cells (RBC) in chronic hypoxia and shifts the O_2 dissociation curve to the right
   C. Rightward shifts mean more unloading of O_2 at a given PO_2; normal PCO_2 at 50% O_2 saturation is approximately 26 mm Hg in a capillary
   D. Deoxygenated Hb can carry more CO_2

CARBON DIOXIDE

I. Transport
   A. Dissolved in blood
      1. In plasma (as HCO_3^-): 85%
      2. In RBCs as carbamino compounds
      3. Carried in physical solution
   B. The measurement of end-expired CO_2 ($ETCO_2$) and $PaCO_2$ permits the calculation of dead space ventilation (VD)

$$VD = \frac{PaCO_2 - ETCO_2}{PaCO_2}$$

CARBON MONOXIDE

I. $Hb + CO \rightarrow COHb$ (carboxyhemoglobin)
II. Carbon monoxide has approximately 210 times the affinity for Hb as O_2
   A. Small amounts of CO can tie up large amounts of Hb, making it unavailable for O_2 carriage
   B. PaO_2 is normal, but O_2 content is dramatically reduced
   C. The oxyhemoglobin curve is shifted to the left, impairing O_2 unloading in tissues

NORMAL pH AND BLOOD GAS VALUES

I. pH = 7.40; range 7.35 to 7.45
II. PaO_2 = 95 mm Hg; range 80 to 110 mm Hg
III. PvO_2 = 40 mm Hg; range 35 to 45 mm Hg
IV. $PaCO_2$ = 40 mm Hg; range 35 to 45 mm Hg
V. $PvCO_2$ = 45 mm Hg; range 40 to 48 mm Hg
VI. HCO_3^- = 24 mEq/L; range 22 to 27 mEq/L (a little higher in horses and ruminants)

THE $PaCO_2$/pH/HCO_3^- RELATIONSHIP		
$PaCO_2$ (mm Hg) (ACUTE CHANGE)	pH	HCO_3^- (mEq/L) (EFFECT)
80	7.2	28
60	7.3	26
40	7.4	24
30	7.5	22
20	7.6	20

VII. Nomenclature
    A. **Acidemia:** pH less than 7.35 (acid blood)
        1. Metabolic or nonrespiratory acidosis: an abnormal physiologic process characterized by a primary gain of acid (H^+) or primary loss of base (HCO_3^-) from the extracellular fluid
        2. Respiratory acidosis: an abnormal process in which there is a primary reduction in alveolar ventilation relative to CO_2 production ($PaCO_2$ increase)
    B. **Alkalemia:** pH greater than 7.45 (alkaline blood)
        1. Metabolic alkalosis or nonrespiratory alkalosis: an abnormal physiologic process characterized by a primary gain in base (HCO_3^-) or loss of acid (H^+) from the extracellular fluid
        2. **Respiratory alkalosis:** an abnormal physiologic process in which there is a primary increase in alveolar ventilation relative to the rate of CO_2 production ($PaCO_2$ decrease)

C. **Compensation:** an abnormal pH is returned toward normal by altering the component not primarily affected; for example, if the $PaCO_2$ is elevated, the HCO_3^- should be elevated (retained) to compensate

1. If the $PaCO_2$ or HCO_3^- values are outside normal limits, but the pH is within the normal range, then the patient is fully compensated

2. Because it takes time for the process of compensation to return the pH to within normal limits, a compensatory process implies a degree of chronicity

   a. Respiratory compensation occurs within a few minutes after primary insult, but a few hours are required to reach highest efficacy

   b. Renal compensation for primary respiratory effects takes at least a few hours, but days are required to reach highest efficacy

3. It is important to determine primary or secondary (compensatory) changes

PRIMARY pH AND BLOOD GAS CLASSIFICATION				
CLASSIFICATION	$PaCO_2$	pH	HCO_3^-	BE
Acute ventilatory failure	↑	↓	N	N
Chronic ventilatory failure	↑	N	↑	↑
Acute alveolar hyperventilation	↓	↑	N	N
Chronic alveolar hyperventilation	↓	N	↓	↓
Uncompensated metabolic acidosis	N	↓	↓	↓
Compensated metabolic acidosis	—↓	N	↓	↓
Uncompensated metabolic alkalosis	N	↑	↑	↑
Compensated metabolic alkalosis	↑	N	↑	↑

↓, Decreased; ↑, increased; *N*, normal.

I. Mixed respiratory and metabolic conditions can coexist; when this occurs, look at the individual values (pH, PCO_2, HCO_3^-) to determine the severity

RAPID QUALITATIVE INTERPRETATION OF pH AND BLOOD GASES

I. Determine pH: acidemia or alkalemia; the pH is the most important value in determining the animal's acid-base status; match subsequent values to it

II. Determine PCO_2
   A. Respiratory alkalosis: less than 35 mm Hg
   B. Respiratory acidosis: greater than 50 mm Hg

III. Determine BE or HCO_3^-
   A. Metabolic alkalosis: BE > +5 mEq/L ($HCO_3^- > 28$ mEq/L)
   B. Metabolic acidosis: BE < −5 mEq/L ($HCO_3^- < 20$ mEq/L)

IV. Determine the primary problem by matching either the P_{CO_2} or BE or both with the pH; determine whether compensation exists (pH near normal)

V. Look more closely at BE
   A. BE can be influenced by four things:
      1. Free water (use $[Na^+]$ as the measure): Na^-, K^+, and Cl^+ are examples of strong ions
      2. $[Cl^-]$
      3. Protein concentration (A_{tot})
      4. Unidentified anion concentrations (e.g., lactic acid)
   B. Abnormalities in all four can exist simultaneously (Fig. 16-3); they can have opposite effects and therefore can offset and mask each other; for example, severe lactic acidosis from shock can be offset by a severe hyper-

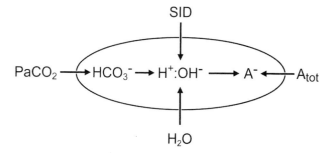

Fig. 16-3
Factors that affect acid-base balance.

chloremic alkalosis from sustained vomiting; the net (observed) BE could be zero

VI. Determine PaO_2

    A. If PaO_2 is less than 80 mm Hg, suspect hypoxemia

    B. 5 g/dl of unoxygenated Hb results in cyanosis in patients with more than 5 g/dl of Hb

PRINCIPLES OF PRACTICE

  I. The HCO_3^- concentration rises approximately 1 to 2 mEq/L for each acute 10 mm Hg increase in $PaCO_2$ above 40; maximum compensatory change in HCO_3^- is approximately 4 mEq/L

  II. The HCO_3^- concentration falls 1 to 2 mEq/L for each acute 10 mm Hg decrease in $PaCO_2$ below 40; maximum compensatory change in HCO_3^- is approximately 6 mEq/L

  III. Acute respiratory and nonrespiratory disorders can be distinguished by their BE, $PaCO_2$, and HCO_3^- values; BE above 5 or below -5 and HCO_3^- above 30 or below 15 mEq/L imply a nonrespiratory (metabolic) component

  IV. During chronic elevation of the $PaCO_2$ (hypercapnea), each 10 mm Hg increase in $PaCO_2$ causes a 4 mEq/L increase in HCO_3^- concentration

  V. An acute 10 mm Hg increase in $PaCO_2$ results in a 0.05 unit decrease in pH; an acute 10 mm Hg decrease in $PaCO_2$ results in a 0.10 unit increase in pH

  VI. Rapid determination of the predicted respiratory pH

    A. Determine the difference between the measured $PaCO_2$ and 40 mm Hg (the respiratory component)

    B. If the $PaCO_2$ is greater than 40, move the decimal two places to the left and subtract half the value from 7.40

    C. If the $PaCO_2$ is less than 40, move the decimal two places to the left and add the value to 7.40

    D. Examples

      1. pH = 7.01; $PaCO_2$ = 75 ($PaCO_2$ > 40 mm Hg)
$75 - 40 = 35; 0.35 \times 0.5 = 0.175$
$7.40 - 0.175 = 7.225$

      2. pH = 7.43; $PaCO_2$ = 23 ($PaCO_2$ < 40 mm Hg)
$40 - 23 = 17$
$7.40 + 0.17 = 7.57$

VII. Rapid determination of the metabolic (nonrespiratory) component
- A. A 10 mEq/L change in HCO_3^- concentration changes pH by 0.15 units; if the pH decimal is moved two places to the right, then a 10:15 or two-thirds relationship exists
- B. The absolute difference between the measured pH and the predicted respiratory pH is the metabolic component of the pH change; moving the decimal point two places to the right and multiplying by two thirds yields an estimate of the mEq/L variation of the buffer baseline (usually assumed as the HCO_3^- concentration change)

VIII. Rapid quantitative clinical determination of acid-base changes
- A. Determine the predicted respiratory component of the pH change
- B. Estimate BE or deficit
- C. Examples:
  1. pH = 7.02; $PaCO_2$ = 75
     Predicted respiratory pH:
     75 − 40 = 35; 0.35 × 0.5 = 0.175
     7.40 − 0.18 = 7.22
     Metabolic (nonrespiratory) component:
     7.22 − 7.02 = 0.02; 20 × 2/3 = 13.3 mEq/L, or 13.3 mEq/L base deficit
  2. pH = 7.64; $PaCO_2$ = 25
     Predicted respiratory pH:
     40 − 25 = 15; 0.15
     7.40 + 0.15 = 7.55
     Metabolic component:
     7.64 − 7.55 = 0.09; 9 × 2/3 = 6 mEq/L, or 6.0 mEq/L BE

IX. Quantitative analysis of metabolic or nonrespiratory acid-base ratio state[*]
- A. Enter the observed BE at the bottom of the Table 16-1
- B. Calculate and enter the expected contributions to BE caused by the following:
  1. Any free water abnormality

---

[*] Modified from Leith DE: Proceedings of the Ninth ACVIM Forum, New Orleans, May 1991.

TABLE 16-1

QUANTITATIVE ANALYSIS OF NONRESPIRATORY ACID-BASE PROBLEMS

Free water abnormalities:	$0.3 ([Na^+] - 140)$	—
Chloride abnormalities:	$102 - [Cl^-]corr$	—
Hypoproteinemia:	$3(6.5 - [P_{tot}])$	—
Unmeasured anions make up the balance:		—
Total, or the observed (reported) BE:		—

([ ] = measured value)
$[Cl^-]corr = [Cl-]obs \times 140/[Na^+]$.
For [Alb] instead of $[P_{tot}]$, use 3.7 (4.5 – [Alb]).

    2. Abnormalities in the corrected $[Cl^-]$

    3. Abnormalities in protein concentrations; be careful about signs (+ or −)

  C. Algebraically sum the values in "B" to determine whether there are unmeasured anions; be careful about sign (+ or −)

  D. Compare "A" and "C"; the observed BE should never be greater than the summed values in "C"; if the observed BE is less, the presence of unmeasured anions (UA⁻) equal in magnitude to the difference of the summed values in B and BE can be inferred

X. Example

  If:

    pH = 7.250, Na^+ = 135

    PCO_2 = 75, Cl^- = 79

    BE = 2; P_{tot} + 8.4

  Then:

    Free water abnormality = − 1.5

    Chloride abnormality = + 20.1

    Hyperproteinemia = −5.7

    Observed BE = 2

  Therefore:

    UA^- = 14.9

    [(12.9) + (2) = 14.9]

This patient has considerable unmeasured ions (14.9 mEq/L), which suggests a severe nonrespiratory acidosis

XI. Summary of acid-base disorders
   A. All acid-base disturbances are caused by changes in $PaCO_2$, SID, and P_{tot}
   B. Because protein concentration is not manipulated clinically, all acid-base disturbances are corrected by changes in $PaCO_2$ and SID

XII. Therapy
   A. Base deficits of less than 10 mEq/L are not routinely treated
   B. pH above 7.20 is not routinely treated unless there is evidence of shock
   C. Because extracellular water is approximately 20% body weight (intravascular fluid 5% and the interstitial fluid 15%), base deficits × body weight (kg) 20% = amount of HCO_3^- needed as replacement, or

$$\frac{\text{Base deficit} \times \text{wt (kg)}}{4} = \text{mEq } HCO_3^- \text{ required}$$

COMMON CAUSES OF ACID-BASE IMBALANCE

I. Respiratory acidosis
   A. Anesthesia or respiratory depressant drugs
   B. Obesity
   C. Pulmonary disease
   D. Rib or thoracic disease; trauma
   E. Airway obstruction
   F. Brain damage
   G. Hypoventilation during artificial ventilation

II. Respiratory alkalosis
   A. Anxiety, fear
   B. Fever
   C. Endotoxemia
   D. Pneumonia, pulmonary embolus
   E. Hypoxemia, anemia
   F. Left-to-right shunts
   G. Heart failure
   H. Central nervous system disease

III. Metabolic acidosis
   A. Renal disease (uremia)
   B. Chronic vomiting

   C. Diarrhea
   D. Exercise fatigue, hypoxia, ischemia, shock, trauma
   E. Diabetes mellitus
   F. Hypoaldosteronism
IV. Metabolic alkalosis
   A. Acute vomiting
   B. Hypokalemia
   C. Excessive use of diuretics
   D. Cushing syndrome
   E. Excessive use of HCO_3^-

ACID-BASE AND ELECTROLYTE INTERRELATIONSHIPS

I. Most CO_2 entering the blood passes into RBCs, where the majority of CO_2 enters into a reversible formation with HCO

$$CO_2 + H_2O \overset{CA}{\leftrightarrow} H_2CO_3 \overset{CA}{\leftrightarrow} H^+ + HCO_3^-$$

The HCO_3^- formed by this reaction diffuses out of RBCs; this movement sets up an electrostatic difference across the cell membrane, which is neutralized by the movement of Cl^- from plasma into the RBC (chloride shift)

II. The location and absolute numbers of positively and negatively charged ions (strong ions) and their difference in combination with CO_2 production, the resultant PCO_2, and the total protein determine pH (H^+) and (HCO_3^-) changes in the body; the principal strong ions are Na^+, K^+, and Cl^-; SID = (Na^+) + (K^+) − (Cl^-) (Fig. 16-3)

III. Changes in strong ions in various body fluids result in changes in SID, which provide the major mechanism for acid-base interactions

IV. To maintain electrical neutrality, electrolyte shifts generally occur simultaneously with acid (H^+) or base (HCO_3^-) shifts; the most important electrolyte shift occurring with acid-base changes is K^+; for example, when HCO_3^- is added to the extracellular fluid, hydrogen ions (H^+) leave cells, causing K^+ to move intracellularly to maintain electrical equilibrium; therefore:
   A. In metabolic alkalosis, suspect hypokalemia
   B. In metabolic acidosis, suspect hyperkalemia

CHAPTER SEVENTEEN

Pain

"Dying is nothing, but pain is a very serious matter."
HENRY JACOB BIGELOW, 1871

OVERVIEW

The definition, recognition, quantitation, and treatment of pain have become central issues in veterinary practice. Providing pain relief is as important as choosing the proper sedative, muscle relaxant, and injectable or inhalant anesthetic. This is particularly true for pain in the perioperative period. Apprehension and stress, produced by fear, can initiate a variety of potentially deleterious neurohumoral reactions (stress response) and can sensitize both the peripheral and central nervous systems to noxious stimuli, which heightens pain awareness. Understanding pain pathways and the mechanisms of action of analgesic therapies helps veterinarians treat pain before it occurs. This practice is called *preemptive analgesia.* The best way to treat pain is to preempt it.

GENERAL CONSIDERATIONS

  I. Definitions
  Acute pain: Pain that disappears when the stimulus is removed or that occurs after some bodily injury; disappears with healing, and tends to be self-limiting
  Allodynia: Pain evoked by a stimulus that does not normally cause pain
  Analgesia: Loss of sensibility to pain
  Analgesic: Any method or drug that relieves pain
  Analgia: Painlessness

323

Breakthrough pain: A transient flare-up of pain in the chronic pain setting, which can occur even when chronic pain is under control

Cancer pain: Pain that can be acute, chronic, or intermittent and is related to the disease itself or to the treatment

Central sensitization: An increase in the excitability and responsiveness of nerves in the central system, particularly the spinal cord

Chronic pain: Pain that lasts several weeks to months and persists beyond the expected healing time, when nonmalignant in origin

Deep pain: Originates in tendons, joints, muscles, and periosteum; it is not unusual for deep pain to cause a drop in blood pressure, a slowing of the pulse, and nausea, vomiting, and sweating; can cause reflex cramping of nearby skeletal muscles

Distress: The state produced when the biologic cost of stress negatively affects biologic functions critical to the animal's well-being. To cause pain or suffering or to make miserable

Epidural: The space above the dura mater

Field or production surgery: Any surgery performed on farm or free-ranging wild animals residing in their natural or production habitat

Hyperalgesia: An increased or exaggerated response to a stimulus that is normally painful (a heightened sense of pain) either at the site of injury (primary) or in surrounding undamaged tissue (secondary or extraterritorial). Stimulated nociceptors respond to noxious stimuli more vigorously and at a lower threshold

Hyperesthesia: Increased sensitivity to sensation

Hyperpathia: A painful syndrome characterized by an increased reaction to a stimulus, especially if it is repetitive

Hypoalgesia: Decreased sensitivity to pain

Hypoesthesia: Decreased sensitivity to stimulation

Institutional Animal Care and Use Committee: A committee whose existence is required by the United States Department of Agriculture and the Department of Health and Human Services at institutions conducting research on animals; consists of veterinarians, practicing scientists, nonscientists, and individuals not affiliated with the institution; responsible for evaluating the institutional animal care and use programs and making recommendations to the administration of the institution; ultimately responsible for approving or disapproving the use of animals in research at the institution on a case-by-case basis

Interventional pain management: Action taken to alter the body's production or transmission of pain signals to the brain. This may involve an invasive procedure to treat or manage pain through an injection of a drug or implantation of a drug delivery device

Local anesthesia: The temporary loss of sensation in a defined part of the body without loss of consciousness

Major surgery: Any surgical intervention that penetrates and exposes a body cavity; any procedure that has the potential for inducing permanent physical or physiologic impairment; any procedure associated with orthopedics or extensive tissue dissection or transection

Minor surgery: Any surgical intervention that produces minimal impairment of physical or physiologic function (e.g., laparoscopy, superficial vascular cutdown, and percutaneous biopsy)

Multimodal analgesia: The use of multiple drugs with different actions to produce optimal analgesia

Myofascial pain: A syndrome of focal pain in a muscle or related tissues, associated with stiffness, muscle spasm, and decreased range of motion

Neuralgia: Pain exhibiting periodic intensification, which extends along the course of one or more nerves

Neuropathic pain: Pain that originates from injury or involvement of the peripheral or central nervous system (CNS), possibly associated with motor, sensory, or autonomic deficits

Neuroleptanalgesia: Hypnosis and analgesia produced by the combination of a neuroleptic drug and an analgesic drug

Nociception: The transduction, conduction, and CNS processing of nerve signals generated by the stimulation of nociceptors. It is the physiologic process that leads to the perception of pain

Nonsurvival/nonrecovery surgery: A surgical procedure performed with the patient under general anesthesia at the conclusion of which the animal is euthanatized without regaining consciousness

Opioid: A drug that is related naturally or synthetically to morphine

Pain: An aversive sensation and feeling associated with actual or potential tissue damage

Pain threshold: The least experience of pain that a patient can recognize

Pain tolerance level: The greatest level of pain that a patient can tolerate

Pathologic pain: Pain that has an exaggerated response beyond its protective usefulness. It is often associated with tissue injury incurred at the time of surgery or trauma

Perception of pain: Only humans report and demand treatment of pain; pain in animals must be inferred by the observation of deviations from normal behavior; pain may manifest itself as a limp or altered gait; withdrawal of an injured part; awkward, abnormal postures; a worried or distressed expression; looking at, licking, scratching, or kicking at the site of perceived pain; these and similar signs are the only clues a veterinarian can use to diagnose the presence and magnitude of pain; it seems likely that the presence of pain in animals is underdiagnosed and, when diagnosed, that its magnitude is underestimated

Perioperative: All events associated with a surgical procedure

Peripheral sensitization: An increase in the activity, excitability, and responsiveness of peripheral nerve terminals

Physiologic pain: The normal response to a noxious stimulus that produces protective mechanisms causing the animal to minimize tissue damage (fight or flight) or to avoid contact with external stimuli during a reparative phase

Preemptive analgesia: The administration of an analgesic before painful stimulation to prevent sensitization of neurons, or windup, thus improving postoperative analgesia

Projected pain: An error in the localization of pain; occurs with superficial pain, which is normally quite accurately located; injury to a nerve containing pain pathways causes a phantom pain to be projected into the uninjured area at the origin of the pain fibers

Referred pain: Pain originating in one part of the body but perceived as occurring in another; occurs as the result of the synapses in the spinal cord of visceral pain fibers with pain fibers from the skin

Regional anesthesia: The loss of sensation in part of the body caused by interruption of the sensory nerves that conduct impulses from that region of the body

Sedation: CNS depression in which the patient is awake but calm; a term often used interchangeably with tranquilization; with sufficient stimuli the patient may be aroused

Somatic pain: Pain that originates from damage to bones, joint, muscle, or skin and is described by humans as localized, constant, sharp, aching, and throbbing

Stoic: Indifferent to pain or pleasure

Stress: The biologic responses of an animal in order to cope with a disruption or threat to homeostasis. A stressor is a physical, chemical, or emotional factor (e.g., pain, trauma, fear) to which an individual fails to make a satisfactory adaptation and that causes physiologic tensions that may be contributory to the development of disease

Subarachnoid: The space above the pia mater and below the arachnoid mater in which cerebrospinal fluid is found. A subarachnoid injection is also referred to as a *spinal*

Superficial or cutaneous pain: Originating on an outer surface (skin) and well localized; it may be sharp or acute or it may be chronic, burning, or aching; may cause an increase in the pulse rate and blood pressure

Surgery: The act of incising living tissue; an operative procedure; the room or facility where an operative procedure is done

Surgical facility: A group of interrelated rooms specifically designed for the conduct of surgery and for preoperative and postoperative functions associated with the conduct of surgery in animals

Survival/recovery surgery: A surgical procedure from which animals recover from the effects of general anesthesia and become conscious

Sympathetic mediated pain: A syndrome in which there is abnormal sympathetic nervous system activity, causing a severe debilitation and often associated with tenderness to a light touch

Tolerance: A shortened duration and decreased intensity of the analgesic, euphorigenic, sedative, and other CNS-depressant effects, as well as marked elevation in the average dose required to achieve a given effect

Tranquilization, ataraxia, neurolepsis: State of tranquility and calmness in which the patient is relaxed, reluctant to move, awake, and unconcerned with its surroundings and potentially indifferent to minor pain; sufficient stimulation will arouse the patient

Visceral pain: Originating from internal organs, visceral pain is poorly localized; small injuries may not cause severe pain, but diffuse foci can produce extremely severe pain; pulling and twisting of viscera, mesenteries, and ligaments can cause pain in an anesthetized patient; visceral pain can be perceived as a pain on the body surface; this error in pain localization is called *referred pain;* if the visceral involvement results in an inflammation that extends to an area of parietal peritoneum, pleura, or pericardium, pain fibers from these areas are also stimulated; pain fibers in the parietal peritoneum or pleura are innervated like the skin and are capable of sensing acute, highly localized pain referring to the corresponding area on the surface of the body; visceral pain can also produce skeletal muscle spasm of the abdominal wall over the affected area; usually involves the parietal peritoneum

Windup: Temporal summation of painful stimuli in the spinal cord. Mediated by C fibers and responsible for "second" or delayed pain

II. Physiology of pain and pain pathways
   A. Peripheral pain receptors
      1. Mechanosensitive
         a. Stress, stretching
         b. Compression, crushing
      2. Thermosensitive; involves temperature change
         a. Heat
         b. Cold

3. Chemosensitive
  a. Neurotransmitters (e.g., Ach, substance P)
  b. Prostaglandins
  c. Autocoids
    (1) Bradykinin
    (2) 5-hydroxytryptamine (5HT)
    (3) Histamine
    (4) Potassium
    (5) Proteolytic enzymes
  d. Acids (e.g., lactic acid)
  e. Cytokines
    (1) Tumor necrosis factor
    (2) Interleukin-1, 6, 8(3) Calcitonin gene-related peptide
  f. Leukotriene
  g. Nerve growth factor
B. Peripheral nerves (Table 4-1)
  1. Myelinated nerve fibers (Aa, Afl, Ag, Ad) transmit acute, accurately localized, (epicritic) sharp and rapid onset pain
  2. Nonmyelinated C nerve fibers transmit chronic, diffuse (protopathic), dull, burning, and aching pain
C. Spinal cord pathways
  1. Peripheral nerves enter the spinal cord through the dorsal roots and then ascend or descend one or two segments in Lissauer's tract
  2. Peripheral nerves terminate in the dorsal horn gray matter (substantia gelatinosa)
  3. Peripheral nerves synapse with nerves of the spinothalamic tract and are carried centrally to the following:
    a. Thalamus: somatosensory cortex
    b. Reticular activating system, which is important in activating the autonomic nervous system, limbic system, amygdala, and locus coeruleus; the following conditions can result:
      (1) Sleep arousal
      (2) Cardiopulmonary changes
      (3) Aversion reaction
      (4) Stress response

4. Spinal cord pain modulators
   a. Facilitatory
      (1) Substance P (neurokinin-1 type)
      (2) Glutamate (N-methyl-D-aspartate [NMDA type])
      (3) Prostanoids
      (4) Serotonin (5-HT$_2$)
      (5) Norepinephrine
      (6) Acetylcholine
      (7) Adenosine triphosphate (ATP)
      (6) BDNF (brain derived neurotrophic factor)
   b. Inhibitory
      (1) γ-Aminobutyric acid-B (GABA)
      (2) Opioids
      (3) α_2-Agonists
      (4) Adenosine (A$_1$-type)
      (5) Serotonin (5-HT$_1$)
      (6) Norepinephrine
      (7) Kainate
5. Central perception
   a. Pain is inferred by observation of deviations from normal behavior and physiologic responses
      (1) Decreased appetite
      (2) Less sleep
      (3) Facial expression
      (4) Altered gait
      (5) Increased locomotion
      (6) Reluctance to move
      (7) Abnormal posture
      (8) Licking, scratching
      (9) Self-mutilation
      (10) Aversion
      (11) Vocalization
      (12) Aggression
   b. Pain in anesthetized animals is inferred by changes in response to manipulation (surgical or otherwise)
      (1) Movement
      (2) Trembling
      (3) Increased heart rate or respiratory rate
      (4) Increased arterial blood pressure

      (5) Autonomic nervous system

      (6) Neuroendocrine

      (7) Immunology

      (8) Hematology

      (9) Metabolites

      (10) Morphology

    c. Pain or stress is inferred by increases in circulating "stress" substances

      (1) Adrenocorticotrophic hormone

      (2) Glucose

      (3) Catecholamines (dopamine, epinephrine, norepinephrine)

      (4) Beta-endorphin

      (5) Leu-enkephalin

      (6) Lactic acid

      (7) Free fatty acids

III. Response to tissue injury (Fig. 17-1)

    A. Classification of pain

      1. Physiologic pain; minimal or nontissue-damaging stimuli that is experienced in everyday life and serves

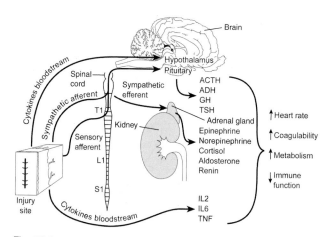

Fig. 17-1

Tissue injury causes significant hemodynamic, hematologic, metabolic, and immune mediated responses.

a protective role from noxious stimuli (e.g., heat, cold, pressure)
   a. Well localized
   b. Transient
   c. High threshold
2. Clinical pain is composed of inflammatory pain and neuropathic pain
   a. Inflammatory pain is caused by peripheral tissue damage (e.g., crushing, surgery)
      (1) Low threshold to pain (allodynia)
      (2) Exaggerated response to noxious stimuli (hyperalgesia)
      (3) Poorly localized (secondary hyperalgesia)
      (4) Initiates peripheral and central sensitization
   b. Neuropathic pain is caused by damage to the peripheral nervous system (e.g., burning, stabbing); characteristics are similar to those of inflammatory pain
3. Clinical pain differs from physiologic pain because of the presence of pathologic hypersensitivity
B. Peripheral and central hypersensitization (Fig. 17-2)
   1. Peripheral sensitization causes a decrease in pain threshold (hyperalgesia)
      a. At the site of injury
      b. In surrounding tissue
   2. Central sensitization
      a. Activity-dependent increase in the excitability of spinal neurons termed *spinal facilitation* or *windup*
         (1) Evokes progressively greater responses in dorsal-horn, wide dynamic-range neurons
         (2) Increases the size of peripheral receptive fields
         (3) Demonstrates continual changes (field plasticity) in spatial, temporal, and threshold qualities that parallel postinjury hyperalgesia
      b. Central sensitization includes "windup" and a prolonged phase of hyperalgesia; mediated by substance P (NK-1) and glutamate (NMDA) receptors
   3. Differences between peripheral and central sensitization
      a. Peripheral sensitization is produced by low-intensity stimuli activating Ad and C nociceptors

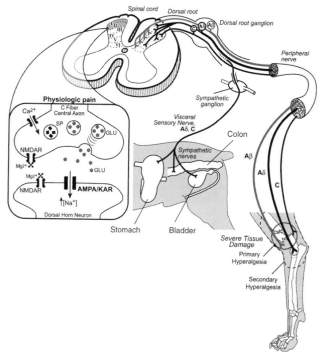

Fig. 17-2

Trauma causes peripheral sensitization that when not treated or inadequately treated can result in central sensitization.

        b. Central sensitization is produced by normal, low-threshold A-β sensory fibers because of changes in central processing from neural inputs

  C. Implications for pain therapy

    1. Complete analgesia is required during surgery intraoperative analgesia can be produced by general anesthesia, local anesthetics, and a variety of analgesic drugs (Table 17-1)

        a. Inhalation anesthetics (isoflurane, sevoflurane, desflurane)

        b. Hypnotics (barbiturates, etomidate, propofol)

TABLE 17-1

INJECTABLE ANALGESIC DRUGS AND THEIR MECHANISM OF ACTION

DRUG	MECHANISM OF ACTION
Opioids (morphine, fentanyl, methadone, meperidine, hydromorphone, oxymorphone, buprenorphine, butorphanol)	Combine with opioid receptors to produce sedation, analgesia, and euphoria
α_2-Agonists (xylazine, detomidine, medetomidine, romifidine)	Combine with α_2-receptors to produce sedation, muscle relaxation, and analgesia
Nonsteroidal antiinflammatory drugs (flunixin meglumine, phenylbutazone, aspirin, carprofen, ketoprofen, etodolac, meloxicam, deracoxib, piroxicam)	Act centrally (CNS) on the hypothalamus; antiinflammatory and analgesic activity mediated by peripheral inhibition of prostaglandins
Local anesthetics (lidocaine, mepivacaine, bupivacaine, ropivacaine)	Block nerve transmission of electrical impulses

CNS, Central nervous system.

    c. Dissociogenic drugs (ketamine, tiletamine)

    d. Local anesthetics (lidocaine, mepivacaine, bupivacaine, ropivacaine)

    e. Opioids (morphine, fentanyl, methadone, meperidine, hydromorphone, oxymorphone, buprenorphine, butorphanol)

    f. α_2-Agonists (xylazine, detomidine, medetomidine, romifidine)

    g. Nonsteroidal antiinflammatory drugs (NSAIDs); (aspirin, phenylbutazone, flunixin meglumine, ketoprofen, carprofen, etodolac, meloxicam, deracoxib, piroxicam)

2. Converting clinical pain to physiologic pain may be sufficient before and after surgery; best accomplished with behavioral modifiers and antiinflammatory drugs

    a. Opioids

   b. α_2-Agonists
   c. NSAIDs
3. Prevent the establishment of pain and central sensitization (Tables 17-2 and 17-3)
   a. Preemptive analgesia; drug combinations (e.g., opioids-tranquilizers) may be needed
   b. Dose and routes of drug administration can produce select effects; intravenous IV), intramuscular, subcutaneous (SQ), and oral (PO) versus epidural, intrathecal, and site-specific administration

NSAIDS (Table 17-3)

I. Reduce inflammation and produce analgesia primarily through inhibition of prostaglandin synthesis
   A. CNS actions not well characterized
   B. Inhibit the activity of cyclooxygenase (COX) peripherally
II. Prostaglandins
   A. During inflammation, prostaglandins:
      1. Cause vasodilation
      2. Increase vascular permeability
      3. Sensitize peripheral pain receptors
      4. Chronically, new blood vessels and granulation tissue are produced
   B. Prostaglandins also help maintain tissues
      1. Protect gastric mucosa
      2. Facilitate platelet aggregation
      3. Regulate renal blood flow
   C. Currently available NSAIDs inhibit all prostaglandin formation
III. COX enzyme isoforms
   A. COX-1
      1. Responsible for basal prostaglandin production for normal homeostasis in many tissues
   B. COX-2
      1. Involved in pathologic process and found in sites of inflammation
      2. Expressed from endothelial cells, smooth muscle cells, chondrocytes, fibroblasts, monocytes, macrophages, and synovial cells

TABLE 17-2
PREEMPTIVE ANALGESIC DRUGS AND DOSES*

DRUG	DOSE (mg/kg)				ROUTES	DOSE INTERVAL (HR)
	DOGS	CATS	HORSES	RUMINANTS†		
Local anesthetics						
Epidural drugs‡						
Lidocaine	1 ml/4.5-6 kg (2%)	1 ml/4.5-6 kg (2%)			—	1-2
Bupivacaine	1 ml/4.5-6 kg (0.75%)	1 ml/4.5-6 kg (0.75%)			—	4-6
Ropivacaine	0.5	0.5			—	4-6
Morphine	0.1	0.1		0.5-1	—	16-24
					—	12
Fentanyl	1-10 μg/kg	1-10 μg/kg			—	3-5
Oxymorphone	0.05-0.1	0.05			—	7-10
Butorphanol	0.25	0.25			—	2-4
Xylazine	0.1-0.4	0.1-0.4			—	3
Medetomidine	10-15 μg/kg	10-15 μg/kg			—	6-7
Opioids						
Agonists						
Morphine	0.4-2	0.1-0.2	0.05-0.1		IV, IM	1-4
		0.1-0.3 mg/kg/hr		0.5-1	IV	12-48
					IV	12

Drug				Route	
Meperidine	1-5	0.5-1		IV, IM	0.5-2
Hydromorphone	0.1-0.4	0.1-0.2		IV, IM	4-6
Oxymorphone	0.1-0.4	0.1-0.2	0.001-0.02	IV, IM	4-6
				IV6	
Methadone	0.5-2	0.1-0.02		IV, IM	2-6
Fentanyl	2-6 µg/kg	1-3 µg/kg		IV	0.2-0.5
	2-5 µg/kg/hr	1-4 µg/kg/hr		IV	12-72
	2-5 µg/kg/hr	2-5 µg/kg/hr		Transdermal patch	8-12 onset of effect; 2-4 days duration
Codeine	0.5-2	0.5-2		PO	4-6
	0.5-2	Contraindicated		PO with paracetamol (acetaminophen)	6-8
	0.5-2	0.5-2		SQ	
Agonist-antagonists					
Butorphanol	0.2-0.8	0.2-0.8		IV, IM	1-2
	0.1-0.3 mg/ kg/hr			IV	6-12
			0.05		
Pentazocine	0.5-4	0.5-2		SQ	6
Nalbuphine	0.5-1 0.2	0.4		IV, IM	2-4
				IV, IM	1-6

Continued

TABLE 17-2

PREEMPTIVE ANALGESIC DRUGS AND DOSES—cont'd

DRUG	DOSE (mg/kg)					ROUTES	DOSE INTERVAL (HR)
	DOGS	CATS	HORSES	RUMINANTS†			
Partial Agonists							
Buprenorphine	0.01-0.04	0.01-0.04	0.01-0.04	0.005 (sheep and goats)		IV, IM IV12 IM	6-12 12
α₂-Agonists							
Medetomidine	0.005-0.02	0.01-0.04	0.01-0.02			IV, IM IV IV, SQ	1-4 12 1-3
Xylazine	0.4-1	0.4-1	0.5-1			IV	12
Romifidine	0.04-0.09	0.09-0.18	0.04-0.08			IM, SQ IV	2-4 12
Detomedine			0.01-0.02			IV	12

*Refer to the text for description of local, regional, intercostal, and intrapleural nerve blocks (bupivacaine and ropivacaine 1to3 mg/kg, for selective nerve blocks). Lidocaine can be administered by infusion (2 to 3 ml/kg/hr [50 mg/kg/min]; IV) as an adjunct to analgesia.

†Refers to adult cattle unless otherwise noted.

‡Drug is diluted in 1 ml of 0.9% saline/5 kg; epidural opioids and local anesthetics are frequently combined (0.1 mg/kg of oxymorphone diluted in 0.75% bupivacaine to a volume of 1 ml/5 kg) to produce longer acting analgesic effects.

NOTE: Morphine (0.1 mg/kg) has been administered intraarticularly for added analgesia after stifle joint surgery in dogs. Magnesium sulfate 6 to 8 mg/kg/hr or 5 to15 mEq/L/hr can be administered as an adjunct to analgesia.

PO, By mouth; *IV*, intravenous; *IM*, intramuscular; *GI*, gastrointestinal.

TABLE 17-3

NONSTEROIDAL ANTIINFLAMMATORY DRUGS AND DOSES

DRUG	DOSE (mg/kg)				ROUTES	DOSE INTERVAL (HR)	APPROVED INDICATIONS	PRECAUTION AND COMMENTS
	DOGS	CATS	HORSES	RUMINANTS				
Salicylates								
Aspirin	10-35	10-15		100	PO	8-12 (dogs); 24-48 (cats)		Gastrointestinal side-effects (ulcers, hemorrhage); renal failure
					PO	12		
Propionic acids								
Carprofen*	4.4				PO (SID)	SID	Pain and inflammation associated with osteoarthritis and pain associated with soft tissue or orthopedic surgery	
	2.2				PO (BID)	BID		
	4.4				SQ			
		2			SQ, PO	10 (dogs); 40 (cats)		
			0.05-1.1		IV	24		

*Nonsteroidal antiinflammatory drugs approved for use in dogs in North America.

Continued

TABLE 17-3

NONSTEROIDAL ANTIINFLAMMATORY DRUGS AND DOSES—cont'd

DRUG	DOSE (mg/kg)				ROUTES	DOSE INTERVAL (HR)	APPROVED INDICATIONS	PRECAUTION AND COMMENTS
	DOGS	CATS	HORSES	RUMINANTS				
Ibuprofen	5-10	Not used			PO	24-48		Gastrointestinal side-effects (ulcers, hemorrhage); renal failure
Naproxen	1-2	Not used			PO	24-72		
Ketoprofen	0.5-2.2	0.5-2.2			IM (dogs), SQ, PO	24; approximately 2 days (cats)		
			1.1-2.2		IV	24		
				2	IV	12		
Etodolac*	10-15	Not used			PO	24 (SID)	Pain and inflammation associated with osteoarthritis	Safety not evaluated in dogs ≤12 months, dogs used for breeding, or pregnant or lactating bitches

Fenamates						
Flunixin meglumine	0.25-1	Not used		IV, IM	24; do not repeat	
				IV	24	
			0.2-1.1	IV	12	
				PO	24	
Meclofenamic acid	1-2	Not used	1			
Pyrazoles						
Phenylbutazone	10-22 (maximum 800 mg/day)	4-20		IV, PO	8-12 (dogs); 24-48 (cats)	
			2-4	IV	24	
			2-4	PO	12	
				PO	24	
				PO	SID	
Tepoxalin*	Loading: 10 or 20, maintenance: 10	Not used	5	PO	SID	Pain and inflammation associated with osteoarthritis	Not evaluated in dogs ≤6 months, dogs used for breeding, or pregnant or lactating bitches

*Nonsteroidal antiinflammatory drugs approved for use in dogs in North America.

Continued

TABLE 17-3
NONSTEROIDAL ANTIINFLAMMATORY DRUGS AND DOSES—cont'd

DRUG	DOSE (mg/kg)				ROUTES	DOSE INTERVAL (HR)	APPROVED INDICATIONS	PRECAUTION AND COMMENTS
	DOGS	CATS	HORSES	RUMINANTS				
Oxicams								
Piroxicam	0.2-0.4	Not used			PO	48		
Meloxicam*†	Loading: 0.2, maintenance: 0.1	Preoperative: 0.3			PO IV, SQ	SID SID	Pain and inflammation associated with osteoarthritis	Loading dose can be administered SQ or IV; not evaluated in dogs ≤6 months, dogs used for breeding, or pregnant or lactating bitches
	Loading: 0.2, maintenance: 0.1				PO SQ, PO	24 (dogs); 11-21 (cats)		

Coxibs

Deracoxib*	Osteoarthritis: 1-2 Postoperative: 3-4	Not used	PO PO	SID SID (7-day limit)	Pain and inflammation associated with osteoarthritis and postoperative pain and inflammation associated with orthopedic surgery	Safety not evaluated in dogs <4 months, dogs used for breeding, or pregnant or lactating bitches
Firocoxib*	5	Not used	PO	SID	Pain and inflammation associated with osteoarthritis	Safety not evaluated in dogs <10 wks, dogs used for breeding, or pregnant or lactating bitches

Phenacetin derivatives

Acetaminophen	10-15	Not used	PO	8-12		Liver failure.

*Nonsteroidal antiinflammatory drugs approved for use in dogs in North America.

†Only nonsteroidal antiinflammatory drug approved for use (preoperative only) in cats in North America.

C. Selective inhibition of certain prostaglandins primarily produced by COX-2 should allow for the therapeutic analgesic and antiinflammatory effects while greatly diminishing the unwanted side effects caused by COX-1 inhibition

---

PRINCIPAL POINTS ■ NSAIDs

- Inhibition of COX and prevent prostaglandin synthesis
- Reduction of inflammation
- Analgesia
- Antipyretic

IV. Minimal acute side effects
V. Toxicity associated with gastrointestinal ulceration and renal papillary necrosis

---

CAUTION · NSAIDs

- Gastrointestinal ulceration
- Renal papillary necrosis
- Use in patients with less blood volume
- Use in patients with significant pulmonary disease

VI. Currently used NSAIDs
   A. Aspirin, Piroxicam, Phenylbutazone
      1. Widely used (PO and IV); Phenylbutazone is used in horses
      2. Primarily COX-1 selective
      3. Used to treat pain and for a variety of musculoskeletal inflammatory conditions
      4. Potentially toxic in dogs, cats, and horses (especially foals) (gastric ulceration, renal necrosis, anemia)
   B. Flunixin meglumine
      1. Used in horses (PO, IV)
      2. Not COX-2 selective
      3. Used for musculoskeletal conditions and mild colic
      4. Counteracts the effects of absorbed endotoxins

     5. Toxic in dogs and cats (single dose occasionally used for ocular inflammation)

C. Carprofen
1. Used in dogs (PO, SQ)
2. COX-2 selective in dogs
3. Indicated for chronic arthritis and mild perioperative pain
4. Liver toxicity reported in Labrador retrievers (resolves with drug withdrawal)

D. Ketoprofen
1. Approved for use in horses (IV)
2. Used in dogs and cats (IV, intramuscular, SQ) for perioperative analgesic

E. Meloxicam
1. Used in dogs and cats (PO, IV, SQ; only SQ in cats)
2. COX-2 selective in dogs
3. Indicated for chronic arthritis and mild perioperative pain in dogs
4. Only once before surgery is approved in cats in the United States

F. Etodolac
1. Used in dogs (PO)
2. Not COX-2 selective
3. Used for chronic osteoarthritis
4. Adverse events on the gastrointestinal tract seem to be limited

G. Tolfenamic acid
1. Used in dogs and cats (PO, SQ)
2. Not COX-2 selective
3. Used for acute and chronic pain management
4. Adverse effects on the gastrointestinal tract seem to be limited

H. Deracoxib
1. Used for dogs and cats (PO)
2. COX-2 selective
3. Used for musculoskeletal conditions

CHAPTER EIGHTEEN

Acupuncture Analgesia

"Medicine is not only a science, but also the art of letting our own individuality interact with the individuality of the patient."

ALBERT SCHWEITZER

OVERVIEW

Acupuncture can be used to induce pain relief (hypoalgesia) in clinical disorders and as a complementary method of pain control during surgical procedures in well-restrained, large and small animal patients. Acupuncture analgesia is best achieved by electrostimulation through acupuncture needles in acupuncture points. Many acupuncture points can be used to induce electroacupuncture analgesia (EAA) in animals. It is not known which point combination is best for a particular operation. Generally, the area of analgesia is related to the site of electrostimulation. The major advantages of EAA are good analgesia in high-risk patients without producing central nervous system (CNS) and respiratory depression, bradycardia, and hypotension commonly observed after the use of sedatives, opioids, and general anesthetics; excellent postoperative pain relief; fast postoperative recovery of appetite and gut and bladder function; and fast postoperative wound healing with minimal infection. The major disadvantages are the need for very good restraint; a long induction period (mean time is 20 minutes) with variable degrees of analgesia; maintenance of sensations to touch, pressure, and traction; poor relaxation of abdominal muscles attributable to "ballooning" of viscera; nausea and/or vomiting attributable to prolonged manipulation of viscera and organs or traction on mesentery; and maintenance of reflexes to sight, sound, and fear in conscious animals.

346

TYPES OF OPERATIONS POTENTIALLY PERFORMED UNDER EAA

I. Dog
   A. Cesarean section with no depressive effects on the fetus
   B. Ovariohysterectomy, including toxic pyometra
   C. Abdominal laparotomy
   D. Gastric and intestinal surgery
   E. Nephrectomy
   F. Splenectomy
   G. Umbilical hernioplasty
   H. Removal of mammary and skin tumors
   I. Ear cropping
   J. Craniotomy
   K. Open reduction and repair of long bone fractures
II. Horses, cattle, sheep, pigs
   A. Castration
   B. Orchidopexy
   C. Reposition of prolapsed uterus
   D. Surgery of anal and vaginal region
   E. Relief of dystocia
   F. Surgery on esophagus and rumen
   G. Repair of navel and umbilical hernia
   H. Surgery on the bladder and urethra
   I. Orthopedic surgery (bones and joints)

EQUIPMENT

I. Acupuncture needles
   A. Human acupuncture needles: 29 to 34 gauge
   B. Veterinary acupuncture needles: 22 to 26 gauge for large animals; 26 to 30 gauge for small animals
   C. The needles are inserted at acupuncture points to the correct depth, taped or sutured firmly in position, and connected in pairs to the output socket of an acupuncture electrostimulator
   D. Each pair of electrodes should be on the same side of the spinal cord. To prevent cardiac fibrillation, any one pair of leads must not cross the spine between the cervical and thoracic vertebrae

E. The leads may be alternated between needles if more needles are used than can be stimulated simultaneously

II. Acupuncture electrostimulators

A. There are many electrostimulators on the market today. They are manufactured in China, Japan, the United States, Canada, Europe, and Australia

B. There is little standardization of equipment. The equipment is expected to have the following characteristics:
1. Strength
2. Portability
3. Battery-operated
4. Outputs for at least six to eight electrodes
5. Delivers a bipolar waveform (+) and (−) at each electrode to prevent electrolytic injury from prolonged use of monopolar waveform
6. Delivers a square or spike wave form biphasic

C. A handheld unit (Pointer Plus, M.E.D. Servi-Systems, Canada Ltd.) to locate and stimulate acupuncture and trigger points, using 10 Hz, 1 to 25 volts, and 1 to 50 milliamps, is shown in Fig. 18-1

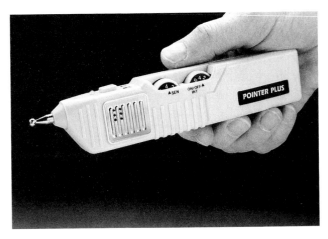

Fig. 18-1
Pointer Plus, a handheld unit for locating and stimulating acupuncture points.

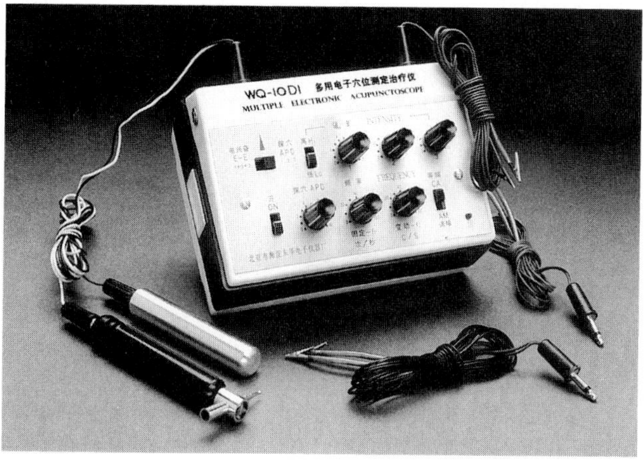

Fig. 18-2
Electronic acupunctoscope for locating and stimulating acupuncture points percutaneously.

D. A multiple electronic acupunctoscope (WQ10C, M.E.D. Servi-Systems, Canada Ltd.) is shown in Fig. 18-2. It possesses the following characteristics:
   1. It detects acupuncture and auricular points
   2. It stimulates three pairs of acupuncture needles for acupuncture analgesia and therapy
   3. The frequency can be varied between 1 and 1000 Hz
   4. It has a constant amplitude and amplitude modulation switch
   5. It operates on 9-volt batteries

RESTRAINT

I. Technique in small animals
   A. Small animals are generally operated on in lateral, dorsal, or ventral recumbency
   B. Dogs are given a sedative/analgesic and small doses of general anesthetics

    C. The animal's elbows and hocks are tied with bandages and secured to the operation table

    D. A tape bandage may be tied around the dog's jaws to prevent biting (Fig. 18-3)

    E. The owner or an attendant should comfort and speak to the dog from time to time during surgery

II. Technique in large animals

    A. Electroacupuncture may be performed in horses and cattle restrained in the standing position or in dorsal, lateral, or ventral recumbency

    B. For a standing animal, usual methods for restraint (stock, chute, cattle crate) as applied for surgery under local anesthesia may be used

    C. Nervous animals may be given a sedative/analgesic intravenously

    D. Recumbency may be induced with a short-acting, intravenous anesthetic

    E. Recumbent animals should be securely restrained with ropes

    F. The operator should keep noise and movement to a minimum

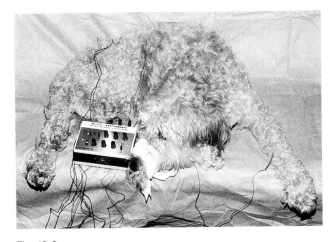

Fig. 18-3
Sedated and restrained dog during electroacupuncture stimulation.

SELECTION OF ACUPUNCTURE POINTS

I. General statements
   A. Point combinations for induction of hypalgesia sufficient for surgery vary with the operative site and the preference and experience of the surgeon
   B. Points are generally chosen based on the channel (meridian) theory of human acupuncture
   C. Acupuncture points in animals have the same name and code as in humans and are transposed from human acupuncture anatomy
   D. Channels have a superficial course (from the first to the last point on the channel), a deep course (going to the organ of the channel), and a collateral course (linking to interior and exterior parts of the body). This may explain why a Liver point is used for operations of the eye, a Heart point for operation of the tongue, and a Kidney point for operation of the ear and bone

II. Acupuncture point selection in the dog. In general, the following points bilateral of the spine are chosen:
   A. For surgery in all areas: BL 23 +/or SP 6; LI 11 + Japanese point In Ko Ten; ST 36 + Japanese point Bo Ko Ku
   B. For surgery on the head, neck, thorax, and front limb: PC 6 + TH 5
   C. For surgery on the abdomen and hindlimbs: SP 6 + ST 36 and paraincisional for ovariohysterectomy
   D. For surgery on high-risk dogs: LI 4 + LI 11 + SP 6 + ST 36
   E. For back surgery: BL 23 + BL 40 + BL 60 + ST 36 + GB 34

III. Anatomic location of acupuncture points in dogs
   A. Fig 18-4 illustrates the location of the various acupuncture points for dogs
   B. The International Veterinary Acupuncture Society describes the abbreviation and location of these points as follows:
      1. LI 4 (large intestine point 4): between the first and second metacarpal bones, approximately in the middle of the second metacarpal bone on the radial side

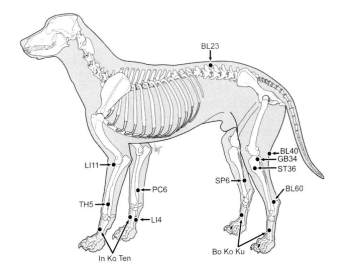

Fig. 18-4
Location of various acupuncture points to induce analgesia in dogs.

2. LI 11 (large intestine point 11): at the end of the lateral cubital crease, halfway between the biceps tendon and the lateral epicondyle of the humerus, with the elbow flexed
3. PC 6 (pericardium point 6): at two ribs-width above the transverse crease of the carpus between the tendons of the flexor digitorum superficialis and flexor carpi radialis
4. TH 5 (triple Heater point 5): at two ribs-width above the carpus, on the cranial aspect of the interosseous space between the radius and ulna
5. In Ko Ten: between metacarpal bones 2 and 3
6. BL 23 (bladder point 23): at one- to two ribs-width lateral to the caudal border of the spinous process of the second lumbar vertebra
7. ST 36 (stomach point 36): at one finger-width from the anterior crest of the tibia, in the belly of the medial tibialis cranialis

8. GB 34 (gallbladder point 34): in the depression anterior and distal to the head of the fibula
9. BL 40 (bladder point 40): in the center of the popliteal crease
10. SP 6 (spleen point 6): at three ribs-width directly above the tip of the medial malleolus, on the posterior border of the tibia
11. BL 60 (bladder point 60): in the depression, between the lateral malleolus and tendon calcaneus, level with the tip of the lateral malleolus
12. Bo Ko Ku: between metatarsal bones 2 and 3

C. The needle penetrates completely from TH 5 to PC 6 between the radius and ulna of both limbs

D. The needle may penetrate completely through the limb at ST 36 and SP 6 of both hindlimbs

IV. Acupuncture point selection in horses (Fig. 18-5, *A, B*) and cattle (Fig. 18-6)

A. For abdominal surgery: LU 1 (lung point 1) + TH 8 (triple heater point 8)

1. Technique: one needle is inserted in LU 1 (caudal to the shoulder in the second intercostal space) for a depth of 3 to 5 cm (positive pole). A second needle is inserted at TH 8 (approximately one hand-width ventral to the elbow joint, on the lateral side) and is advanced ventromedially caudal to the radius/ulna to reach PC 4.5, subcutaneously dorsal to the "chestnut" (negative pole). A third needle is inserted at small intestine point 10 (SI 10, approximately on the caudal border of the deltoids and between the long and lateral heads of the triceps brachii). A fourth needle is inserted in the center depression between the bulbs of the heel on the forelimb

B. For abdominal, vaginal, and hindlimb surgery: Bai Hui (main point) + Wei Gan (secondary point) + San Tai (tertiary point) + Tian Ping (minor point) + added points on or near the spinal nerves supplying the surgical site

1. Technique: one needle is inserted in acupuncture point Bai Hui (GV 3a point) at the dorsal midline of the lumbosacral space, 3 to 5 cm deep. A second needle is inserted in Wei Gan (at the dorsal midline of the

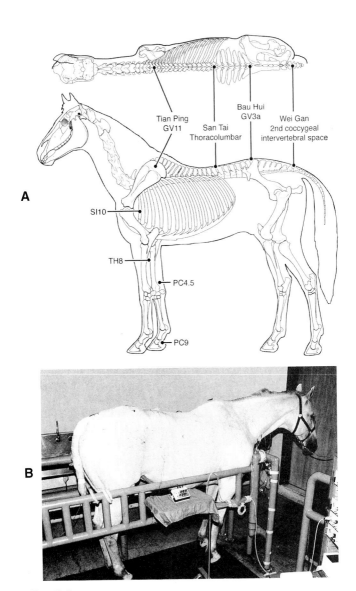

Fig. 18-5

A, Location of various acupuncture points to induce analgesia in horses. **B,** Percutaneous electrical nerve stimulation of various acupuncture points in a 560-kg Thoroughbred mare, which is well sedated (detomidine 5 mg intramuscularly) and physically restrained.

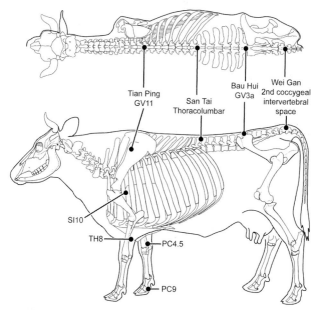

Tian Ping
GV11

San Tai
Thoracolumbar

Bau Hui
GV3a

Wei Gan
2nd coccygeal
intervertebral
space

SI10

TH8

PC4.5

PC9

Fig. 18-6
Location of various acupuncture points to induce analgesia in cattle.

second coccygeal intervertebral space), 1 to 1.5 cm deep. A third needle is inserted in San Tai (at the dorsal midline of the thoracolumbar intervertebral space), 2 to 4 cm deep. A fourth needle is inserted at Tian Ping (at the dorsal midline of the fourth or fifth thoracic intervertebral space, GV 11 point) and advanced cranioventrally 6 to 8 cm

V. Acupuncture point selection in pigs
  A. The Akita Veterinary Acupuncture Research Unit in Japan tested many point combinations in pigs, including LU 1 and TH 8 penetrating to PC 4.5
  B. The most effective points for producing hypoalgesia are located in the midline of the thoracolumbar space (point Tian Ping) and lumbosacral spaces (Bai Hui) penetrating almost to the dura mater spinalis

NEEDLE PLACEMENT

I. The needles are inserted deeply into the acupuncture points
   A. The points are palpated at precise anatomic landmarks
   B. Point finders (Figs. 18-1 and 18-2) are helpful in localizing acupuncture points
II. The needles are taped or sutured in position to prevent dislodgment

ELECTROACUPUNCTURE STIMULATION (EAA)

I. Voltage, current, frequency
   A. The power controls of the stimulator are set at zero
   B. The pairs of needles are attached to each circuit of the electrostimulator with alligator clips
   C. The power switch is turned on and the electrical stimulation frequency is set at 2 to 15 Hz
   D. The output voltage is increased slowly until the needles begin to twitch in time with the frequency of the stimulator at 2 to 15 Hz
   E. At higher frequencies (more than 15 Hz), the muscle goes into local spasm, and the needle vibration is not obvious
   F. The output voltage from each control is first increased to maximum tolerance of anesthesia mode, dense-disperse waveform
   G. The output is then reduced to a level the animal can tolerate without obvious discomfort or pain (e.g., restlessness, struggling, vocalization)
II. Onset and duration of hypoalgesia
   A. Induction time for hypoalgesia ranges from 10 to 40 minutes; 20 minutes is the duration most commonly reported
   B. The surgery site is tested for analgesia by grasping the skin with toothed forceps or clamps or pricking the skin with needles or pins every 5 minutes after the onset of electrical stimulation
   C. The electroacupuncture stimulation is continued during the entire surgery
   D. Inadequate or excessive electroacupuncture stimulus produces little or no analgesia

ADVANTAGES OF ELECTROACUPUNCTURE STIMULATION

I. EAA can induce hypoalgesia sufficient for surgery
   A. It can be used in "balanced anesthesia" to greatly reduce the dose of sedatives/analgesic and anesthetic drugs
   B. It is advantageous in Cesarean sections because it has no depressive effects on the fetus
   C. It is suitable for animals that are in shock, debilitated, or toxic

II. EAA is suitable for prolonged surgery (up to 10 hours)
   A. Autonomic functions remain stable

III. When compared with general anesthesia:
   A. The technique is relatively simple and inexpensive
   B. There is less hemorrhage
   C. Postoperative recovery of appetite and gastrointestinal and bladder function are faster
   D. Postoperative healing is faster; attributable to no chemical interference with wound healing
   E. Postoperative infection is less
   F. Postoperative pain is reduced

DISADVANTAGES OF ELECTROACUPUNCTURE STIMULATION

I. An induction period of 10 to 40 minutes (average is 20 minutes) is necessary

II. To facilitate surgery, sedatives and anesthetics are needed in 50% to 95% of cases

III. Intrathoracic surgery cannot be performed

IV. Physical restraint is necessary
   A. The amount of restraint needed depends on the skill of the surgeon and tolerance of the patient

V. Muscle relaxation may be inadequate
   A. Poor relaxation of abdominal muscles can cause "ballooning" of viscera

VI. All sensory inputs except pain are present
   A. Manipulation of viscera and organs or traction of mesentery can induce nausea, vomiting, and shock

VII. Certain body regions are more sensitive to pain than others
- A. The skin, serosa (peritoneum, pleura), periosteum, and nerves are very sensitive
- B. Incision of such organs requires the frequency and output voltage to be increased to counteract the pain
- C. The success rate for intestinal surgery is higher than for limb surgery

VIII. Pain thresholds vary among species
- A. Cattle and sheep are the most tolerant, followed by dogs, pigs, and horses

IX. Temperaments vary among species
- A. Nervous animals may be tolerant but are easily frightened and difficult to restrain, even with good analgesia

MECHANISMS OF ACUPUNCTURE ANALGESIA

I. The mechanisms of acupuncture analgesia have been reviewed in the medical literature*

II. Modern theories attribute the effects of EAA to:
- A. Inhibition of ascending (sensory) pain signals at the peripheral, spinal ("pain inhibition gates"), and central level
- B. Activation of descending brain-based pain inhibition mechanism, especially the midbrain and hypothalamus

III. Sensory nervous system components involved in pain sensation include A-delta and C fibers
- A. Acupuncture points are cutaneous areas with high concentrations of nerves (particularly A-delta fibers), mast cells, capillaries, venules, and lower electrical resistance than surrounding areas
- B. Acupuncture stimuli are transmitted to the spinal cord by peripheral nerves
- C. A-delta fibers are 10 times thicker, transmit impulses 10 times faster, have a lower threshold, and are associated with milder pain sensation than C fibers
- D. The "gate" theory suggests that A-delta fibers carry nonpainful sensations rapidly to the spinal cord where

---

*Kho H-G, Robertson EN: The mechanisms of acupuncture analgesia: review and update, *Am J Acupunct* 25 (4):261-281, 1997.

inhibitory neurons are stimulated and prevent slower pain impulses from reaching higher pain centers of conscious perception

IV. Neurotransmitters involved in acupuncture therapy and pain inhibition include:
  A. Endorphins (beta-endorphin, enkephalins, dynorphin)
  B. Serotonin
  C. Norepinephrine
  D. Acetylcholine

V. Other neurotransmitters that potentiate acupuncture analgesia include:
  A. Parasympathomimetics
  B. Substance P
  C. Histamine
  D. Cyclic guanosine monophosphate

VI. Frequency of stimulation affects fibers and neurotransmitters involved in pain perception response
  A. <5 Hz: A-delta fibers and enkephalin
  B. >100 Hz: C fibers and dynorphin
  C. >200 Hz: analgesia via serotonin and norepinephrine

VII. Duration of stimulation may change the mechanism of analgesia from opiate to nonopiate
  A. Segmental acupuncture analgesia usually occurs rapidly
  B. Generalized opiate effects take 20 to 40 minutes

VIII. Intensity of stimulation (voltage) traditionally is increased until muscle fasciculation is seen at 1 to 5 Hz. This produces the following conditions:
  A. General analgesia with prolonged induction
  B. Prolonged analgesia after cessation of stimulation
  C. Endorphin-mediated analgesia
  D. Analgesia that is reversible by naloxone

IX. High-frequency/low-intensity stimulation results in local segmental analgesia, which is irreversible by naloxone

ACUPUNCTURE SUPPLIES

M.E.D. Servi-Systems
8 Sweetnam Drive
Stittsville, Ontario
Canada K2S 1G2

1-800-267-6868 (Canada and United States)
1 (613) 836-3004 (worldwide)
1 (613) 831-0240 (fax)
http: //www.medserv.ca

Lhasa OMS, Inc.
230 Libbey Parkway
Weymouth, Massachusetts 02189
1-800-722-8775
(781) 340-1071
(781) 335-5779 (fax)
http://www.lhasaoms.com/home.ccml

PROFESSIONAL ORGANIZATIONS

The International Veterinary Acupuncture Society (IVAS)
PO Box 271395
Ft. Collins, Colorado 80527
(970) 266-0666
(970) 266-0777 (fax)
office@ivas.org (e-mail)
http: //www.ivas.org

The American Academy of Veterinary Acupuncture (AAVA)
100 Roscommon Drive, Suite 320
Middletown, Connecticut 06457
(860) 635-6300
(860) 635-6400 (fax)
office@aava.org (e-mail)
http: //www.aava.org

CHAPTER NINETEEN

Anesthetic Procedures and Techniques In Dogs

"Come now let us reason together."
LYNDON BAINES JOHNSON

OVERVIEW

Anesthetic procedures and techniques for dogs are designed to produce calming, sedation, and unconsciousness safely, effectively, and economically. Techniques using single drugs have largely been abandoned in favor of techniques producing sedation, analgesia, and anesthesia by combining different types of drugs in reduced doses, reducing unwanted side effects and toxicity. The advantage of combination drug therapy over single-drug therapy is a more controlled anesthetic state by manipulation of hypnosis, analgesia, and muscle relaxation. Combination drug therapy requires a comprehensive knowledge of the pharmacology of anesthetic drugs, their interactions, and potential side effects.

GENERAL CONSIDERATIONS

I. A variety of anesthetic procedures and techniques can be used to safely produce chemical restraint and anesthesia in dogs. Local anesthetic techniques (see Chapter 7) should be considered to augment analgesia

II. The choice of anesthetic regimen is influenced by the following characteristics:
   A. Breed and size (weight)
   B. Temperament
   C. Health and physical condition
   D. The procedure (medical; surgical)

    E. The duration of anesthesia

    F. The familiarity of personnel with the drugs being used

    G. Concurrent medication

    H. Available assistance

III. Whenever possible, drugs that are reversible should be used

IV. Endotracheal intubation should be performed whenever possible to ensure a patent airway

V. Careful monitoring is mandatory to recognize and treat untoward drug effects

VI. Food and water should be withheld for approximately 4 to 6 hours before surgery, except in very small, very young, or diseased dogs

PREANESTHETIC EVALUATIONS (SEE CHAPTER 2)

I. Review history and current drug therapy

II. Perform a physical examination

III. Review available laboratory data

IV. Formulate a specific anesthetic plan (Fig. 19-1)

    A. Determine whether additional preoperative tests are needed

    B. Choose appropriate drugs

V. Intravenous catheter placement is recommended in case of emergency

VI. Gather appropriate equipment and supplies

    A. Mouth gag or speculum

    B. Endotracheal tube

        1. Select diameter of cuffed endotracheal tube based on dog size, breed, and procedure; brachycephalic breeds usually have smaller diameter trachea (Table 19-1); a reinforced tube (kink resistant) should be used for procedures that require severe curvature of the neck (e.g., ophthalmic surgeries)

        2. Check cuff for leaks by inflating with air

        3. Use a stylet for small-diameter, endotracheal tubes and reinforced tubes

        4. Use an uncuffed endotracheal tube in very small animals (Fig. 19-2)

        5. Use a small amount of sterile lubricant

PREANESTHETIC EVALUATION

ANESTHETIST:_____
DATE:_____
CLINICIAN:_____
WARD/CAGE OR STALL #:_____

PROCEDURE: ....

BODY WEIGHT: .... **AGE:**.................

TEMPERAMENT:

OBJECTIVE FINDINGS
Temp_____ Pulse_____ Resp. _____
Cardiac auscultation_____
Pulse quality _____
Mucous membrane color_____
Capillary refill time_____
Respiratory auscultation _____

ASSESSMENT: Physical status I II III IV V E
Reasons:

CBC
  WBC_____ TP_____ PCV_____
  Fibrinogen _____
SERUM CHEMISTRIES
  BUN_____ GLUCOSE_____
  AST(SGOT)_____
  ALT(SGPT)_____
URINE SPECIFIC GRAVITY_____
OTHER RESULTS _____
PRIOR ANESTHESIA _____

COMPLICATIONS ANTICIPATED   pre op, intra op, post op: consider age , body wt.,
breed, position, surgical procedure, physical status.

Plan   Anesthesia regimen (include reasons as related to this animal)
(Include premeds, induction agent, inhalation agent, O_2 flow rate, post op analgesics)

DRUG   ROUTE   DOSE/#   MG   ML   REASONS OR JUSTIFICATION

MONITORING: Esophageal stethoscope, Doppler, ECG, Temp. Probe, Blood gas, Arterial Line,
Other_____

IV FLUID TYPE_____ Dose: MLS/HR_____ DROPS/MIN_____

ADMINISTRATION SET: MINI DRIP (60 drops/ml)   MAXI DRIP (10 drops/ml)

Approved_____

Fig. 19-1
Anesthetic plan.

C. Laryngoscope (Fig. 19-3)
1. Aids intubation by allowing visualization, illumination, and manipulation of tongue and laryngeal structures

TABLE 19-1
ENDOTRACHEAL TUBE SIZE FOR DOGS

BODY WEIGHT (KG)	TUBE SIZE (MM, ID)
2	5
4	6
7	7
9	8
12	8
14	9
20	10
30	12
40	14

2. May be optional, depending on anatomy and dog size
D. Anesthetic machine and breathing system
    1. Size and type of system determined by dog size
        a. Use a small-animal anesthetic machine (adult human anesthetic system) for dogs
           (1) Use the circle system for dogs weighing more than 3 kg

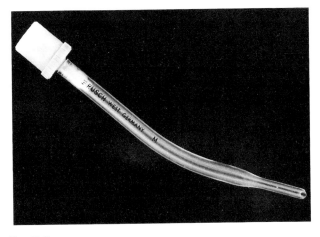

Fig. 19-2
A tapered uncuffed endotracheal tube (Cole catheter) for intubating smaller animals.

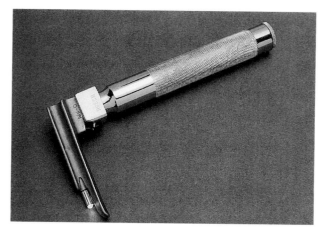

Fig. 19-3
A laryngoscope facilitates visualization and illumination for intubation.

(2) Use the non-rebreathing system for dogs weighing less than 3 kg
2. Rebreathing bag should be approximately five times the tidal volume. Tidal volume is 10 to 15 ml/kg (e.g., 5 kg × 10 ml/kg = 50 ml V_T)
3. Refill carbon dioxide absorbent canister if material is exhausted (discolored or dry)
4. Evaluate anesthetic system for possible malfunctions (see Chapter 13)
   a. Fill vaporizer and check operation
   b. Turn on flowmeters and check for free movement of indicator balls or slides
   c. Close pressure relief valve and pressurize the system using oxygen flush valve to 20 to 30 cm water and maintain for 15 seconds; check for leaks (Fig. 19-4)
5. Connect the waste gas scavenging system to the anesthetic circle or non-rebreathing system
E. Fresh gases
1. Oxygen
   a. Connect to "house" oxygen system, if present

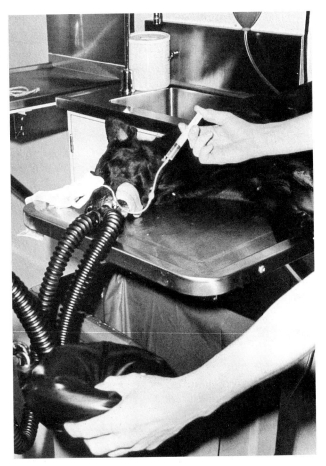

Fig. 19-4
Escape of gas from around the endotracheal tube can be eliminated by inflating the endotracheal tube cuff (right hand) until no gas escapes from the mouth during rebreathing bag compression (left hand) to 20 to 30 cm H_2O.

      b. Attach smaller (E) tanks to machine; change oxygen tank if pressure gauge reads less than 500 psi

    2. Nitrous oxide (used to produce analgesia)

      a. Optional

      b. Change tank if pressure gauge reads less than 750 psi

  F. Intravenous (IV) administration supplies

    1. IV catheter (16- to 23-gauge)

    2. Appropriate IV fluids

    3. Solution administration set (standard set 10 drops/ml, pediatric 60 drops/ml). Use 60 drop/ml on dogs less than 5 kg. Administer at 5 to 20 ml/kg/hr

    4. Fluid infusion pump (Fig. 19-5)

  G. Drugs

    1. Calculate appropriate drug dose and volume

    2. Draw drugs into labeled syringes

  H. Monitoring equipment (see Chapter 15)

    1. Electrocardiographic monitor

    2. Doppler or oscillometric blood pressure monitor

    3. Pulse oximeter

    4. Thermometer

    5. Esophageal stethoscope

    6. End-tidal gases (O_2, CO_2, inhalant)

  I. Ancillary supplies

    1. 4×4-inch gauze sponges

    2. Adhesive tape

    3. Roll gauze

    4. Flashlight

PREANESTHETIC MEDICATION (SEE CHAPTER 3)

I. Choice of drug determined by the dog's preoperative condition and any other special considerations pertinent to the procedure

II. Drugs given intramuscularly (IM) or subcutaneously (SQ) should be administered 10 to 20 minutes before catheterization and induction

III. Drugs used as premedications

  A. Anticholinergics

    1. Atropine 20 to 40 µg/kg IM, IV, or SQ

    2. Glycopyrrolate 5 to 10 µg/kg IM, IV, or SQ

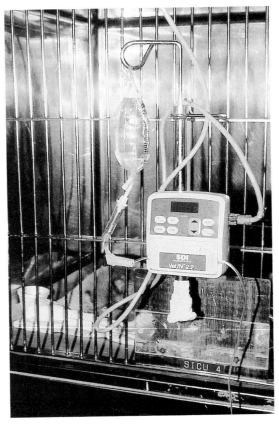

Fig. 19-5
Examples of infusion pumps. **A,** Infusion pump that uses a fluid administration set.

B. Tranquilizer
  1. Acepromazine 0.1 to 0.2 mg/kg IM, maximum total dose 4 mg
  2. Diazepam or midazolam 0.2 to 0.4 mg/kg IV, maximum total dose 5 mg; diazepam or midazolam is usually administered in conjunction with opioids; a single-drug use is recommended for old or depressed

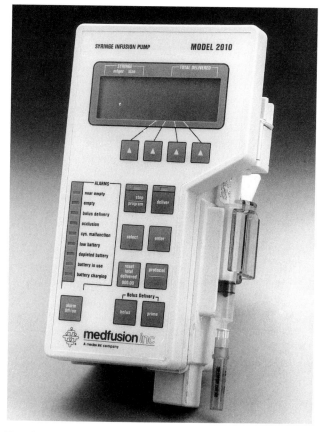

Fig. 19-5, cont'd
B, Infusion pump that uses a syringe.

dogs; young and healthy dogs may become excited (release of suppressed behavior)
C. Opioids (frequently used with tranquilizers)
   1. Morphine 0.1 to 0.3 mg/kg IM
      a. Epidural morphine (0.1 mg/kg, qs with 0.9% NaCl to a volume of 1 ml/5 kg)
   2. Hydromorphone 0.05 to 0.1 mg/kg IM

      3. Oxymorphone 0.1 to 0.3 mg/kg IM
      4. Butorphanol 0.2 to 0.4 mg/kg IM
      5. Buprenorphine 5 to 20 µg/kg IM
   D. α_2-Agonists
      1. Xylazine 0.2 to 1 mg/kg IM or IV (low end)
      2. Medetomidine 5 to 20 µg/kg IM or IV
      3. Romifidine 20 to 40 µg/kg IM or IV
   E. Tiletamine/zolazepam (Telazol®) 2 to 10 mg/kg IM or IV
      1. Vicious or mean dogs: Add 4 ml of 100 mg/ml ketamine and 1 ml of 100 mg/ml xylazine or 1 mg/ml medetomidine to a 5 ml bottle of Telazol®
         a. Dose 0.1 ml per 5 to 10 kg, IM
   F. Nonsteroidal antiinflammatory drugs
      1. Carprofen 4 mg/kg IM
      2. Meloxicam 0.2 mg/kg IM
      3. Deracoxib 0.5-1 mg/kg PO

INDUCTION

  I. IV
   A. Catheterize vein (s) (generally the cephalic vein)
   B. Start IV fluid administration to ensure catheter patency
      1. Lower fluid bag or bottle below the dog's thorax to allow blood to siphon back into catheter to confirm catheter placement
   C. Inject drug (s) at an appropriate rate (s), allowing time (15 to 30 seconds) for equilibration before administering further increments
   D. Specific IV induction drugs (see Chapter 8)
      1. Propofol 4 to 10 mg/kg IV (Table 19-2)
      2. Ultrashort-acting barbiturates
         a. Thiopental 2% to 5%; 8 to 20 mg/kg IV
         b. Methohexital 2%; 3 to 8 mg/kg IV
      3. Etomidate 0.5 to 2 mg/kg IV
      4. Ketamine 5 to 10 mg/kg IV
      5. Short-acting barbiturates
         a. Pentobarbital 10 to 30 mg/kg IV
      6. Injectable drug combinations
         a. Diazepam-lidocaine-thiopental: diazepam 0.2 mg/kg IV, lidocaine 2 mg/kg IV, and thiopental 4 mg/kg IV; do not mix in single syringe

TABLE 19-2

INJECTABLE ANESTHESIA TECHNIQUE INCLUDING INFUSION IN DOGS

PREMEDICATION	INDUCTION	MAINTENANCE	COMMENTS
Acepromazine 0.05 mg/kg IM	Propofol 4 mg/kg IV + fentanyl 2 µg/kg IV + atropin 40 µg/kg IV	Propofol 0.2-0.4 mg/kg/min IV + fentanyl 0.1-0.5 µg/kg/min IV	Whining or paddling may occur in recovery
—	Propofol 5 mg/kg	Propofol 0.4 mg/kg/min CRI	Provide a light plane of anesthesia, use of ventilatory support is recommended
Acepromazine 0.025 mg/kg IM + Atropine 0.02 mg/kg IM	Propofol 4 mg/kg (Greyhound) 3.2 mg/kg (non-Greyhound)	Propofol 0.4 mg/kg/min CRI	Muscle tremors may occur

CRI, Constant rate infusion.

(1) Useful in animals with central nervous system and/or cardiovascular depression

(2) Stabilizes myocardium

(3) Lidocaine reduces amount of thiopental required

b. Diazepam-ketamine: diazepam 0.25 mg/kg IV and ketamine 5 mg/kg IV. Maximum effect reached 60 to 180 seconds after drug administration

(1) Mix equal parts of diazepam (5 mg/ml in stock vial) and ketamine (100 mg/ml in stock vial) to yield a mixture that is 2.5 mg/ml diazepam and 50 mg/ml ketamine

(2) Use 1 ml of mixture per 10 kg; add 0.1 ml medetomidine for added analgesia and sedation

c. Ketamine-midazolam-butorphanol/oxymorphone: ketamine (7.5 mg/kg IV) and midazolam (0.375 mg/kg IV) with or without the 10-minute previous administration of butorphanol (0.2 mg/kg IV) or oxymorphone (0.1 mg/kg IV)

(1) Use with butorphanol or oxymorphone to improve induction

d. Thiopental-lidocaine: thiopental 11 mg/kg IV and lidocaine 2 to 4 mg/kg IV (do not combine in same syringe)

(1) Less cardiopulmonary depression than thiopental alone

(2) Shorter duration than thiopental alone

e. Oxymorphone/hydromorphone-diazepam: oxymorphone (0.05 mg/kg IV)/hydromorphone (0.1 mg/kg IV) and diazepam (0.2 mg/kg IV)

(1) Introduction effect is evident within 1 minute

(2) Additional amounts (same dose) of oxymorphone/hydromorphone (IV) may be necessary for intubation

II. Inhalant anesthesia

A. Sevoflurane or isoflurane produces optimal control of anesthesia. The odor of sevoflurane is less offensive than isoflurane and induction is faster (lower blood/gas partition coefficient)

1. Face mask

a. Be aware of potential for vomiting and possible aspiration

      b. Ensure adequate physical restraint
      c. Environmental pollution is significant
  2. Induction chamber
      a. For very small aggressive dogs
      b. Use high fresh-gas flow rates (4 to 5 L/min)
      c. Monitor closely for loss of righting reflex, then remove from box and complete induction with a mask
      d. Not recommended for routine use because control of anesthetic delivered is poor and atmospheric pollution with anesthetic gases is very significant

ENDOTRACHEAL INTUBATION

  I. Dogs are usually intubated in sternal recumbency
 II. Open the dog's mouth and manipulate the tongue to the side with the endotracheal tube; grasp the tongue with a gauze sponge, straighten the head and neck, and extend the tongue between the lower canine teeth to hold the mandible open (Fig. 19-6, *A*)
III. Locate the larynx and insert the endotracheal tube
    A. Direct visualization
    B. Use a laryngoscope to facilitate visualization of the larynx and reflect epiglottis rostral and ventral (Fig. 19-6, *B, C*)
    C. Potential difficulties
      1. Laryngospasm (0.1 ml lidocaine sprayed on the laryngeal cartilages reduces spasms)
        a. Larynx sensitized
        b. Dog not adequately anesthetized
      2. Soft-palate displacement prevents rostroventral movement of the epiglottis; push the soft palate dorsally with the endotracheal tube to visualize the epiglottis
      3. Mass involving the larynx or pharynx; may need a smaller tracheal tube or tracheotomy
    D. Turn on oxygen flowmeter
    E. Secure the tube to the dog and connect the breathing system to the endotracheal tube (Fig. 19-6)
    F. Monitor heart rate, pulse, and respirations
      1. If pulses are present, turn on the vaporizer and nitrous oxide if desired

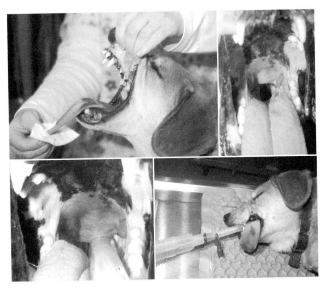

Fig. 19-6
Placing an endotracheal tube into the trachea of a dog is facilitated by extending the head and neck, widely opening the dog's mouth, pulling out the dog's tongue, and visualizing the larynx.

2. If pulses are weak, leave oxygen on. Diagnose the cause of the weak pulses and resuscitate; do not start inhalation drugs (see Chapter 29)
3. Spontaneous ventilation should be 4 to 6 breaths/min minimum (assist ventilation if required)
4. Apnea or dyspnea
   a. Anesthetic induction drugs may depress ventilatory drive; begin manual ventilation (2 to 4 breaths/min) using the breathing system
   b. Endotracheal tube may be obstructed or kinked (dyspnea)
   c. If bronchial intubation has occurred, withdraw the tube into the trachea
   d. Pneumothorax or pneumomediastinum
      (1) Remove intrathoracic air by percutaneous needle insertion
      (2) Evaluate hemodynamic status

G. Set the vaporizer to desired maintenance concentration and adjust as necessary

H. Connect monitors (e.g., electrocardiogram, pulse oximeter, blood pressure)

MAINTENANCE ANESTHESIA

I. Monitoring (see Chapter 15)

II. Record doses and time of drug administration; readjust doses according to response, depth of anesthesia, and amount of analgesia needed

III. Check patency of airway frequently
A. Blocked or kinked tube
B. Tube impinging at bifurcation of trachea
C. Do not overinflate lungs (P_I = 15 to 20 cm H_2O; V_T = 10 to 15 ml/kg)

IV. Maintain the endotracheal tube, head, and neck in a natural, slightly curved position to prevent kinking of the tube; position the dog to avoid excessive flexion of neck, abduction of limbs, and pressure on thorax

V. Calculate IV fluids needed and adjust fluid flow rate (approximately 5 to 20 ml/kg/hr); record all fluids (the infusion rate, total volumes), electrolytes, and other drugs administered

VI. Complete anesthetic record (Fig. 19-7)
A. Note the effects of preanesthetic findings and drug effects
B. Note the start and end of the anesthetic period
C. Note the start and end of surgery
D. Note all major surgical events (number 1 → x)
E. Note all changes in dog status, cardiorespiratory variables, and anesthetic technique
F. Note all laboratory results during anesthesia (e.g., pH and blood gases, electrolytes, packed cell volume [PCV], total protein [TP], hemoglobin)

VII. Turn off the vaporizer immediately if cardiopulmonary emergency occurs

VIII. Nitrous oxide: turn off N_2O 5 to 10 minutes before the end of anesthesia to hasten recovery and prevent diffusion hypoxia (see Chapter 10)

IX. Turn off the inhalant anesthetic at the end of surgery or earlier, depending on the depth of anesthesia

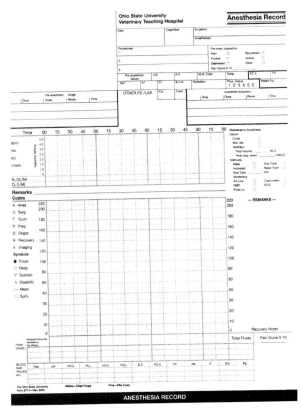

Fig. 19-7
The anesthetic record is used to record all anesthetic and related events.

X. Oxygen: deliver (20 ml/kg or more) during the recovery period; empty the rebreathing bag to dump anesthetic gases and hasten recovery

THE RECOVERY PERIOD

I. Deflate the endotracheal tube cuff; remove it when the animal swallows and/or coughs

II. Pull out the animal's tongue frequently to check its mucous membrane color and administer oxygen if necessary (endotracheal tube, mask, oxygen cage) to maintain oxygenation

III. Position the animal in sternal recumbency with its head extended

IV. Observe the animal until it can maintain sternal recumbency

V. Keep the airway free of secretions (use postural drainage, sponges, and suction tubes)

VI. Check temperature ($>36°$ C); raise and maintain body temperature using towels, heating pads, or warm air blankets

VII. Change the animal's positions frequently and stimulate it by rubbing its body, rolling from side to side, and flexing and extending its limbs

VIII. Additional tranquilizers or analgesics may be needed if the animal becomes excited, delirious, or is in pain during recovery

IX. Maintain IV fluids as needed
  A. Occasionally cardiovascular support may be required (see Chapter 29)
    1. Dopamine 1 to 5 $\mu g/kg/min$
    2. Dobutamine 1 to 5 $\mu g/kg/min$

X. Consider drug antagonists
  A. Opioids: naloxone
  B. α_2-Agonists: yohimbine, tolazoline, and atipamezole
  C. Benzodiazepines: flumazenil
  D. Respiratory depression: doxapram
  E. Bradycardia: atropine, glycopyrrolate

CHAPTER TWENTY

Anesthetic Procedures and Techniques in Cats

"Again I must remind you that a dog's a dog—a cat's a cat."
T. S. ELIOT

OVERVIEW

Cats are not small dogs. Some preanesthetic drugs (acepromazine, diazepam, butorphanol) administered as single drugs do not consistently produce a calm, tractable animal amenable to physical restraint as they may in dogs. Combining different types of drugs in reduced doses should be considered to increase predictability and reduce unwanted side effects. Combination drug therapy requires a comprehensive knowledge of the pharmacology of anesthetic drugs, their interactions, and potential side effects. Because of their size, cats are prone to hypothermia. so measures should be used to reduce anesthetic duration and provide external warming.

GENERAL CONSIDERATIONS

I. A variety of anesthetic procedures and techniques can be used to safely produce sedation, analgesia, and anesthesia in cats. Local anesthetic techniques should be considered to provide additional analgesia

II. The choice of anesthetic regimen is influenced by the following characteristics:
   A. Age, size, breed
   B. Temperament
   C. Health and physical condition
   D. The purpose of chemical restraint and anesthesia
   E. The duration of anesthesia
   F. The familiarity of personnel with the drugs being used

      G. Concurrent medication

      H. Available assistance

III. Drugs that are reversible are preferred

IV. Endotracheal intubation should always be performed whenever possible to ensure a patent airway

V. Careful monitoring is mandatory to recognize and compensate for drug-related effects

VI. Food and water should be withheld for approximately 6 and 2 hours before surgery, respectively, except in very small, very young, or diseased cats

PREANESTHETIC EVALUATION (SEE CHAPTER 2)

  I. Review history and current drug therapy

 II. Perform a physical examination

III. Review available laboratory data

IV. Formulate a specific anesthetic plan (Fig. 20-1)

      A. Determine whether additional preoperative tests are needed

      B. Choose appropriate drugs

  V. Intravenous catheter placement is recommended in case of emergency

VI. Gather appropriate equipment and supplies

      A. Endotracheal tube

          1. Select endotracheal tube diameter based on patient size (usual range 2 to 5 mm, ID: Table 20-1)

          2. If using a cuffed endotracheal tube, check cuff for leaks by injecting air

          3. Use a rigid or flexible stylet for small-diameter, flimsy tubes

          4. Use an uncuffed tube in very small animals (refer to Fig. 19-2 in Chapter 19)

          5. Use a small amount of sterile lubricant

      B. Laryngoscope (refer to Fig. 19-3 in Chapter 19)

          1. Aids intubation by allowing visualization, illumination, and manipulation of the tongue and laryngeal structures

      C. Anesthetic machine and breathing system

          1. Size and type of anesthetic system (rebreathing; nonrebreathing [see Chapter 13]) determined by body weight

PREANESTHETIC EVALUATION

ANESTHETIST:_____
DATE:_____
CLINICIAN:_____
WARD/CAGE OR STALL #:_____

PROCEDURE: ....

BODY WEIGHT: .... **AGE:** ....

TEMPERAMENT:

OBJECTIVE FINDINGS
Temp_____ Pulse_____ Resp. _____
Cardiac auscultation_____
Pulse quality _____
Mucous membrane color_____
Capillary refill time_____
Respiratory auscultation _____

ASSESSMENT: Physical status I II III IV V E
Reasons:

CBC
WBC_____ TP_____ PCV_____
Fibrinogen _____
SERUM CHEMISTRIES
BUN_____ GLUCOSE_____
AST(SGOT)_____
ALT(SGPT)_____
URINE SPECIFIC GRAVITY_____
OTHER RESULTS _____
PRIOR ANESTHESIA _____

COMPLICATIONS ANTICIPATED   pre op, intra op, post op: consider age , body wt.,
breed, position, surgical procedure, physical status.

Plan   Anesthesia regimen (include reasons as related to this animal)
(Include premeds, induction agent, inhalation agent, O_2 flow rate, post op analgesics)

DRUG	ROUTE	DOSE/#	MG	ML	REASONS OR JUSTIFICATION

MONITORING: Esophageal stethoscope, Doppler, ECG, Temp. Probe, Blood gas, Arterial Line,
Other_____

IV FLUID TYPE_____ Dose: MLS/HR_____ DROPS/MIN_____

ADMINISTRATION SET: MINI DRIP (60 drops/ml)   MAXI DRIP (10 drops/ml)

Approved_____

Fig. 20-1
Anesthetic plan.

    a. Use a small-animal anesthetic machine (adult human anesthetic system)

      (1) Use a pediatric circle system for cats weighing more than 3 kg

      (2) Use the non-rebreathing system for cats weighing less than 3 kg

TABLE 20-1
ENDOTRACHEAL TUBE SIZE FOR CATS

BODY WEIGHT (KG)	TUBE SIZE (MM, ID)
1	3
2	4
5	5

2. The rebreathing bag should be at least five times the tidal volume. The tidal volume (V_T) is usually between 10 to 15 ml/kg (e.g., 5 kg $\times$ 10 ml/kg = 50 ml V_T)
3. Refill carbon dioxide absorbent canister if material is exhausted (discolored or dry)
4. Evaluate anesthetic system for possible malfunctions (see Chapter 13)
   a. Fill vaporizer and check operation
   b. Turn on flowmeters and check for free movement of indicator balls or slides
   c. Connect the non-rebreathing system or circle system to anesthetic machine and check for leaks or close the pop-off valve and pressurize (increase the O_2 flow) the system to 20 to 30 cm water and maintain for 15 seconds; check for leaks
5. Connect waste gas scavenging system to the non-rebreathing system or the circle breathing circuit

D. Fresh gases
   1. Oxygen
      a. Connect to "house" oxygen system, if present
      b. Attach smaller (E) tanks to machine; change oxygen tank if pressure gauge falls below 500 psi
   2. Nitrous oxide (used to produce analgesia)
      a. Optional
      b. Change tank if pressure gauge falls below 750 psi
E. Intravenous (IV) administration equipment
   1. IV catheters (18- to 23-gauge)
   2. Appropriate volume of IV fluids
      a. Balanced electrolyte solutions (e.g., LRS, Plasma-lyte®)
      b. Use 250 ml bags or smaller to prevent fluid overload
      c. Administer 5 to 20 ml/kg/hr

3. Solution administration set (mini-drip; 60 drops/ml)
4. Fluid infusion pump (refer to Fig. 19-5 in Chapter 19)

F. Drugs
  1. Calculate appropriate drug dose and volume
  2. Draw drugs into labeled syringes

G. Monitoring equipment (see Chapter 15)
  1. Electrocardiographic monitor
  2. Indirect blood pressure (Doppler; oscillometric)
  3. Pulse oximeter
  4. Thermometer
  5. Esophageal stethoscope
  6. End-tidal CO_2

H. Ancillary supplies
  1. 4×4-inch gauze sponges
  2. Adhesive tape
  3. Roll gauze
  4. Forced hot air blanket

PREANESTHETIC MEDICATION (SEE CHAPTER 3)

I. Choice of drug determined by the cat's preoperative condition and the surgical procedure to be performed

II. Intramuscular (IM) or subcutaneous (SQ) drugs should be administered 10 to 20 minutes before catheterization and induction of anesthesia

III. Drugs used before anesthesia
  A. Anticholinergics
    1. Atropine 20 to 40 µg/kg IM, IV, or SQ
    2. Glycopyrrolate 5 to 10 µg/kg IM, IV, SQ
  B. Tranquilizer
    1. Acepromazine 0.05 to 0.2 mg/kg IM
    2. Diazepam or midazolam 0.1 to 0.2 mg/kg IV
      a. Benzodiazepines can produce restlessness, apprehension, and disorientation in cats, making them more difficult to restrain
    3. Single-drug use is recommended for only old or depressed cats
  C. Opioids (give in combination with tranquilizers)
    1. Butorphanol 0.2 to 0.4 mg/kg IM
    2. Buprenorphine 5 to 20 µg/kg IM

      3. Hydromorphone 0.05 mg/kg IM

      4. Oxymorphone 0.1 to 0.3 mg/kg IM

      5. Morphine 0.1 to 0.2 mg/kg IM

      6. Fentanyl patch 25 μg/kg/hr

  D. α_2-Agonists

      1. Medetomidine 5 to 40 μg/kg IM or IV

      2. Xylazine 0.2 to 1 mg/kg IM or IV

      3. Romifidine 0.09 to 0.18 mg/kg IM or IV

  E. Ketamine 5 to 10 mg/kg IM (give in combination with tranquilizer or an α_2-agonist)

  F. Telazol® 2 to 10 mg/kg IM or IV

  G. Popular preanesthetic drug combination in cats

      1. Medetomidine (60 to 80 μg/kg) with ketamine (5 mg/kg) and butorphanol (0.2 mg/kg)

        a. Mix and give IM to healthy cats

      2. Acepromazine (0.2 mg/kg) with hydromorphone (0.05 to 0.1 mg/kg)

        a. Mix and give IM or SQ

      3. Midazolam (0.2 mg/kg) with hydromorphone (0.05 to 0.1 mg/kg)

        a. Mix and give IM or SQ

  H. Nonsteroidal antiinflammatory drugs

      1. Meloxicam 0.3 mg/kg SQ

      2. Carprofen 2 mg/kg SQ, one time

INDUCTION

  I. Intravenous

    A. Catheterize vein(s) (generally the cephalic or medial saphenous vein)

    B. Start IV fluid administration to ensure catheter patency

      1. Lower fluid bag or bottle below cat's thorax to allow blood to siphon back into catheter; this confirms catheter placement within the vein

    C. Inject induction drug(s) slowly (15 to 30 seconds), allow time for equilibration before administering further increments

    D. Specific IV induction drugs (see Chapter 8)

      1. Ketamine 2 to 6 mg/kg IV

      2. Propofol 3 to 10 mg/kg IV (Table 20-2)

TABLE 20-2
INJECTABLE ANESTHESIA TECHNIQUE INCLUDING INFUSION IN CATS

INDUCTION	MAINTENANCE	COMMENTS
Propofol 6.6 mg/kg/min CRI	Propofol 0.22 mg/kg/min CRI or Propofol 0.14 mg/kg/min CRI + ketamine 23 µg/kg/min CRI (loading dose 2 mg/kg)	Stable hemodynamics
Propofol 5 mg/kg/min CRI	Propofol 0.05-0.1 mg/kg/min CRI or Propofol 0.025 mg/kg/min CRI + ketamine 23 or 46 µg/kg/min	

CRI, Constant rate infusion.

3. Ultrashort-acting barbiturates
   a. Thiopental 2% to 5%; 8 to 20 mg/kg IV
   b. Methohexital 2% 3 to 8 mg/kg IV
4. Etomidate 0.5 to 2 mg/kg IV
5. Short-acting barbiturates
   a. Pentobarbital 25 mg/kg IV
6. Popular injectable drug combinations
   a. Diazepam-ketamine: diazepam 0.2 mg/kg IV and ketamine 5 mg/kg IV
      (1) Mix equal parts of diazepam (5 mg/ml in stock vial) and ketamine (100 mg/ml in stock vial) to yield a mixture that is 2.5 mg/ml diazepam and 50 mg/ml ketamine
      (2) Add an additional 0.1 ml of medetomidine (10 µg/kg) if the cat is healthy and fractious
      (3) 0.1 ml/kg of mixture IV
   b. Tiletamine (50 mg/ml), zolazepam (50 mg/ml), ketamine (80 mg/ml), and xylazine (20 mg/ml)
      (1) Mix and give 0.24 ml/cat IM

(2) Cats can be spayed or neutered with single injection

NOTE

Drug combination for feral cats:
TKM
Add 4 mL of 100 mg/mL ketamine and 1 mL of 1 mg/mL of medetomidine to a 5 mL bottle of Telazol®
Dose: 0.1-0.2 mL/5-10 kg IM

II. Inhalant anesthetic induction
   A. Sevoflurane or isoflurane can be used for mask or chamber induction in cats. Sevoflurane's odor is less offensive than isoflurane and induction is faster (lower blood/gas partition coefficient)
      1. Face mask (Fig. 20-2)
         a. Be aware of the potential for vomiting and possible aspiration
         b. Provide adequate physical restraint
      2. Induction chamber (Fig. 20-3)
         a. Use high, fresh-gas flow rates (4 to 5 L/min)

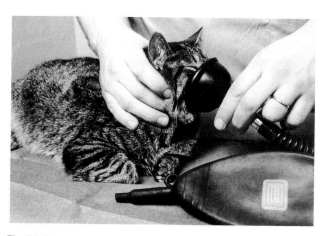

Fig. 20-2
A face mask is often used to induce cats and small dogs to anesthesia.

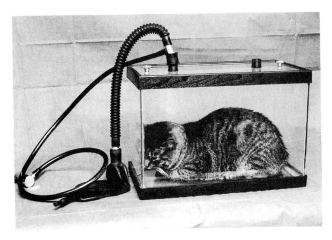

Fig. 20-3
An induction chamber is used to confine cats and small animals for induction to general anesthesia with an inhaled anesthetic.

    b. Monitor cat closely for loss of righting reflex, then remove from chamber and complete induction with a mask

    c. Not recommended for routine induction because atmospheric pollution with anesthetic gases is very significant

ENDOTRACHEAL INTUBATION

  I. Open the cat's mouth and manipulate the tongue to the side with the endotracheal tube; grasp the tongue with a gauze sponge, straighten the head and neck, and extend the tongue between the lower canine teeth to hold the mandible open

  II. Locate the larynx and insert the endotracheal tube (Fig. 20-4)

    A. Direct visualization

    B. Use a laryngoscope to facilitate visualization of the larynx and reflect the epiglottis rostral and ventral

    C. Potential difficulties

      1. Laryngospasm (0.1 ml 2% lidocaine sprayed onto the laryngeal cartilages reduces spasms)

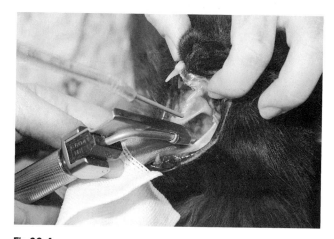

Fig.20-4
A stylet to stiffen the endotracheal tube is frequently used to place an endotracheal tube in the trachea of cats.

NOTE

Do NOT! use cetacaine (methemoglobinemia).

---

     a. Cat not adequately anesthetized
     b. Larynx sensitized
  2. Small tubes may be too pliant to easily place. Use a stylet to stiffen them
  3. Soft-palate displacement prevents rostroventral movement of the epiglottis; push the soft palate dorsally with the endotracheal tube to release epiglottis
  4. Mass involving the pharynx and larynx; may need a smaller tracheal tube or tracheotomy
D. Turn on oxygen (be careful not to overinflate lungs)
E. Connect the breathing system (Y-piece or elbow) to the endotracheal tube, and secure the tube to the cat
F. Monitor heart rate, pulse, and respirations
  1. Normal heart rate and pulse: turn on the vaporizer and nitrous oxide (if desired)

2. Low heart rate or weak pulse: leave oxygen on, diagnose the cause of the weak pulses, and resuscitate; do not start inhalation drugs (see Chapter 29)
3. Spontaneous ventilation: minimum of 4 to 6 breaths/min (assist ventilation if required)
4. Apnea or dyspnea
   a. Anesthetic induction drugs may have depressed the cat's ventilatory drive; begin manual ventilation (2 to 4 breaths/min) using the breathing system

---

NOTE

Do not overinflate lungs: PI = 15 to 20 cm HO; V_T = 10 to 15 ml/kg); may cause pneumomediastinum, pneumothorax.

---

   b. Endotracheal tube may be obstructed or kinked
   c. If bronchial intubation has occurred, withdraw the tube into the trachea
G. Set the vaporizer to a maintenance concentration determined by monitoring responses
H. Connect monitors (e.g., Doppler, electrocardiogram, pulse oximeter, temperature)

LOCAL ANESTHETIC TECHNIQUES (SEE CHAPTER 7)

I. Declaw procedure
   A. Use 0.2% ropivacaine or 0.25% bupivacaine (total dose 1 mg/kg)
   B. Perform a ring block at the level of the carpus (refer to Figure 7-3 in Chapter 7)
II. Epidural anesthesia

MAINTENANCE OF ANESTHESIA (SEE CHAPTER 19)

THE RECOVERY PERIOD (SEE CHAPTER 19)

I. Check respirations, pulse, and temperature (>36° C) at frequent intervals until in sternal recumbency

CHAPTER TWENTY-ONE

Anesthetic Procedures and Techniques in Horses

"The little neglect may breed mischief ... for want of a nail the shoe was lost; for want of a shoe the horse was lost; and for want of a horse the rider was lost."

BENJAMIN FRANKLIN

OVERVIEW

Horses may be the most difficult domestic species to safely anesthetize. Current mortality rates for horses are significantly higher than for cats and dogs: ranging from up to 2% in horses compared with approximately 0.1% in dogs and cats. The ability to anticipate drug effects and drug actions in a given patient is the single most important asset of a good equine anesthetist. Individual equine temperament varies considerably and has significant influence on the dose of drug required and selection of the best anesthetic technique. Boluses and infusions (total intravenous anesthesia) of anesthetic drugs are combined with physical restraint to induce general anesthesia in horses. Anesthetic techniques are designed to produce rapid and safe induction to and recovery from recumbency and to maximize muscle relaxation and analgesia while maintaining optimal cardiopulmonary status. Horses frequently benefit from assistance in regaining and maintaining a standing position after general anesthesia.

GENERAL CONSIDERATIONS

I. Preparation of the equine surgical patient
   A. Withhold food for approximately 4 to 8 hours before surgery if possible; do not withhold water

B. Perform a complete physical examination with emphasis on cardiorespiratory function

C. Weigh each animal and note body type (e.g., lean/racing, conditioned, draft)

D. Groom the horse and wipe it with a moist cloth to remove dander; place an intravenous (IV) catheter before induction

E. Clean the feet before induction; pull or pad all shoes to prevent injury; clip the surgical site before induction to anesthesia (if possible)

F. Give each animal preanesthetic medication approximately 5 to 20 minutes before induction of anesthesia

G. Rinse the mouth with water before induction

II. All horses develop some degree of acid-base disturbance under anesthesia, particularly respiratory acidosis ($\uparrow$ $PaCO_2$, end-tidal CO_2)

III. Proper positioning and appropriate padding of the head, shoulder, and hip minimize the incidence of neuropathies and myopathies

IV. Assisted or controlled ventilation can be used to maintain normal arterial carbon dioxide concentrations during prolonged anesthesia in the horse

V. Prevention of hypotension and hypoxemia helps avoid postoperative complications, including myopathy

VI. Horses should be watched closely during the recovery period and, if needed, assisted to a standing position

A. Nasotracheal intubation may be required in horses that snore or demonstrate signs of upper airway obstruction in the recovery period

PREANESTHETIC EVALUATION

I. Review patient history

II. Conduct a physical examination

A. Determine age, weight, sex

B. Judge the temperament of the horse and health status (see Chapter 2)

C. Emphasize the cardiopulmonary system; check for subclinical respiratory disease

    D. Determine the degree of lameness or ataxia
    E. Review the concurrent or previous drug history
    F. Assess the procedure to be performed
    G. Prepare an anesthetic care plan
III. Conduct a laboratory evaluation
    A. Routine evaluation
      1. Complete blood count (packed cell volume, hemoglobin)
      2. Total protein
      3. Fibrinogen
    B. Suggested further evaluation
      1. Serum electrolytes
      2. Serum chemistry
      3. Acid-base balance

PREANESTHETIC MEDICATIONS

I. Xylazine (used to produce sedation, analgesia, and muscle relaxation)
    A. Dose: 1 to 2 mg/kg intramuscularly (IM), 0.4 to 1 mg/kg IV
    B. Onset of action: within 2 to 3 minutes after IV administration and within 10 to 15 minutes after IM administration
    C. Duration: 30 minutes after IV administration and 60 minutes after IM administration
    D. Sinus bradycardia and first- and second-degree atrioventricular block may occur
II. Detomidine (similar to xylazine)
    A. Dose: 20 to 40 μg/kg IM
       10 to 20 μg/kg IV
       60 μg/kg sublingual
    B. Approximately 2 times longer duration of action than xylazine
III. Medetomidine (similar to xylazine)
    A. Dose: 10 to 40 μg/kg IM
       5 to 20 μg/kg IV
    B. More pronounced and longer effects than xylazine but shorter than detomidine

IV. Romifidine (similar to xylazine)
  A. Dose: 90 to 120 µg/kg IV
     80 to 120 µg/kg IM
  B. Reduced ataxia and head drop compared with xylazine with a longer duration
V. Acepromazine (used to produce a calming effect)
  A. Dose: 20 to 80 µg/kg IM; 10 to 40 µg/kg IV
  B. Onset of action: within 10 to 20 minutes
  C. Duration: 2 to 3 hours
  D. Hypotensive effect may last for 12 hours
IV. Chloral hydrate (infrequently used to produce or enhance sedation); 20 to 100 mg/kg IV

ANESTHETIC EQUIPMENT

I. Collect the necessary equipment
  A. Endotracheal tubes
    1. Choose the largest tube possible (30, 26, 20, or 15 mm); most tube size designations are related to internal diameter
    2. Check the endotracheal tube cuff for leaks
    3. Use lubricating jelly for the endotracheal tube
    4. Use 25- to 60-ml syringe to inflate the endotracheal tube cuff
    5. Use 5-cm polyvinylchloride plumber's pipe as a speculum
  B. Commercially available 10-, 12-, and 14-gauge, 13-cm catheters are used for IV anesthetic drug and fluid administration (Fig. 21-1)
  C. Pressure bag for administration of IV fluids or drugs (e.g., guaifenesin)
  D. Cotton ropes for restraining front legs (Fig. 21-2)
  E. Proper padding (Fig. 21-2)
  F. Monitoring equipment (see Chapter 15)
    1. Electrocardiographic monitor
    2. Blood pressure monitoring device
    3. End expired gas monitor (% O_2; end-tidal CO_2; inhaled anesthesia)
    4. pH and blood gases (PO_2; PCO_2)

      G. Infusion pump for controlled infusion of additional drugs (e.g., lidocaine; dobutamine)

II. Before induction of general anesthesia

      A. The anesthetic machine should be examined to be sure the vaporizer has an adequate anesthetic level; the circle system should be tested for leaks

          1. The anesthetic system can be checked for leaks by occluding the Y piece, closing the pop-off valve, and flushing the anesthetic circuit with oxygen; if pressure is maintained for more than 15 seconds, the system is not leaking

          2. The circle system should be capable of maintaining a pressure of approximately 30 cm of H_2O

      B. Check gas pressures in the tanks

          1. Oxygen tank pressure should be 500 psi or greater

      C. Fresh carbon dioxide absorbent should be placed in the canister after approximately 6 hours of use

      D. Fresh gas flow rate

          1. Oxygen: 5 to 10 ml/kg; high flow rates (up to 20 mL/kg) are used during induction and recovery to rapidly increase inhalant concentrations and denitrogenate and remove anesthetic vapors, respectively

      E. Check scavenger system

INDUCTION

I. Ketamine

      A. Dose: 1.5 to 2 mg/kg IV after xylazine, detomidine, romifidine, medetomidine, or guaifenesin (see Chapter 3)

      B. Usually administered with diazepam (0.1 mg/kg IV), but after an α_2-agonist

      C. 10% contains 100 mg/ml

      D. Short-acting (10 to 15 minutes)

      E. Causes apneustic breathing pattern

II. Guaifenesin: centrally acting skeletal muscle relaxant

      A. Dose: 50 to 100 mg/kg to produce recumbency; 50 mg/kg to produce ataxia and relaxation

      B. 5% to 10% solution (50 to 100 mg/ml): >15% concentrations may cause hemolysis

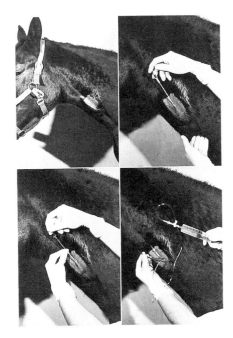

Fig. 21-1
A, Placement of IV catheter.

    C. Can be administered before or in solution with thiopental
       sodium or ketamine

    D. Duration: 15 to 25 minutes

    E. Causes minimal analgesia and sedation by itself

    F. Toxic signs include the following:
        1. Apneustic breathing pattern (inspiratory hold) or apnea
        2. Muscle rigidity
        3. Hypotension

III. Diazepam (muscle relaxant)

    A. Dose: 0.04 to 0.1 mg/kg IV

    B. Administered before thiopental or with ketamine

    C. Duration: 5 to 15 minutes

    D. No analgesia, minimal sedation

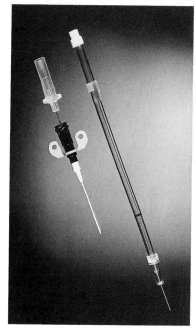

Fig. 21-1, cont'd
B, Types of IV catheters.

   IV. Midazolam (similar to diazepam)
      A. Dose: 0.04 to 0.1 mg/kg IV
    V. Thiopental sodium
      A. Dose: combined with guaifenesin (5 mg/ml in 5% guaifenesin), given IV to effect
      B. Ultrashort-acting (5 to 15 minutes)
      C. Causes cardiorespiratory depression and may cause transient apnea (dose-dependent)
  VI. Telazol® (tiletamine/zolazepam)
      A. Dose: 0.5 to 1.5 mg/kg IV
      B. Similar to ketamine and used in the same manner
      C. Greater muscle relaxation
      D. Longer duration of action

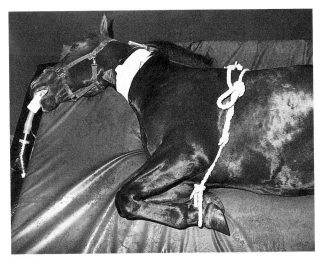

Fig. 21-2
During general anesthesia, horses are usually positioned on large foam rubber pads or on air or water mattresses with their front legs restrained. Once the horse is properly positioned, the halter should be removed.

  E. Greater respiratory depression
  F. Longer and poorer recovery than ketamine-diazepam
VII. Halothane, isoflurane, sevoflurane: 3% to 7% concentration and high oxygen flow rate can be used for induction in foals after placement of a nasotracheal tube or mask

ENDOTRACHEAL INTUBATION

 I. Endotracheal intubation (Fig. 21-3)
  A. Two clean endotracheal tubes and a speculum or mouth gag should be available for intubation
  B. Intubation is performed blindly
   1. Place a bite block between the incisors
   2. Extend the head and neck
   3. Advance the tube over the base of the tongue into the pharynx

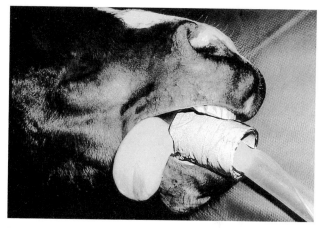

Fig. 21-3
Endotracheal intubation is performed blindly in horses and foals.

  4. Rotate the tube as it is advanced into the trachea
  5. Repeat if unsuccessful
C. Make sure that the tube is in trachea, not in esophagus; water vapor on tube during exhalation and air movement
D. If the tube appears too small, choose a larger one
E. Do not advance the endotracheal tube tip past the thoracic inlet
F. Secure the tube with gauze, if necessary
G. Nasal intubation can be performed in adult horses and foals (Fig. 21-4)
H. Connect the endotracheal tube to the anesthetic system; the rebreathing bag size should be at least five times the tidal volume; 15-L to 30-L bags are standard
I. Inflate the endotracheal tube cuff, and check to see that it does not leak by squeezing the rebreathing bag, expanding the animal's lungs
  1. Do not overinflate the cuff; generally, 50 to 75 ml is adequate to inflate the cuff of an endotracheal tube in a 500-kg patient (Fig. 21-5)

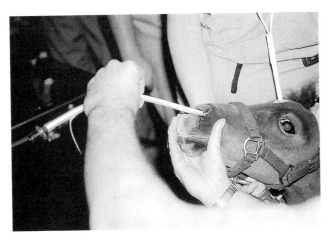

Fig. 21-4
Nasal intubation is easily performed in adult horses and foals.

J. Pull the dependent forelimb toward horse's head immediately after induction to prevent neuropathy and myopathy of the down forelimb

MAINTENANCE OF ANESTHESIA

I. Total intravenous anesthesia (TIVA): a mixture of 500 ml of 5% guaifenesin and 500 mg of ketamine with or without 250 to 500 mg of xylazine can be mixed together and delivered to effect (Table 21-1)
II. Inhalation anesthesia
   A. Isoflurane: 1% to 3%
   B. Sevoflurane: 2% to 5%
III. Analgesia
   A. Morphine 0.04 to 0.1 mg/kg IM
IV. Monitoring (see Chapter 15)
   A. Body temperature
      1. Changes very little but usually decreases in adult horses during anesthesia
      2. Decreases in foals
      3. May increase if muscle relaxation is inadequate

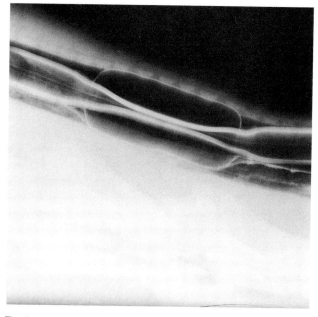

Fig. 21-5
Accidental overinflation of the endotracheal tube cuff can result in tube occlusion.

    B. Chart all anesthetic and surgical events and the animal's response (Fig. 19-8)

    C. Monitor all vital signs (i.e., cardiovascular, respiratory) and the depth of anesthesia (i.e., unconsciousness, eye signs)

    D. Measure and maintain arterial blood pressure directly (especially important); mean arterial blood pressure greater than 60 mm of Hg; if hypotensive:

        1. Administer fluids

        2. Reduce anesthetic delivery if possible

        3. Administer dobutamine (1 to 3 µg/kg/min) or a bolus of ephedrine (0.05 to 0.1 mg/kg IV)

IV. Administration of fluids (see Chapter 26)

TABLE 21-1
TOTAL INTRAVENOUS ANESTHESIA TECHNIQUE IN HORSES

DRUG CONCENTRATION	COMBINATIONS (mg/ml)	INFUSION DOSE
Xylazine	1	1-2 ml/kg/hr to effect
Guaifenesin	100	
Ketamine*	2	
Detomidine	0.02	1-2 ml/kg/hr to effect
Guaifenesin	100	
Ketamine*	2	
Medetomidine	0.02	1-2 ml/kg/hr to effect
Guaifenesin	100	
Ketamine*	2	
Romifidine	0.06	1-2 ml/kg/hr to effect
Guaifenesin	100	
Ketamine*	2	

Butorphanol (20 μg/kg) may be added to enhance analgesia.
Ketamine is generally infused at rates of 50 to 150 μg/kg/min after adequate muscle relaxation.
*4 mg/ml ketamine reduces infusion to 0.8 ml/kg/hr.

THE RECOVERY PERIOD

I. Turn off the anesthetic before the oxygen
II. Administer oxygen until the patient is swallowing, if possible; then extubate
III. Oxygen is routinely administered by the following:
   A. O_2 humidifier (minimum flow rate 15 L/min)
   B. O_2 demand valve (Fig. 21-6)
IV. Keep tranquilizers, ropes, and emergency drugs available in case of rough recoveries
   A. Make sure the cuff on the endotracheal tube is deflated
   B. Keep the animal's head and muzzle down to allow drainage
   C. Assist the animal to a standing position, if necessary
   D. Administer sedative (50 mg xylazine IV) to adult horses if they demonstrate any of the following:
      1. Excessive nystagmus or oculogyric activity
      2. Excessive muscle tremors
      3. Uncoordinated limb movements; paddling
      4. Delirium

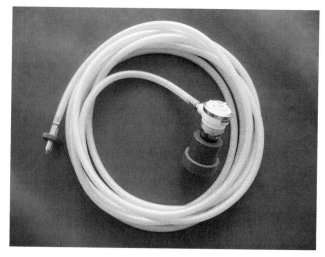

Fig. 21-6
An oxygen flush valve (demand valve) can be used to deliver high flows (50 L/sec) of oxygen into a face mask or an endotracheal tube.

COMMON ANESTHETIC PROBLEMS

   I. Hypotension (mean arterial blood pressure less than 60 mm Hg)
  II. Hypoventilation ($PaCO_2$ greater than 55 mm Hg)
 III. Hypoxemia (PaO_2 less than 60 mm Hg)
       A. PaO_2 should be greater than 150 mm Hg when breathing 100% O_2
  IV. Bradycardia (heart rate less than 25 bpm)
   V. Difficulty maintaining adequate anesthetic depth
  VI. Nonrespiratory (metabolic) acidosis
 VII. Overhydration (>50 ml/kg fluids within 3 hours)
VIII. Nasal congestion and/or upper airway obstruction
  IX. Poor or prolonged recovery
   X. Neuropathy and/or myopathy

CHAPTER TWENTY-TWO

Anesthetic Procedures and Techniques in Ruminants

"You've got to stop and eat the roses along the way."
ANONYMOUS PHILOSOPHER

OVERVIEW

Physical restraint and local anesthetic techniques are frequently used in ruminants to provide immobility and analgesia. General anesthesia techniques are similar to those for dogs, cats, or horses. Regurgitation of rumen contents and bloat (distention of the rumen) are potential hazards not usually encountered in dogs, cats, or horses. Close observation and monitoring of palpebral and ocular reflexes, eyeball position, and pupil size can be used to monitor the depth of anesthesia in ruminants. Recovery from anesthesia is generally quiet and uneventful and does not routinely require assistance.

GENERAL CONSIDERATIONS

I. Preparation of the ruminant for anesthesia and surgery
   A. The most important factor in decreasing the risk of regurgitation is to decrease rumen size and pressure before anesthesia
      1. Withhold food for 12 to 18 hours in large ruminants
      2. Withhold water for 8 to 12 hours in large ruminants
      3. Withhold food for 12 to 18 hours in sheep and goats; there is no need to withhold water
      4. Withhold food for 2 to 4 hours in calves, lambs, and kids; when these animals are less than 1 month of age,

they are essentially monogastric and are less prone to regurgitation during anesthesia

B. Side effects of withholding food are minimal
   1. Mild metabolic alkalosis is observed in healthy animals
   2. Bradycardia in adult cattle results from increased vagal tone
C. Endotracheal and rumen tubes should be placed when appropriate to avoid bloat and aspiration of rumen contents

II. Most surgical techniques in cattle can be performed with local or regional anesthesia (see Chapter 5)

III. General anesthesia is required if local or regional anesthetic techniques are inadequate; light stages of anesthesia may predispose the animal to stress, which may result in tachycardia and hypertension

PREANESTHETIC EVALUATION

I. Preanesthetic evaluation is very similar to that in horses (see Chapter 21)
   A. Patient history
   B. Physical examination
   C. Basic laboratory tests
      1. Packed cell volume or hemoglobin
      2. Plasma total protein

PREANESTHETIC MEDICATION

I. Preanesthetic drugs are used to calm or sedate ruminants or to decrease the dose of a more potent intravenous (IV) or inhalation anesthetic drug

II. Tranquilizers are not approved for use in food animals; drug residues in milk and meat products are problematic

III. Popular preanesthetic medications include the following drugs:
   A. Xylazine
      1. One tenth the IV dose used in horses: 0.1 mg/kg or less IV; 0.1 to 0.6 mg/kg intramuscular (IM)

2. Only low-concentration xylazine is recommended (20 mg/ml)
3. A moderate dose of 0.02 to 0.1 mg/kg IV generally induces recumbency and depresses or abolishes pharyngeal and laryngeal reflexes, thus allowing easy intubation and inhalation anesthesia without additional medication
4. Side effects
   a. Cardiovascular depression
   b. Respiratory depression
   c. Rumen atony with bloat
   d. Hyperglycemia from decreased plasma insulin
   e. Diuresis
   f. Decreased packed cell volume
   g. Premature delivery in late pregnancy
5. Antagonists
   a. Nonspecific antagonists:
      (1) Doxapram 1 mg/kg IV can be used as a respiratory stimulant
   b. Specific antagonists:
      (1) Atipamezole 20 to 60 µg/kg IV
      (2) Yohimbine 0.12 mg/kg IV
      (3) Tolazoline 0.5 to 2.0 mg/kg IV
B. Detomidine or medetomidine
   1. Dose is similar to other species: 10 to 20 µg/kg IM
   2. Effects are similar to xylazine
   3. Antagonists: see section on xylazine
C. Acepromazine (to produce a calming effect)
   1. Not frequently used because of prolonged elimination
   2. Dose: 40 to 90 µg/kg IM; 10 to 20 µg/kg IV
   3. Onset of tranquilization is within 10 to 20 minutes
   4. Duration of tranquilization is 2 to 4 hours
D. Atropine, glycopyrrolate
   1. Not frequently used
   2. Saliva flow is best controlled by pointing the animal's head downward and placing an endotracheal tube with an inflatable cuff
   3. Anticholinergics increase the viscosity of the saliva (without significantly decreasing the volume of saliva)

4. Atropine sulfate, 40 µg/kg IM or subcutaneous, may be useful in preventing bradycardia and hypotension during manipulation of viscera
5. The duration of action of atropine in ruminants is short
6. Anticholinergics increase the incidence of bloat because of a decrease in intestinal motility and an accumulation of gas from bacterial fermentation

INDUCTION

I. Barbiturates
   A. Thiopental sodium (Pentothal) is an ultrashort-acting (10 to 15 minutes) barbiturate with predictable effects
      1. Doses of 7 to 13 mg/kg of thiopental will achieve light surgical anesthesia within 12 to 15 seconds
      2. Less barbiturate is needed if the animal is premedicated or induced with guaifenesin
      3. Barbiturates should be used with caution in animals less than 3 months of age
      4. Barbiturates rapidly cross the placental barrier and depress fetal respiration
II. Guaifenesin
   A. Dose: 50 to 100 mg/kg IV in small increments until effective, followed by thiobarbiturates or ketamine
   B. 5% solution (50 mg/ml) in water or with 5% dextrose; more concentrated solutions (more than 7%) may cause hemolysis
   C. Can be used in combination with xylazine, thiopental, ketamine, or Telazol®
III. Xylazine-ketamine combination
   A. Dose: 40 µg/kg xylazine and 2 mg/kg ketamine IV
      1. Both drugs can be administered in the same syringe
      2. When given IV, immobilization occurs in approximately 45 to 90 seconds, supplying anesthesia for 20 to 30 minutes; standing recovery occurs 2 hours or more after the initial injection
      3. When given IM, induction time is 3 to 10 minutes; anesthesia and recovery times are increased

4. Decreases heart rate, respiratory rate, and temperature; an apneustic respiratory pattern and salivation are seen in ruminants

IV. Xylazine-ketamine-guaifenesin combination ("triple drip")
  A. Dose: 30 to 50 mg xylazine + 500 mg ketamine in 500 ml of 5% guaifenesin given in small increments to effect, approximately 1 to 2 ml/kg IV; anesthesia can be continued at a rate of 2 ml/kg/hr
    1. All three drugs are soluble in water
    2. Induction is gradual and generally uneventful but may require some physical restraint
    3. Anesthesia is adequate for periods of 30 to 90 minutes; respiration may need to be assisted
    4. Drug overdose causes apnea and hypotension

V. Ketamine-guaifenesin combination ("double drip")
  A. Dose: 500 mg ketamine in 500 ml of 5% guaifenesin given in small increments to effect, approximately 1 to 2 ml/kg IV; anesthesia can be continued at a rate of 2 ml/kg/hr
    1. Both drugs are water-soluble
    2. Induction is gradual and generally uneventful but may require some physical restraint
    3. Anesthesia is adequate for periods of 30 to 90 minutes; respiration may need to be assisted
    4. Drug overdose causes apnea and hypotension
    5. Can be used in calm animals

VI. Ketamine-diazepam
  A. Ketamine (1 ml; 100 mg/ml) mixed 50:50 with diazepam (1 ml; 5 mg/ml) 0.05 to 0.1 ml/ kg is used in small ruminants

VII. Ketamine or Telazol®
  A. Dose: ketamine, up to 2 mg/kg IV or 2 to 7 mg/kg IM; Telazol®, 1 to 4 mg/kg IV or 2 to 6 mg/kg IM
  B. Previous administration of xylazine (0.1 to 0.2 mg/kg IM) decreases ketamine or Telazol® dose by one half
  C. Produce excellent, short-term (20 to 30 minutes) surgical anesthesia
  D. Ocular, pharyngeal, and laryngeal reflexes are depressed
  E. Compatible with inhalation anesthetics

    F. Side effects
       1. Respiratory depression
       2. Hypotension
VIII. Masking down with an inhalation anesthetic: animals under 70 kg can be induced with a mask induction technique with 3% isoflurane, or 4% to 6% sevoflurane; the animal is intubated and maintained at 1% to 2%

ENDOTRACHEAL INTUBATION

  I. Intubation should immediately follow the induction of anesthesia
  II. Several techniques are useful
    A. A dental speculum or mouth gag can be placed in the mouth
    B. Method 1: insert an arm into the oral cavity of the adult cow, reflect the epiglottis forward manually, and guide the endotracheal tube into the larynx
    C. Method 2: extend the patient's head and neck and gently advance the tube into the trachea during inspiration
    D. Intubation may be facilitated by a long-blade laryngoscope and endoscopic light (Fig. 22-1)

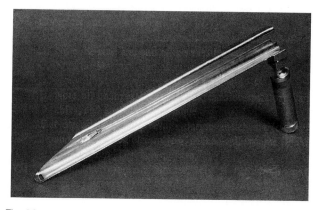

Fig. 22-1
Endotracheal intubation in cattle, sheep, and goats can be facilitated with a long-blade laryngoscope.

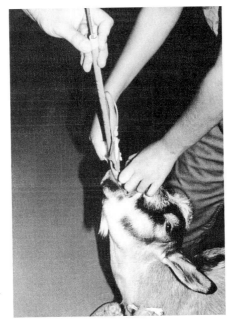

Fig. 22-2
To facilitate intubation in small ruminants, a steel dowel can be placed in the trachea and the endotracheal tube slid over it.

    E. In small ruminants, a long, small-diameter dowel made of wood, steel, or plastic may be placed into the trachea first; the endotracheal tube can then be passed over it (Fig. 22-2)
    F. Intubation should be done quickly to avoid regurgitation and aspiration of fluid
    G. A tracheostomy may be performed if necessary

MAINTENANCE OF ANESTHESIA

    I. Total intravenous anesthesia (see Table 21-1)
      A. Triple drip (see guaifenesin-ketamine combination)
    II. Inhalation anesthetic drugs produce general anesthesia very effectively, particularly for prolonged surgical procedures

III. Analgesia
   A. Butorphanol 0.1 mg/kg IM
   B. Morphine 0.04 mg/kg IM
IV. Induction is completed with 2% to 4% isoflurane, or 4% to 6% sevoflurane
V. A surgical plane of anesthesia may be maintained at 1% to 2% isoflurane, or 3% to 4% sevoflurane
VI. If surgical procedures last longer than 1 hour or blood carbon dioxide concentrations are greater than 60 mm Hg, ventilate ruminants to minimize respiratory acidosis

MONITORING

I. The position of the eyeball provides a useful guide to anesthetic depth
   A. Ocular reflexes are good indicators of anesthetic depth; the corneal reflex should be present throughout anesthesia and the palpebral reflex depressed by inhalation anesthesia
   B. The eyeball often rotates medioventrally when the patient is in a light surgical plane of anesthesia (Fig. 22-3)
   C. The iris and pupil are centered when the patient is in a deep surgical plane of anesthesia or awake; dilated pupils are a sign of anesthetic overdose when using inhalation anesthesia
   D. The auricular artery, located on the dorsal surface of the ear, can be cannulated to monitor arterial blood pressure
II. See Chapter 15
III. Administration of fluids (see Chapter 26)

THE RECOVERY PERIOD

I. Ruminants are allowed to breathe 100% oxygen for several minutes before being disconnected from the anesthetic machine
II. Leave the endotracheal tube in place with the cuff partially inflated until the laryngeal reflex returns to prevent aspiration of regurgitated material
III. Position the patient's head to allow drainage before the endotracheal tube is pulled

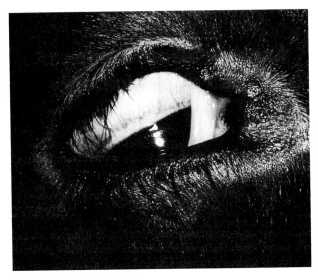

Fig. 22-3
The bovine eye rotates ventromedially during light planes of anesthesia.

IV. Leave the cuff inflated while the endotracheal tube is removed
V. Pass a stomach tube before removing the endotracheal tube to decompress the rumen if the animal has bloated
VI. To avoid regurgitation, position ruminants on their right side or in sternal recumbency once the tube is pulled
VII. Cattle do not usually require assistance during inhalation anesthesia recovery

COMMON ANESTHETIC PROBLEMS

I. The most frequently encountered problems associated with sedation and general anesthesia include the following:
A. Regurgitation
B. Bloat
C. Inadequate oxygenation
D. Respiratory depression and apnea

    E. Pulmonary aspiration

    F. Injury

II. Regurgitation is caused by a vagal effect on reticular contractions and parasympathetic effects on pharyngoesophageal and gastroesophageal sphincters

    A. Anesthetic drugs increase the risk of regurgitation in the following ways:

        1. By relaxing the pharyngoesophageal sphincter

        2. By relaxing the gastroesophageal sphincter

        3. By depressing the swallow reflex

    B. Recumbency also increases the risk of regurgitation; especially left lateral recumbency

    C. Rumen tube should be placed to avoid pulmonary aspiration

CHAPTER TWENTY-THREE

Anesthetic Procedures and Techniques in Pigs

"It is a bad plan that admits of no modification."
PUBLILIUS SYRUS

OVERVIEW

Anesthesia of pigs is a unique challenge. Swine have few superficial veins that are easily accessible, other than those on the dorsal surface of the ear. Ear veins may be difficult to use because of identification and tagging procedures; therefore most chemical restraining drugs are administered intramuscularly (IM). Pigs are difficult to intubate because of their small oral cavity, large tongue, and the presence of a pharyngeal diverticulum. Respiratory depression and elevations of body temperature are frequently associated with chemical restraint and general anesthesia. Respiratory depression may be caused by the combined respiratory-depressant effects of chemical restraining drugs and the limited expansion of the chest wall because of abnormal body positioning and body fat. Elevation in body temperature occurs because of the relatively low body surface area to body mass ratio, the relative absence of sweat glands, and inefficient thermoregulatory mechanisms. Hyperpyrexia and malignant hyperthermia have been reported in genetically predisposed pigs and can be triggered by intravenous (IV) (ketamine) and inhalation (halothane) anesthetics. Physical restraint combined with sedatives, tranquilizers, and local anesthetic techniques are the usual methods for simple surgical procedures in pigs. General anesthesia with inhalation anesthetics provides excellent, stable anesthesia for prolonged or complicated surgical procedures.

GENERAL CONSIDERATIONS

I. Surgical preparation of the pig
   A. Obtain a complete history and do a complete physical examination; pay particular attention to the respiratory system
   B. Withhold food for 6 to 10 hours in adults, 1 to 3 hours in neonates
   C. Do not withhold water
   D. Avoid stressing the pig; leave it with other pigs until it is tranquilized

II. The preanesthetic evaluation (see Chapter 2)
   A. Physical examination
   B. Basic laboratory tests, including a complete blood count

III. Injection sites
   A. IM injections should be made in the cervical region
   B. IV injections can be accomplished with the use of auricular veins if necessary

PREANESTHETIC MEDICATIONS

I. Azaperone (availability is limited)
   A. Butyrophenone tranquilizer
   B. The most effective tranquilizer in pigs
   C. Dose: 2.5 mg/kg IM
      2 mg/kg in older pigs, 8 mg/kg in large pigs
   D. Rapid onset: 5 to 10 minutes after IM
   E. Duration: 30 minutes after IM
   F. Disturbances after induction (especially first 20 minutes) may trigger excitement
   G. Large doses may induce deep sedation and hypotension

II. Diazepam
   A. Produce sedation and muscle relaxation in pigs
   B. Dose: 1 to 10 mg/kg IM
      0.5 to 2 mg/kg IV

III. Midazolam (similar to diazepam)
   A. Dose: 0.1 to 0.5 mg/kg IV or IM; approximately twice as potent as diazepam

IV. Xylazine
   A. Does not produce potent sedation as in other species
   B. Dose: 1 to 2 mg/kg IM
V. Acepromazine
   A. Does not produce potent sedation as in other species; use with xylazine is more effective
   B. Dose: 0.1 to 0.2 mg/kg IV or IM

ANESTHETIC PROCEDURES

I. Telazol®-ketamine-xylazine combination
   A. Formulation: reconstitute 500 mg of Telazol® powder with 2.5 ml of xylazine (100 mg/ml) and 2.5 ml of ketamine (100 mg/ml)
   B. Administer the combination IM at 1 to 2 ml/25 kg body weight
   C. Provides useful restraint and short-term anesthesia
   D. Endotracheal intubation can be performed
   E. Compatible with inhalant agents
   F. Duration of action is 20 to 30 minutes; recovery occurs in 60 to 90 minutes
II. Lumbosacral epidural or spinal anesthesia is a commonly used local anesthetic technique in pigs (see Chapter 5)
   A. The major advantages are minimal systemic effects and the minimal effect on the fetuses during cesarean section
   B. Disadvantages include lack of unconsciousness, necessitating physical restraint of the forelimbs
   C. A 3- to 12-cm, 18-gauge spinal needle is used to facilitate administration of 2% lidocaine hydrochloride
      1. The dose varies from 0.04 to 0.1 ml/kg, with the higher dose providing anesthesia cranially to the paralumbar fossa; spinal doses are one half of epidural doses
III. Intratesticular injection
   A. Large boars can be castrated by using physical restraint and the injection of 15 to 30 mg/kg of sodium pentobarbital into each testicle
   B. Anesthesia occurs in approximately 5 minutes
   C. As soon as the testicles are removed, the source of anesthetic is removed

IV. Atropine-acepromazine-ketamine combination
  A. Dosage: 40 µg/kg atropine and 0.1 to 0.4 mg/kg acepromazine IM, followed in 20 minutes by 10 mg/kg IM ketamine
  B. Useful for minor surgical or medical procedures, such as detusking or castration of large boars
  C. Advantages
      1. Ease of administration
      2. Some analgesia and muscle relaxation within 5 minutes; lasts 10 to 15 minutes
  D. Disadvantages
      1. Additional analgesia is required with a local anesthetic
      2. A 20-minute waiting period between administration of drugs is necessary
      3. Hypotension
V. Atropine-xylazine-ketamine combination
  A. Dosage: 40 µg/kg atropine and 2 to 6 mg/kg xylazine IM, followed in 10 minutes with 10 mg/kg IM ketamine
  B. Advantages
      1. Ease of administration
      2. Some analgesia and muscle relaxation within 5 minutes; lasts 10 to 15 minutes
  C. Disadvantages
      1. Xylazine has a short duration of action because it is rapidly metabolized
      2. Muscle movement is involuntary during the anesthetic period
VI. Xylazine-ketamine-guaifenesin combination
  A. Dosage: 500 mg xylazine + 500 mg ketamine mixed in 500 ml 5% guaifenesin; given IV in small increments until effective, approximately 1 to 2 ml/kg IV
  B. Advantages
      1. Gradual induction
      2. Stable hemodynamics
      3. Good muscle relaxation
  C. Disadvantages
      1. Respiratory depression may require assisted ventilation

VII. Xylazine-Telazol®

    A. Dosage: xylazine 0.2 to 2 mg/kg IM followed in 5 minutes by Telazol® 2 to 6 mg/kg IM

    B. Advantages

        1. Ease of administration

        2. Good analgesia and muscle relaxation

        3. Minimal cardiovascular depression

    C. Disadvantages

        1. Occasional respiratory depression

        2. Light plane of anesthesia

        3. Short duration of action; may need to be supplemented

        4. Pigs may remain drowsy for 24 hours

        5. Increased salivation

VIII. Inhalation anesthesia

    A. The inhalation anesthetic drugs, halothane, isoflurane, or sevoflurane, are administered

        1. For induction (by mask) to anesthesia

        2. For maintenance of anesthesia after the pig is induced with other drugs

    B. Inhalation anesthetic drugs can be administered in the following ways (Fig. 23-1):

        1. Through a face mask

        2. Through nasal tubes, which are made from human nasal tube adapters and small-animal endotracheal tubes (6 to 8 mm)

        3. Through endotracheal intubation, which is preferred; more difficult than other species; laryngoscope or long, rigid dowel rods can be used to pass the endotracheal tube (Fig. 23-2)

            a. Open the patient's mouth, grasp the tongue with a gauze sponge, and retract the tongue between the lower canine teeth to hold the mandible open

            b. Extend the head but not excessively; too much extension makes it more difficult to identify the arytenoid cartilages and may occlude the airway

            c. Use a laryngoscope and spray lidocaine to relieve laryngeal spasm; laryngeal spasm is usually induced after induction of anesthesia

            d. Place a long, small-diameter dowel made of steel or plastic into the trachea

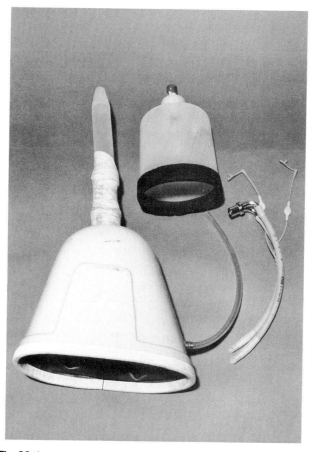

Fig. 23-1
Face masks and nasal endotracheal tubes can be used as an alternative to endotracheal intubation in pigs.

      e. Pass the endotracheal tube over the dowel; rotate the tube 180° when it meets resistance (the tip contacts the pharyngeal diverticulum)

C. Advantages
    1. Good control of anesthesia
    2. Excellent muscle relaxation
    3. Ease of administration

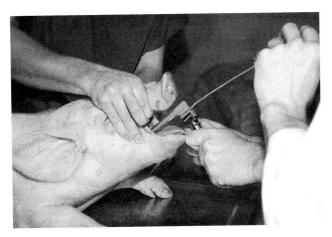

Fig. 23-2
A laryngoscope and stylet to stiffen the endotracheal tube are frequently used to place an endotracheal tube in the trachea of pigs.

ENDOTRACHEAL TUBE SIZES FOR PIGS	
WEIGHT OF PIGS (kg)	**INSIDE DIAMETER OF ENDOTRACHEAL TUBE (mm)**
<10	3-5
10-15	5-7
20-50	8-10
100-200	10-14
>200	16-18

    D. Disadvantages
        1. Expensive equipment required
        2. Not generally suited for field conditions
        3. Halothane can induce hyperthermia in pigs
IX. Analgesia
    A. Most opioids provide excellent analgesia in pigs
        1. Butorphanol 0.1 to 0.2 mg/kg IM
        2. Morphine 0.05 to 0.1 mg/kg IM

MONITORING

I. Monitoring anesthesia in pigs is similar to that for other species (see Chapter 5); the auricular artery, located on the dorsal surface of the ear, can be cannulated to monitor arterial blood pressure

II. Signs of malignant hyperthermia
  A. Extreme muscle rigidity
  B. Increased temperature (more than 107° F); hot to the touch
  C. Tachycardia, arrhythmia
  D. Hypotension
  E. Cyanosis
  F. Tachypnea
  G. Increase in $PaCO_2$
  H. Metabolic acidosis
  I. Myoglobinuria
  J. Myoglobin-induced acute tubular necrosis

III. Treatment of hyperthermia in pigs
  A. Dantrolene: 2 to 6 mg/kg IV; 20 mg/kg by mouth
  B. Termination of anesthesia
  C. Supportive treatment
    1. Cool fluids
    2. Bicarbonate
    3. Steroids
    4. Oxygen
    5. Hyperventilation
    6. Body cooling
    7. Exchange of anesthesia system; especially CO_2 absorbent
    8. Diuresis drugs

THE RECOVERY PERIOD

I. Administer oxygen and/or assist ventilation if necessary

II. Position the pig in sternal recumbency

III. Place the pig in a well-ventilated and quiet environment

IV. Assess vital signs periodically

COMMON ANESTHETIC PROBLEMS

I. Respiratory depression is a frequent sequela to the administration of depressant drugs in pigs
  A. Estimate the size of the pig's trachea before drug administration; it may be very narrow
    1. Use a laryngoscope and preplace a stiff polyethylene stylet
  B. Be prepared for respiratory emergencies
    1. Have a variety of endotracheal tube sizes available
    2. Be prepared to do a tracheotomy
      a. No. 10 blade and scalpel
      b. Hemostat
      c. Cuffed tracheostomy tube
      d. Respiratory stimulants, such as doxapram, may be necessary

II. Increases in body temperature are frequently associated with inhalant anesthesia in pigs
  A. The pig has a low body surface area relative to body mass
  B. The pig has relatively poor thermoregulatory mechanisms and relatively few sweat glands
  C. Depolarizing neuromuscular blocking agents and inhalation anesthetics can trigger malignant hyperthermia
    1. Several strains of pigs (e.g., Landrace, Poland China) are genetically predisposed to malignant hyperthermia
    2. Dantrolene (2 mg/kg IV) is the only truly effective therapy for malignant hyperthermia

CHAPTER TWENTY-FOUR

Anesthesia for Cesarean Section

"The hand that rocks the cradle is the hand that rules the world."

WILLIAM ROSS WALLACE

OVERVIEW

Anesthetic drugs used in pregnant animals affect the fetus. Generally, the effects of anesthetic drugs are more pronounced and longer lasting in the fetus than in the mother. Drugs that cross the placental barrier slowly, or not at all, are preferred. Anesthetic drugs may induce or inhibit parturition by altering uterine function. This chapter describes the changes that occur in maternal physiology during advanced pregnancy and the effects of anesthetic drugs in pregnant animals.

GENERAL CONSIDERATIONS

I. Pregnancy, especially the immediate preparturient period, causes significant alterations in maternal physiology
   A. Altered pharmacokinetics and pharmacodynamics
   B. Changes in hemodynamics
      1. Increased heart rate
      2. Increased cardiac output
      3. Increased blood volume
      4. The weight of the gravid uterus causes aortocaval compression during dorsal recumbency; cardiac reserve is decreased because of increased cardiac output and aortocaval compression

421

5. Central venous pressure and systemic blood pressure remain relatively unchanged but may increase during labor

C. Changes in respiration
1. Increased breathing rate
2. Decreased functional residual capacity (FRC)
3. The gravid uterus may restrict breathing by cranially displacing the diaphragm

II. Anesthetic drug and technique considerations
A. Providing optimal analgesia for surgery
B. Preventing maternal hypoxemia or hypotension
C. Minimizing fetal depression
D. Minimizing postoperative maternal depression
E. Neither inducing nor preventing uterine contractions

CHANGES IN MATERNAL PHYSIOLOGY IN ADVANCED PREGNANCY

I. Central nervous system (CNS)
A. Increased progesterone concentration decreases inhalant anesthetic requirement
B. Vascular engorgement decreases the size of the epidural space; decreased volume of local anesthetic is required for epidural anesthesia

II. Respiratory system
A. Alveolar ventilation is increased because of increased respiratory center sensitivity to CO_2, which is progesterone-induced; increased alveolar ventilation and decreased FRC result in a more rapid alveolar rate of rise in inhalation anesthetics
B. FRC is decreased because of anterior displacement of diaphragm
1. Relative anemia refers to the pregnant patient not tolerating blood loss as well as the nonpregnant patient
2. Patients with a history of heart disease may decompensate
C. Small airways constrict at higher lung volumes; airway closure and decreased FRC cause greater ventilation perfusion mismatches, which may result in decreased oxygenation

III. Cardiovascular system
   A. Maternal blood volume is increased by approximately 30%
   B. Packed cell volume and plasma-protein concentration are decreased
   C. Cardiac output is increased 30% to 50% because of increases in stroke volume and heart rate
IV. Gastrointestinal system
   A. Placental gastrin secretion increases gastric acidity
      1. Increases the chance of regurgitation and aspiration pneumonia
      2. Increases the need for a properly fitting cuffed endotracheal tube
   B. The stomach is displaced cranially, and the tone to the lower esophageal sphincter is altered
V. Other changes: decreased plasma cholinesterase (pseudo-cholinesterase)
   A. Prolonged duration of action of succinylcholine
   B. Prolonged duration of action of ester-linked local anesthetics

DRUG TRANSFER ACROSS THE PLACENTA

I. Factors influencing drug transfer
   A. Surface area and diffusion characteristics of the placenta; the surface area of the placenta is large, and diffusion distance is small in all species
   B. Diffusion properties of drugs
      1. High lipid solubility, which increases diffusibility
      2. Lower molecular weight, which increases diffusibility
      3. Decreased degree of ionization and protein binding, which increases diffusibility
   C. Relative maternal and fetal drug concentrations
      1. Discrete bolus doses of drugs result in rapid transfer of drug to the fetus initially and rapidly declining maternal concentrations
      2. Continuous infusion, repeated bolus administration, and the administration of inhalation anesthetics result in continuously high maternal drug concentration and continual drug transfer to the fetus

UTEROPLACENTAL CIRCULATION AND FETAL VIABILITY

I. Conditions that decrease circulating maternal blood volume can decrease placental perfusion, resulting in fetal hypoxia and acidosis; this includes maternal dehydration, hemorrhage (shock), and drug-induced hypotension
   A. Dehydration
      1. Prolonged labor
      2. Concurrent disease
   B. Hemorrhage and shock
      1. Prolonged labor
      2. Supine positioning: decreases venous return
      3. Anesthetic drugs
      4. Surgically related hemorrhage
      5. Hemorrhagic or endotoxic shock
   C. Drugs: anesthetic drugs cause peripheral vasodilation and hypotension

MATERNAL AND FETAL EFFECTS FROM ANESTHETIC DRUGS USED FOR CESAREAN SECTION

I. Anticholinergics—drug effects
   A. Both atropine and scopolamine pass placental barriers rapidly
      1. Fetal tachycardia noted within 10 to 15 minutes
      2. Fetal disorientation or excitement may be caused by central action of atropine or scopolamine
      3. Fetal effects may vary, depending on the amount of drug absorbed
   B. Glycopyrrolate does not cross the placenta in significant quantities because of its large molecular size and charge
   C. Anticholinergics can reduce placental activity
II. Local anesthetic drugs
   A. Drug effects
      1. Local anesthetic drugs administered by any route cross the placental barrier
         a. Drug effects depend on the total dose, the interval between final dose and delivery, and whether epinephrine is used

b. Doses of local anesthetics used clinically usually do not produce significant depression in the fetus

B. Lidocaine

1. Lidocaine is the preferred local anesthetic for cesarean section because of clinical experience and relatively low toxicity
2. Appears in umbilical venous blood of the fetus within 2 to 3 minutes
3. No correlation has been found between the degree of neonatal depression and the umbilical venous concentration of lidocaine

III. Preanesthetic (sedatives, tranquilizers, opioids) drug effects

A. Drug effects: preanesthetic drugs reduce the amount of potentially more dangerous anesthetic drugs

1. Phenothiazines (acepromazine)

a. Rapidly appear in fetal blood
b. Produce little to no apparent effect on the newborn when used in clinical doses
c. α-Adrenergic blockade may produce hypotension in stressed animals, resulting in decreased uterine blood flow and fetal hypoxia
d. Decrease uterine tone

2. Benzodiazepines (diazepam, midazolam)

a. Concentrations higher in fetal blood than in maternal blood
b. Produce minimal respiratory and cardiovascular depression
c. Duration of action depends on redistribution away from the CNS

3. α_2-Agonists (xylazine, detomidine, medetomidine, romifidine)

a. Respiratory depression may be severe in both the mother and fetus
b. Use in low doses and be prepared to administer an antagonist (yohimbine, tolazoline, atipamezole)
c. α_2-Agonists increase uterine pressure in cattle; may be abortifacients; effects in other species are unknown

4. Opioids
   a. Frequently used as preanesthetic medication for sedation and analgesia or administered epidurally
   b. Readily cross the placenta
   c. Concentrations may be higher in the fetus than in the mother because of a lower fetal pH
   d. Moderate maternal doses do not produce serious CNS depression in neonates; the effect can be reversed by opioid antagonists (naloxone)
   e. Because naloxone has a shorter duration of action than most opioids, neonates should be observed for several minutes and redosed as needed
   f. Specific opioid drugs
      (1) Meperidine (Demerol)
          (a) Reaches the fetal circulation rapidly
          (b) No significant depression is apparent if birth is within the first hour
      (2) Morphine
          (a) Causes observable clinical CNS depression in the newborn
          (b) Has a direct vasoconstrictor effect on placental vessels
      (3) Oxymorphone (Numorphan)
          (a) Better analgesia and sedation than meperidine or morphine but has a shorter duration of effect
          (b) Can produce neonatal depression
      (4) Fentanyl (Sublimaze); 100 times more potent as an analgesic than morphine, with respiratory depression of shorter duration

IV. Injectable anesthetic drugs
   A. Dissociogenic agents (ketamine, tiletamine)
      1. Produce restraint and analgesia
      2. Produce poor muscle relaxation
      3. Rapidly cross the placenta, producing fetal depression within 5 to 10 minutes
      4. Specific dissociogenic drugs
         a. Ketamine
            (1) Good restraint in queens with minimal fetal depression when used intravenously or intra-

muscularly in low doses (2 mg/kg intravenous-ly; 10 mg/kg intramuscularly)
  - (2) Poor muscle relaxation and questionable ability to block deep pain
  - (3) May increase uterine tone and decrease uterine blood flow, leading to fetal hypoxia
      - (4) Fetal blood levels reach 70% of those in the mother
      - (5) Minimal clinical CNS depression is evident in the neonate
  - b. Telazol® (tiletamine-zolazepam)
    - (1) Similar to ketamine but produces better muscle relaxation
    - (2) Greater respiratory depression
- B. Propofol
  - 1. Used for induction of anesthesia in parturients
    - a. Single bolus (2 to 7 mg/kg intravenously) followed by inhalant anesthetic
  - 2. Crosses the placenta readily but produces short-duration effects on the fetus
  - 3. Large volume of distribution causes plasma concentrations to fall rapidly
  - 4. Fetal respiratory depression is a concern
- C. Barbiturates
  - 1. Readily crosses the placenta into fetal circulation
  - 2. Phenobarbital should be avoided because of prolonged fetal CNS depression and reduced fetal ability to metabolize drugs
  - 3. Dose of barbiturates that does not produce anesthesia in the mother can completely inhibit fetal respiratory movements
  - 4. Ultrashort-acting barbiturates (thiopental)
    - a. Thiobarbiturates cross the placenta readily and achieve equilibrium within 5 minutes
    - b. A single dose of 9 mg/kg at induction produces only modest placental transfer and does not endanger the normal fetus
      - (1) Because of a dependence on redistribution for their duration of action, the use of small doses of an ultrashort-acting barbiturate has not been

associated with a significant degree of fetal CNS depression
   (2) Redosing is discouraged
   (3) Peak drug concentrations occur in the fetus within 10 minutes
V. Peripheral muscle relaxants: neuromuscular blocking drugs include succinylcholine, pancuronium, atracurium, and vecuronium
   A. These drugs are highly ionized with a high molecular weight, resulting in minimal and poor placental transfer
   B. No analgesia is produced; used only in combination with other drugs
   C. There is no demonstrable effect on the newborn
   D. Succinylcholine metabolism is reduced because of a decrease in pseudocholinesterase
VI. Inhalation anesthetic drugs
   A. All inhalation anesthetic drugs readily cross the placenta because of their low molecular weight and lipid solubility
   B. The degree of fetal CNS depression depends on the depth and duration of maternal anesthesia
   C. Specific inhalation drugs
      1. Nitrous oxide
         a. Rapidly crosses the placenta
         b. Administration exceeding 15 minutes may result in fetal CNS depression
         c. Diffusion hypoxia, which may occur in the fetus, can be minimized with oxygen therapy
         d. When used in the mother with adequate amounts of oxygen, there is minimal effect on the neonate
      2. Isoflurane
         a. Quickly appears in fetal circulation
         b. Rapid and potent uterine relaxant
         c. If used for cesarean section, the procedure should be performed as quickly as possible
            (1) The degree of fetal CNS depression does not correlate with maternal blood concentration
            (2) Neonatal respiratory depression may be severe, requiring postparturient ventilation

      d. Rapid elimination of this agent with ventilation may be an advantage

   3. Sevoflurane and desflurane are similar to isoflurane; desflurane's rapid onset and elimination minimize the duration of maternal and fetal CNS depression

ANESTHETIC TECHNIQUES

  I. General principles

    A. The choice of a particular anesthetic technique should be influenced by familiarity with the technique or drug and avoidance of excessive fetal CNS depression

    B. Intubation is desirable in all patients

    C. Use local and regional analgesic techniques when possible

    D. Presurgical preparation and oxygenation should be completed before the administration of anesthetic drugs

    E. Avoid excessive physical restraint: sedatives, tranquilizers, and other drugs that can be antagonized are preferred over excessive physical force and subsequent maternal-fetal distress

    F. Avoid dorsal recumbency, if possible; left lateral recumbency may be the safest method

 II. Anesthetic techniques by species (Table 24-1)

III. Analgesia (Tables 24-2 and 24-3)

TABLE 24-1
ANESTHETIC TECHNIQUES BY SPECIES

SPECIES	DRUG/TECHNIQUE	DOSAGE	COMMENTS
Local techniques			
Dog, cat	Epidural with 2% lidocaine or morphine	0.3 ml/kg body weight lidocaine; 0.2 mg/kg body weight morphine	Requires assistant for physical restraint; use sedative/tranquilizer in all but extremely tractable patients
General techniques			
	Diazepam-ketamine induction	0.25 mg/kg diazepam plus 5 mg/kg ketamine IV	Single-bolus dose depresses fetus minimally Diazepam-ketamine good in patients who are depressed and in shock
	Telazol® induction	0.5-2 mg/kg IV	Single administration causes minimal fetal CNS depression
	Maintenance		
	Isoflurane, or sevoflurane in 50% N_2O and oxygen followed by muscle relaxant (atracurium, pancuronium) if needed	See Chapters 9, 10, and 11	Administer inhalation agent as late into procedure as possible

Intractable animal

	1. Premedication Dogs: acepromazine- oxymorphone	1 mg/kg of each; maximum 4 mg of each	Controlled ventilation necessary when using relaxants
	2. Dogs or cats: diazepam- ketamine induction	1 ml of a 50:50 mixture per 5 kg, IM	Sedative-hypnotics generally increase fetal CNS depression; therefore use sparingly
	3. Telazol®	6-10 mg/kg IM	
Horse	Premedication: acepromazine, - xylazine, detomidine, or romifidine	Acepromazine: 0.04 mg/kg IV	Adjust dosage for physical condition of mother; rely on guaifenesin to produce relaxation and to allow less ketamine to be used
		Xylazine: 0.2-0.7 mg/kg IV Detomidine: 10-20 µg/kg Romifidine: 80-160 µg/kg	
	Induction: guaifenesin plus ketamine	Guaifenesin: 50-100 mg/kg Ketamine: 1.5-2 mg/kg	
	Maintenance: sevoflurane, isoflurane		
Local techniques			
Cow	Standing paravertebral analgesia, line block, inverted L block	2% lidocaine (see Chapter 5 for techniques)	Suitable for tractable animals without a sedative Suitable for animals in good physical condition

Continued

IV, Intravenously; *IM*, intramuscularly.

TABLE 24-1
ANESTHETIC TECHNIQUES BY SPECIES—cont'd

SPECIES	DRUG/TECHNIQUE	DOSAGE	COMMENTS
Local techniques—cont'd			
Cow—cont'd	Anterior epidural	2% lidocaine, 2 ml/kg at Co_1-Co_2 junction	Induces recumbency and sensory block anterior to umbilicus Watch for hypotension Intubate if possible
General techniques			
	Guaifenesin-ketamine-xylazine	500 mg ketamine 25 mg xylazine 500 ml of 5% guaifenesin + 0.5-1 mg/kg until effective for maintenance	Intubate; copious salivation Moderate to poor muscle relaxation
Sheep, goat	Guaifenesin-ketamine	500 ml 5% guaifenesin containing 500 mg ketamine 0.5-2 mg/kg induction maintenance until effective	Can add 25 mg xylazine to mixture, but fetal CNS depression is greater Use for induction to gas or as IV technique

Guaifenesin-ketamine induction; sevoflurane, isoflurane	50 mg/kg guaifenesin	Guaifenesin allows small bolus doses of ketamine
Diazepam-ketamine	2 mg/kg ketamine; 1 ml diazepam plus 1 ml ketamine	
	Administer 1 ml/15 kg	Useful in sick, toxic animals and when fetal viability is not a concern
Mask induction isoflurane or sevoflurane	Until effective	
Maintenance		
Pig		
Isoflurane or sevoflurane		
Epidural	2% lidocaine (see Chapter 4 for technique)	Restraint of sow's head and front legs necessary
Xylazine plus ketamine	1 mg/kg, 6-11 mg/kg	Good chemical restraint; however, relatively more fetal CNS depression than with epidural
Xylazine 2.5 ml ketamine 2.5 ml in Telazol®	1 ml/25 kg, IM	Excellent short-term restraint
500 mg ketamine plus 500 mg xylazine in 500 ml 5% guaifenesin	2 ml of mixture per kg until effective for maintenance	Requires placement of IV catheter

IV, Intravenously; *IM*, intramuscularly.

TABLE 24-2
ANALGESIC DOSES FOR PREGNANT CATS AND DOGS (mg/kg)

OPIOID AGONISTS (NARCOTICS)	DOSE	ROUTE OF ADMINISTRATION	DOSING INTERVAL (hr)
Morphine	**Dog**		
	0.1-0.5	Very slow IV bolus	1-4
	0.1-0.5	IV/hr	CRI
	0.5-1	IM, SQ	1-4
	0.1-0.3	Epidural	4-8
	0.5-2	PO titrate to effect	4-6
	Cat		
	0.05-0.2	Very slowly IV, IM, SQ	2-6
	0.5-1	PO titrate to effect	8-12
Hydromorphone	**Dog**		
	0.04-0.2	IV	4-6
	0.05-0.2 (extreme cases)	IM, SQ	4-6
	Cat		
	0.02-0.1 (extreme cases)	IV	4-6
	0.05-0.1	IM, SQ	4-6

Methadone	**Dog and cat** 0.1-0.5	IV, IM, SQ	2-4
Codeine	**Dog** 1-2	PO titrate to effect	6-8
	Cat 0.5-1	PO titrate to effect	12

IV, Intravenously; *IM*, intramuscularly; *SQ*, subcutaneously; *PO*, by mouth; *CRI*, constant rate infusion.

TABLE 24-3

ANALGESIC DOSES FOR NURSING BITCHES AND QUEENS (mg/kg)

OPIOID AGONISTS (NARCOTICS)	DOSE	ROUTE OF ADMINISTRATION	INTERVAL (hr)
Morphine	**Dog**		
	0.1-0.5	Very slow IV	1-4
	0.1-0.5	IV/hr	CRI
	0.5-1	IM, SQ	1-4
	0.1-0.3	Epidural	4-8
	0.5-2	PO titrate to effect	4-6
	Cat		
	0.05-0.2	IV very slowly	2-6
		IM, SQ	
	0.5-1	PO titrate to effect	8-12
Hydromorphone	**Dog**		
Increased temperature may be noted with administration in cats	0.04-0.2	IV	4-6
	0.05-0.2	IM, SQ	4-6
	Cat		
	0.04-0.1	IV	4-6
	0.05-0.1	IM, SQ	4-6

Methadone	**Dog and cat**		
	0.1-0.5	IV, IM, SQ	2-4
Fentanyl	**Dog and cat**		
	1-5+ μg/kg	IV loading	0.5-1
	1-5 μg/kg	IV/20-60 min	CRI
	50 μg/kg for anesthesia	IV 60 min	CRI
Fentanyl transdermal patch	Should be avoided because of potential ingestion by puppies or kittens		
Codeine	**Dog**		
	1-2	PO titrate to effect	6-8
	Cat		
	0.5-1	PO titrate to effect	12

IV, Intravenously; *IM,* intramuscularly; *SQ,* subcutaneously; *PO,* by mouth; *CRI,* constant rate infusion.

CHAPTER TWENTY-FIVE

Anesthetic Procedures in Exotic Animals

"The time has come,' the walrus said, 'to talk of many things."

LEWIS CARROLL

OVERVIEW

The number of exotic animals being maintained as pets and for profit is increasing. Anesthesia for nontraditional species is accomplished by using the same techniques and drugs used in domestic animals. Because exotic species demonstrate idiosyncrasies and widely varying sensitivities to drugs, it is frequently necessary to make modifications. This chapter is an overview of the basic information needed to successfully immobilize exotic animals that are likely to be encountered by general practitioners.[*]

GENERAL CONSIDERATIONS

   I. Preanesthetic considerations

      A. Discussions with owners

---

[*]For more detailed descriptions of chemical restraint and anesthesia in laboratory animals, including primates, refer to the following articles: Flecknell PA: *Laboratory animal anesthesia: a practical introduction for research workers and technicians,* ed 2, San Diego, 1996, Academic Press; Kohn DF, et al: *Anesthesia and analgesia in laboratory animals (American College of Laboratory Animal Medicine Series),* San Diego, 1997, Academic Press; Fox JG, et al., *Laboratory animal medicine (American College of Laboratory Animal Medicine),* ed 2, San Diego, 2002, Academic Press; *Veterinary Clinics of North America: Exotic Animal Practice—analgesia and anesthesia.* 2001; Jan:4(1), Philadelphia, WB Saunders, *Journal of Exotic Pet Medicine,* October 2005 (Vol. 14, Issue 4) Anesthesia and Analgesia. Glenn R. Pettifer (Ed.)

      1. Ensure that the client has realistic expectations

      2. Detail prognosis and risks; owners may not understand that exotic animals respond differently to immobilization than domestic animals

      3. Determine the aftercare provider; owners may not be able to administer treatments to exotic pets

      4. Discuss costs

B. Reduce the animal's stress; exotic animals have high sympathetic drive; excessive stress can induce complications that include arrhythmias, hypertension, and hyperthermia, which can result in death

C. Presurgical evaluation and patient selection

      1. Physical examination:

          a. Quiet observation of animals in their cage will provide a great deal of information (e.g., awareness of and attention to its surrounding environment, body form and posture, skin or feather condition, respiratory rate)

          b. Contraindications to anesthesia

              (1) Abnormally slow recovery rate (the amount of time an animal needs to return to normal respirations after 2 minutes of physical restraint or pursuit); a normal amount of time is less than 3 to 5 minutes

              (2) Shock; septicemia; acidosis

              (3) Anemia or cyanosis

              (4) Prolonged clotting

              (5) Cachexia; obesity

              (6) Animal has not fasted (if regurgitation is likely)

              (7) Severe weakness and central nervous system depression

              (8) Dehydration

              (9) Ascites

      2. Laboratory evaluation

          a. The volume of blood required for the sample should not exceed 10% of the patient's blood volume (e.g., the blood volume of a 30 g (body weight) gerbil is 2.3 mL and 10% of this volume is 0.2 mL)

BLOOD VOLUMES OF EXOTIC SPECIES	
GENUS	BLOOD VOLUME (ml/kg)
Chickens	60
Reptiles	90.8
Frog	95
Fish	17-28
Mouse	50-60
Rat	60
Gerbil	78
Syrian hamster	78
Guinea pig	60-65
Chinchilla	65
Rabbit	55-65
Ferret	60

b. Contraindications to anesthesia
(1) If packed cell volume is low, a blood transfusion may be needed

PERILOUSLY LOW PACKED CELL VOLUMES IN EXOTIC SPECIES	
GENUS	PACKED CELL VOLUME (%)
Avian	<25
Reptile	<17 to 20
Amphibian	<20
Rodent/lagomorph	<20
Mustelid	<25
Felid	<15
Swine	<20
Camelid	<20

(2) If packed cell volume is high, fluids may be needed

PERILOUSLY HIGH PACKED CELL VOLUMES IN EXOTIC SPECIES

GENUS	PACKED CELL VOLUME (%)
Avian	>50 to 60
Reptile	>50 to 60
Amphibian	>60
Rodent/lagomorph	>55 to 60
Mustelid	>60
Felid	>50
Swine	>50
Camelid	>50

(3) If total protein is less than 3 g/dl, amino acid or plasma supplementation may be needed; refractometers and colorimetric tests frequently used at diagnostic laboratories for mammalian blood often register falsely low proteins in nonmammalian species; the biuret method is the most accurate in avian species

(4) If glucose is low, administer 5% dextrose or delay anesthesia

PERILOUSLY LOW BLOOD GLUCOSE LEVELS IN EXOTIC SPECIES

GENUS	GLUCOSE (MG/DL)
Avian	<150
Reptile	30-100
Amphibian	<50
Rodent/lagomorph	<80-100
Mustelid	<80-100
Felid	<80
Swine	<60
Camelid	<60

(5) If calcium is less than 8 mg/dl, correct the level

(6) If potassium is less than 3.5 mg/dl, correct the level

3. Further evaluation
   a. Oral/fecal gram stains in nonmammalians
   b. Culture and sensitivity

      c. Fecal/urinalysis

      d. Complete hemogram/serum profile

      e. Radiographs/ultrasound

      f. Clotting profile

      g. Electrocardiogram/echocardiography

II. Preanesthetic fasting

    A. Hypoglycemia can occur within a few hours in very small mammals

TIME FOR PREANESTHETIC FOOD WITHDRAWAL IN EXOTIC SPECIES	
	TIME (HR)
Avian <100 g	0
Large psittacine	1 to 2
Raptor, ratite, fowl, waterfowl	12 to 24
Carnivorous reptile ingesting whole prey	>5 days
Reptile <200 g	2 to 4
Reptile 200 to 500 g	12
Reptile >500 g	24+
Amphibian	24
Fish	24
Rodent <200 g	0-2
Rodent >200 g/lagomorph	>6
Guinea pig	6-8
Mustelid	12
Ferret	4-12 <2 hr in ferrets with insulinoma
Rabbit	0-24
Felid	24
Swine	24
Camelid	24 to 48

III. Maintenance of homoiothermy

    A. Hypothermia depresses the respiratory control system

        1. Small animals are predisposed to hypothermia; they lose heat rapidly as a result of high surface area-to-volume ratios

2. Ectotherms (reptiles, fish, and amphibians) do not generate their own heat; they require external heat sources to maintain their body temperature; hypothermia depresses the immune system and slows healing

3. Hypothermia can result in brain damage, shock, electrolyte imbalances, and disseminated intravascular coagulation

   a. Well-insulated small animals such as rabbits, chinchillas, water birds, and birds in winter plumage are susceptible to hyperthermia

   b. Ungulates are prone to malignant hyperthermia; stress, high ambient temperature, and high relative humidity during immobilization increase the likelihood of hyperthermia

B. Methods of monitoring core body temperature (skin temperature is not reliable)

  1. Esophageal thermometer

  2. Rectal/cloacal thermometer

C. Heat sources and keeping heat

  1. To avoid iatrogenic burns and hyperthermia, always monitor heat sources

   a. Skin temperature

   b. Surface temperature where the patient's body contacts

   c. Ambient temperature in incubators

  2. Water-circulating heating pad

   a. Very safe

   b. High maintenance cost if punctured

  3. Electric heating pads

   a. Likely to cause iatrogenic burns

   b. Inexpensive

   c. Should never be set on high

  4. Incubators

   a. Must be preheated

   b. Useful before and after anesthesia

   c. Must be escape-proof

  5. Hot water bottles

   a. Very safe

   b. Act as a heat sink after they are cool

6. Warm air blankets (Bair Hugger; made by Augustine Medical)
   a. Very safe
   b. Blankets warm immediate surroundings
   c. Patient temperature must be monitored
7. Prevention of heat diffusion
   a. Aluminum foil
   b. Plastic bubble wrap
   c. Minimize the amount of hair clipped
   d. Use warm prep solutions and warm surgical flush
   e. Quickly cover the exposed surface with a drape
   f. Minimize the duration of anesthesia

IV. Fluids
   A. Perioperative hypovolemia must be prevented to decrease postoperative morbidity and mortality
   B. Preheat to 80° F to 95° F (26° C to 35° C) for animals weighing less than 1 kg and for all ectotherms
      1. Incubator
         a. Even, reliable temperature must be maintained
         b. Microbial growth may occur
      2. Warm water bath
         a. Even, reliable temperature must be maintained
         b. Water must be kept warm
      3. Microwave fluids
         a. Frequently have hot spots
         b. Should be well mixed
      4. Placing intravenous (IV) tubing in warm water bath
         a. Quick method to warm fluids in emergency
         b. Effluent temperature must be carefully monitored
      5. Fluid heating devices (Hotline, SMIS Level 1)
         a. Warms IV fluids to above 104° F (40° C)
   C. Administration (route) (Table 25-1)
      1. IV or intraosseous (IO) administration is best; the humerus in all birds and the femur in many birds are pneumatic bones; placing IO catheters in these bones causes iatrogenic drowning
      2. Subcutaneous (SQ) fluids (usually 5% to 10% of body weight) are given before induction of anesthesia to allow absorption and volume expansion
      3. Intraperitoneal fluids

TABLE 25-1

SITES FOR PARENTERAL ACCESS OR INJECTION IN BIRDS AND SMALL MAMMALS

SPECIES	SITES FOR PARENTERAL ACCESS OR INJECTION	COMMENTS
Birds	IM, IO, IV: basilic, jugular, medial metatarsal	
Rats and mice	SQ, IM, IP, IO, IV: jugular, lateral tail	Lateral tail veins on mice are difficult to obtain blood from except by capillary action
Gerbils	SQ, IM, IP, IO, IV: lateral tail, saphenous, metatarsal	25-gauge needle
Hamsters	SQ, IM, IP, IO (tibial crest), IV: lateral tarsus, cephalic, lingual, dorsal penile	IV: access is difficult, use 27 to 30-gauge needle IM: maximal volume 0.25 ml IO: use 22-gauge spinal needle
Chinchillas	SQ, IM, IP, IO, IV: femoral, cephalic, lateral saphenous, jugular, auricular, dorsal penile, lateral abdomen, tail	IM: 23-gauge or smaller and maximum 0.3 ml IV: 25-gauge or smaller needle
Guinea pigs	SQ, IM, IP, IO (trochanteric fossa), IV: marginal ear, medial saphenous, lateral saphenous, proximal to hock, dorsal penile, jugular	Self-mutilation can occur with IM injections, usually vascular access is difficult with short, mobile, friable veins
Rabbits	SQ, IM, IP, IO (trochanteric fossa), IV: marginal ear, cephalic, lateral saphenous, jugular	Blood clots quickly, external jugular is primary drainage for head (swelling occurs if catheter remains in place)
Ferrets	SQ, IM, IP, IO, IV: cephalic, jugular, lateral saphenous, lateral tail	

SQ, Subcutaneous; *IM,* intramuscular; *IP,* intraperitoneal; *IO,* intraosseous; *IV,* intravenous.

a. More rapidly absorbed than SQ fluids
b. Could cause peritonitis
c. Must be warmed to body temperature
d. Not in birds
e. Not in pregnant animals
f. Bladder should be expressed before administration
4. Colonic fluids
a. Isotonic, warmed solution may be given as an enema
b. Fluids are often absorbed more rapidly across the mucosa of the colon than from the SQ space
D. Fluid rates
1. Standard maintenance: 40 to 100 ml/kg/24 hr; the higher end of the range is used for neonates, birds, and animals with high metabolic rates
2. Intraoperative: 10 to 20 ml/kg/hr
3. Shock: 30 to 80 ml/kg in 20 minutes
E. Fluid rate control
1. Rates less than 10 ml/hr require an IV fluid infusion pump to ensure accuracy
2. Rates of 10 to 50 ml/hr are accurately measured with in-line flow controls or burette fluid chambers
3. Rates greater than 50 ml/hr are accurately measured off of most fluid containers
F. Fluid choice (see Chapter 26)
G. Blood transfusion (see Chapter 26)
1. Ethylenediamine tetra-acetic acid (EDTA) should not be used in small patients to avoid hypocalcemia
2. Heparin is the anticoagulant of choice for birds
3. Birds can receive one interspecies or genera transfusion if a donor of the same species is not available, but survival of red blood cells over 24 hours is limited; intraspecific or at least intragenera transfusions are preferred
a. Pigeons are the most common donors
b. Transfusions should not be repeated for at least 3 weeks
H. Blood substitutes
1. Oxyglobin (Biopure Corp.) can be used in most species as a blood substitute (10 to 30 ml/kg)

V. Premediation
- **A.** If necessary, administer antibiotics to achieve adequate serum levels before induction of anesthesia
- **B.** Select appropriate preanesthetic medication
- **C.** Avian (Table 25-2)

TABLE 25-2
INJECTABLE SEDATIVE AND ANALGESIC DRUGS FOR USE IN BIRDS (mg/kg)

DRUG	DOSE
Atropine	0.01-0.02 IV, 0.02-0.08 IM
Glycopyrrolate	0.01-0.02 IV, IM
Alphaxalone/alphadolone	10-14 IV
Buprenorphine	0.01-0.1 IM
Butorphanol	0.1-4 IM
Codeine	30 IM
Fentanyl	0.2 IM
Morphine	0.1-3 IV, 2.5-30 IM, SQ
Diazepam	0.05-0.15 IV, 0.2-0.5 IM
Midazolam	0.05-0.15 IV, 0.1-0.5 IM, 7.3 mg/kg intranasally
Detomidine	12 mg/kg intranasally
Ketamine >1 kg	15-20 mg/kg IM
<1 kg	30-40 mg/kg IM
Ketamine/midazolam	20-40 mg/kg IM+ 4 mg/kg IM
Ketamine/xylazine	10-30 mg/kg IM+ 2-6 mg/kg IM
Ketamine/midazolam/xylazine	40-50 mg/kg + 3.65 mg/kg + 10 mg/kg intranasally
Propofol	10 slow IV infusion to effect Up to 3 mg/kg increments for supplemental doses
Etomidate	10-20 mg/kg IM
Betamethasone	0.1 IM
Dexamethasone	2-4 IV, IM
Methylprednisolone	0.5-1
Prednisolone sodium succinate	0.5-1 IV, IM
Ketoprofen	5-10 IM, 2 SQ
Flunixin meglumine	1-10 IV, IM
Phenylbutazone	3.5-7 IV
Carprofen	2-10 IM, 1 SQ

IV, Intravenous; *IM*, intramuscular; *SQ*, subcutaneous.

1. Atropine is not indicated in the presence of respiratory secretions, because it makes them more viscous
2. Preanesthetics are rarely indicated if the bird is small enough to be manually restrained
   a. Most are overridden
   b. They may delay recovery
   c. They may depress respirations
   d. Diazepam/midazolam is the most efficacious and safe—0.05 to 0.15 mg/kg IV, 0.2 to 0.5 mg/kg intramuscularly (IM), 7.3 mg/kg intranasally
      (1) Can be reversed with flumazenil 0.13 mg/kg
   e. Detomidine 12 mg/kg intranasally
   f. Combination of midazolam (3.65 mg/kg), xylazine (10 mg/kg), and ketamine (40 to 50 mg/kg) intranasally
3. Because their long legs are susceptible to trauma, ratites, storks, and long-legged wading birds weighing more than 15 kg may benefit from sedation before capture and/or restraint
   a. Xylazine: 0.2 to 0.4 mg/kg IM
   b. Tiletamine-zolazepam (Telazol®): 2 to 5 mg/kg IM
D. Reptile
   1. Atropine is not indicated in the presence of respiratory secretions, because it makes them more viscous
   2. Preanesthetics are rarely indicated, except in large, aggressive, and/or venomous reptiles
E. Amphibian: preanesthetics are not routinely used
F. Fish: preanesthetics are not routinely used
G. Rodent/rabbit
   1. Atropine or glycopyrrolate is useful for decreasing airway secretions and maintaining heart rate
   2. Rabbits have atropinase, therefore making the use of atropine of questionable value—use glycopyrrolate instead
   3. Acepromazine and diazepam are effective preanesthetics
   4. Acepromazine is not recommended in gerbils, because it may potentiate seizures
   5. Hamsters require up to 5 mg/kg of acepromazine
   6. Combination of fentanyl and fluanisone (hypnorm) produces sedation and immobilization for approximately 30 to 60 minutes; analgesic effects may persist

H. Mustelid (ferrets)
   1. Atropine is given as needed to maintain heart rate and decrease secretions
   2. Diazepam or midazolam provides light tranquilization but no analgesia
   3. Acepromazine provides light to moderate tranquilization but also no analgesia; should be avoided in hypovolemic or very sick animals
   4. Xylazine or medetomidine produces dose-dependent sedation, immobilization, and analgesia
   5. Opioids potentiate sedation and provide analgesia; usually given in combination with other sedatives or tranquilizers
   6. Ketamine produces dose-dependent sedation; muscle relaxation is poor if it is given alone
I. Felid
   1. Preanesthetics are not routinely used
   2. Atropine can be used at standard domestic cat doses
      a. Atropine: 0.02 to 0.04 mg/kg SQ, IM, IV
      b. Glycopyrrolate: 0.005 to 0.01 mg/kg SQ, IM, IV
J. Guinea pigs
   1. Hypnorm alone produces sedation and immobilization for approximately 30 to 60 minutes; analgesic effects may persist
K. Swine (see Chapter 23)
L. Camelid
   1. Xylazine 1 to 3 mg/kg IM
   2. Medetomidine 20 µg/kg IM
VI. Monitoring plane of anesthesia
   A. Generalities
      1. Pulse rate and character: a decrease in the heart rate to less than 80% of the stabilized rate after induction indicates that anesthesia should be lightened
      2. Respiratory rate, volume, and character (e.g., apneustic)
         a. A decreasing respiratory rate or apneustic/erratic patterns indicate that anesthesia should be lightened
         b. Ectotherms normally develop apnea at surgical planes of anesthesia; plan to administer positive-pressure ventilation at least four to six times per minute

3. Body temperature
   a. Body temperature can drop as much as 10° C in 15 to 20 minutes
4. The level of anesthesia
   a. Reflexes are a good index of anesthetic depth; the signs vary between the species
      (1) Auricular reflex is useful in rabbits

B. Equipment
   1. Electrocardiogram modifications
      a. To protect delicate skin or to penetrate thick skin, attach clips to steel sutures or metal hubbed needles placed through the skin at lead sites
      b. Attach clips to alcohol-soaked pads placed at the usual lead sites
      c. Wings are used for forelimb lead sites in birds
      d. Place one clip cranial and one caudal to the heart in legless animals
   2. Doppler placement
      a. Over the heart in small animals
      b. Over the peripheral artery
         (1) Avian: medial metatarsal, brachial
         (2) Reptile: tail artery
         (3) Rodent/lagomorph: ear, femoral, saphenous, foot pad
         (4) Mustelid: tail, foot pad, saphenous
   3. Pulse oximeter
      a. Measures oxygenation in addition to heart rate
      b. Placement: tongue, esophageal
         (1) Measures across any nonpigmented capillary bed
         (2) Mucous membranes are excellent sampling sites: oral or nasal mucosa, cloaca, vulva
         (3) Measures through nonpigmented skin: ear, wing web, thin skin of flank or abdomen
   4. Heart rate monitors must be suited for high heart rates and be able to read up to 350 beats/min in rabbits and more than 600 beats/min in mice
   5. Respiratory monitor must be sensitive enough to detect small tidal volumes

AVIAN ANESTHESIA (LESS THAN 15 KG)

I. Attainment of surgical anesthesia
   A. Toe, tail, and cloacal pinches should induce slow withdrawal
   B. Most birds have a slow third-eyelid response; the loss of this response in birds indicates that anesthesia should be deepened
   C. Response is not present in response to pinpricks to the cere
   D. Respirations are slow, deep, and regular

II. Anesthetic procedure recommendations (Tables 25-2 and 25-3)
   A. Preanesthetic agents can be used if needed

TABLE 25-3
AVIAN ANESTHESIA (mg/kg)

SPECIES	DRUG	IM DOSES
Birds >250 g	Ketamine	10
	Ketamine	20-40
	Diazepam	1-1.5
Birds <250 g	Ketamine	30
Parakeet	Ketamine	30
	Xylazine	6.5
Cockatiel	Ketamine	25
	Xylazine	2.5
Amazon	Ketamine	10-20
	Xylazine	1-2
African Grey	Ketamine	15-20
	Xylazine	1.5
Cockatoo	Ketamine	20-30
	Xylazine	2.5-3.5
Macaw	Ketamine	15
	Xylazine	1.5-2
Hawk, falcon	Ketamine	25-30
	Xylazine	2
Owl	Ketamine	10-15
	Xylazine	2
Great horned Owl	Propofol	4.5 (induction)
		0.48 mg/kg/min (maintenance)

B. Inhalation anesthesia is preferred over injectable anesthesia
   1. The safety and efficacy of injectable anesthetics vary among species and individual animals
   2. It is extremely difficult to titrate the dose of injectable anesthetics; therefore inhalants are preferred
   3. Injectable agents can be used for restraint for short diagnostic procedures, minor surgeries, or for induction before the use of inhalation anesthesia
C. Oxygen flow rates
   1. Greater than 200 ml/min/kg in small birds
   2. 0.5 to 2 L/min; maximum dose is 3 to 4 L/min
D. Use a non-rebreathing system for all birds weighing less than 7 kg
   1. Restrain the bird by hand or use toweling
   2. Place the bird's head inside a clear plastic bag taped to the end of the Y- or T-piece while oxygen and anesthetic gas are flowing
   3. Hold the bird until it is relaxed and then maintain anesthesia with a mask or intubation
E. Endotracheal intubation is recommended for all birds
   1. Birds weighing less than 100 g should be intubated for procedures longer than 30 minutes or for procedures involving the coelomic cavity; small face masks are commercially available or can be fashioned from 35- to 60-ml syringe cases and rubber gloves
      a. Very-small-gauge silicone endotracheal tubes sized 1.0 mm and 1.5 mm (internal diameter) are useful (noncuffed endotracheal tubes-silicone V-PAT-10, V-PAT-15; Cook Veterinary Product)
   2. The glottis is easily visualized at the base of the tongue
      a. The trachea is composed of nonexpansible, complete tracheal rings; cuffs are not recommended
      b. Tissue swelling caused by tube-induced tracheitis can occlude the trachea in birds weighing less than 100 g
      c. Small endotracheal tubes can be fashioned from catheters, the hub end of butterfly catheters, or red rubber feeding tubes; the hubs of these items fit into adapters made for commercially available 3.5- to 4.5-mm endotracheal tubes

d. Making the tubes just long enough to ensure secure placement can minimize dead space

e. Tubes should be taped securely to the bird's beak to avoid the sensitive cere

f. Tubes should be monitored for occlusion; mucous plugs and kinking are common; always have a replacement tube immediately available

3. If the trachea is occluded, the caudal thoracic air sacs can be cannulated at the site usually used for surgical sexing with a red rubber feeding tube cut to 2 to 5 cm in length; suture the tube in place; use the tube in the same fashion as an endotracheal tube; use aseptic technique to prevent life-threatening air sacculitis

4. Birds do not tolerate apnea

a. Positive-pressure ventilation is required at least two times per minute to assist self-ventilating birds; ventilate 8 to 25 times per minute in apneic birds, higher rates (30 to 40 breath/min) may be required for smaller species

b. Tidal volume is approximately 15 ml/kg; do not exceed 15 to 20 cm of H_2O during inspiration

c. Birds have no pulmonary reserve; air is stored in the air sacs, which have no gas exchange capability

F. Isoflurane, sevoflurane, and nitrous oxide are the anesthetics of choice in birds (Table 25-4)

1. Induce isoflurane 3% to 4%; sevoflurane 4% to 5%

TABLE 25-4
MINIMUM ALVEOLAR CONCENTRATION (MAC) OF VARIOUS INHALANT ANESTHETICS

SPECIES	INHALANT	MAC (%)
Ducks	Halothane	1.04
	Isoflurane	1.3
Chickens	Sevoflurane	2.21
Rabbits	Halothane	0.8
Ferret	Enflurane	1.99
	Halothane	1.01
	Isoflurane	1.52
Alpaca	Sevoflurane	2.33
Llama	Isoflurane	1.05
	Sevoflurane	2.29

2. Maintain isoflurane 0.5% to 2.5%; sevoflurane 3% to 4%
3. Induction usually takes less than 5 minutes
   a. Induction is more rapid in birds than in mammals because of the cross-current system of the blood and air capillaries in addition to the greater proportional surface area of the lung; this makes the gas exchange in birds more efficient than in mammals
   b. Small changes in the vaporizer setting can cause rapid and dramatic changes in the plane of anesthesia; monitoring the level of anesthesia is critical
   c. Recovery is rapid (usually less than 5 minutes for a procedure less than 45 minutes); hold the bird in a towel until it is able to walk
   d. Apnea is an important signal to lighten anesthesia immediately; cardiac arrest often follows within 2 to 5 minutes of onset of apnea; the endotracheal tube should always be checked for occlusion
4. Nitrous oxide can be used in most species of birds because the air sacs are not a closed compartment
   a. Should not be used in birds with physiologic SQ air pockets (e.g., pelicans)
G. Injectable anesthetics (Table 25-3)
   1. Accurate body weight in grams is critical
   2. Effects of injectable anesthetics vary significantly among species and individual birds
   3. Recommended doses are only guidelines
   4. Administer IM injections in the pectoral muscles only
   5. Use of ketamine alone produces poor relaxation and turbulent recoveries; should be used with benzodiazepines; ketamine does not produce acceptable anesthesia in most waterfowl, owls, and hawks
   6. Xylazine, detomidine, and medetomidine cause excellent muscle relaxation and produce calm recoveries, but they are significant respiratory depressants; avoid using them in ill birds; may not be recommended to use in pet birds
      a. Can be reversed with tolazoline 15 mg/kg, yohimbine 0.1 to 1.0 mg/kg, or atipamezole 5 to 10 μg/kg

7. Benzodiazepines have significantly variable effects; when they are not overridden, they produce safe sedation and muscle relaxation; they decrease stress-induced cardiovascular changes during induction
   a. Can be reversed with flumazenil 0.05 mg/kg (half IV and half IM or SQ)
8. Propofol can be used in birds
   a. Severe respiratory depression and apnea may occur
   b. Dose for induction is 20 mg/kg; 3 mg/kg boluses are required to maintain anesthesia
9. The combination of ketamine with xylazine or a benzodiazepine given IM usually produces adequate anesthesia for minor procedures
   a. Diazepam: 0.5 to 1 mg/kg; ketamine: 10 to 50 mg/kg IM; use higher doses for smaller birds
   b. Xylazine and ketamine
   c. Tiletamine/zolazepam: 4 to 25 mg/kg IM
      (1) Parakeet: 15 to 20 mg/kg IM
      (2) Duck: 5 to 10 mg/kg IM
   d. If a deeper plane of anesthesia is needed
      (1) After waiting 10 minutes, readminister one fourth to one half of the ketamine dose
   e. If the plane of anesthesia is still inadequate, postpone the procedure for 24 hours before attempting anesthesia again
10. Recovery from injectable anesthetics is variable, but it usually takes more than 45 minutes after a 45-minute procedure
11. Use one fourth to one half of the IM dose if administering drugs IV

H. Anesthetic emergencies
   1. Apnea
      a. Positive-pressure ventilation; if no endotracheal tube is available, lift and compress the sternum
      b. Flush system free of anesthetic gas; administer 100% O_2
      c. Doxapram: IV, IO, or IM at 5 mg/kg
      d. Reverse α_2-agonists and benzodiazepines

2. Cardiac arrest
   a. Epinephrine 5 to 10 µg/kg IV, IO, or intratracheally
   b. Lift and compress sternum
   c. Perform a laparotomy and use fingertips or cotton-tipped applicators to perform internal cardiac massage
   d. See Chapters 28 and 29 for additional information on treating anesthetic emergencies
I. Recovery
   1. Continue monitoring the patient until it has recovered
   2. Provide warmth; continue after recovery as necessary, but hyperthermia must be avoided
   3. Place the bird in a warm, dark, and quiet recovery area
   4. Monitor hydration and energy needs
   5. Reduce the incidence and severity of self-induced trauma
      a. Wrap the bird in a towel to control its wings
      b. If the bird panics, hold it until it completely recovers
J. Analgesia (Table 25-2)
   1. In contrast to domestic mammals, birds indicate pain in a less obvious manner and tend to respond to noxious stimuli with a fight-or-flight and/or conservation-withdrawal response that may be difficult for practitioners to interpret
   2. Pain-associated behavior
      a. Acute pain: wing flapping and/or vocalization, decreased head movement, increased heart and respiratory rate, and increased blood pressure
      b. Prolonged pain: inappetence, inactivity, and a "puffed-up" appearance are often demonstrated

AVIAN ANESTHESIA (MORE THAN 15 KG; LONG-LEGGED)

I. The same general principles apply as for smaller birds
II. Unless they are very weak, these birds are large enough to require chemical sedation before induction of inhalant anesthesia
   A. Large ratites (ostriches) are extremely dangerous; they should never be approached from the front; a forward kick can disembowel a person

B. Using large sheets of wood as shields, herd large ratites into a corner or chute from the sides and rear (head first)

C. Long-billed birds, such as storks and herons, strike swiftly with their beaks; it is *imperative* that eye protection be worn; first restrain these birds from over the back by their wings and neck; a second person should then grasp and protect the legs; if the likelihood of hyperthermia is low, the beak may be taped partially shut by placing padding between and over the upper and lower tips of the beak

D. If the head can be reached safely, hood it with soft material to help calm and restrain the bird; ensure that the mouth and nares are open to the air to decrease the likelihood of hyperthermia

E. Capture myopathy, compartmental syndrome, hyperthermia, and leg fractures resulting from violent recoveries are complications associated with anesthesia in large, long-legged birds

  1. Adequate padding, maintenance of blood pressure, and oxygenation during these procedures is critical

  2. Exertional myopathies can develop in long-legged birds, especially if their legs have been maintained in a flexed position for a long period during surgery or recovery

  3. Reduce the handling needed to administer sedatives to a minimum; keep the induction and recovery areas as quiet and dark as possible

  4. Well-padded induction and recovery areas are desirable; a recovery stall slightly larger than a recumbent bird often makes it feel secure; after the bird has completely recovered, the hood can be removed and the crate opened for the bird's release; give it time to stand on its own; if a bird becomes agitated before it is fully recovered, inject it with 0.1 to 0.2 mg/kg of diazepam

F. If the bird has not fasted, carefully inflate the cuff on the endotracheal tube to prevent aspiration; regurgitation is common in birds that have not fasted

III. Injectable anesthetics are useful for short procedures and for induction of inhalant anesthesia

A. IV injections can be administered in the brachial veins in standing animals (e.g., ostriches and emus); some calm birds tolerate jugular injections; rheas have poor brachial veins but are small enough to be manually restrained for inhalant anesthesia after an IM sedative

   B. Brachial, jugular, and medial metatarsal veins are excellent sites for indwelling IV catheters

   C. Ratites (ostriches, emus, moas, kiwis)
1. Xylazine: 0.5 to 1 mg/kg IM, followed by ketamine, 2 to 4 mg/kg IV after 15 minutes
2. Xylazine: 0.25 mg/kg and ketamine, 2.2 mg/kg IV
3. Tiletamine/zolazepam: 4 to 10 mg/kg IM
4. Tiletamine/zolazepam: 2 to 6 mg/kg IV
5. Diazepam: 0.2 to 0.3 mg/kg and ketamine, 2.2 mg/kg IV

REPTILE ANESTHESIA

I. Hypothermia (refrigeration)
   A. Depresses bodily functions, including the immune system, and delays healing
   B. It is questionable whether it provides enough analgesia
   C. Delays recovery from anesthesia
   D. Preferred optimal temperature during perianesthetic period
1. Temperate and aquatic reptiles: 25° to 30°C
2. Tropical reptiles: ≥30° C

II. Premedication (Table 25-5)
   A. Phenothiazines should be avoided because of their prolonged clearance
   B. α_2-Agonists alone produce minimal to no sedation and questionable restraint; their combination with dissociative anesthetics produces chemical immobilization
   C. Midazolam
1. Midazolam 1.5 mg/kg IM sufficiently relaxes most red-eared slider turtles to allow manual extension of the head and neck and opening of the mouth without resistance
2. Midazolam alone produces poor to no sedation in snapping turtles and painted turtles
3. Combination with ketamine can produce more reliable sedation and anesthesia

TABLE 25-5
PREANESTHETICS AND ANALGESIC DRUGS FOR REPTILES (mg/kg)

DRUGS	ROUTE	DOSES
Preanesthetics		
Glycopyrrolate	IV, IM, SQ	0.01-0.04
Acepromazine	IM	0.1-0.5
Medetomidine	IM, IV	0.05-0.1 (tortoises) 0.15-0.3 (aquatic turtles)
Atipamezole	IM, IV	0.5
Midazolam	IM	1.5-2
Ketamine	IM, IV	5-20 (in combination with α_2-agonist or benzodiazepine)
Tiletamine/zolazepam	IM	3.5-10
Isoflurane*	Inhaled	2%-3% (on vaporizer)
Sevoflurane	Inhaled	4%-5% (on vaporizer)
Analgesics		
Butorphanol*	IM	1
Buprenorphine*	IM, IV, SQ	0.4-1
Ketamine	IM, IV, SQ	10-100
Meloxicam*	IM, IV, PO	0.1-0.2 q 24 hr
Carprofen*	IM, IV, SQ	2-4 followed by 1-2 q 24-72 hr
Lidocaine (2%)*	Local infiltration	Toxic dose unknown, recommended <5 mg/kd
Bupivacaine (0.5%)*	Local infiltration	Toxic dose unknown, recommended <2 mg/kd

IV, Intravenous; *IM*, intramuscular; *SQ*, subcutaneous.
*Dose anecdotal or determined by extrapolation from other species.

III. Induction of anesthesia
  A. Excitement is followed by loss of motor control; loss of the righting reflex is followed by muscle relaxation; surgical anesthesia is attained when toe, tail, and vent pinches do not elicit a withdrawal
  B. Most reptiles with third eyelids retain this reflex; a decrease in heart rate to less than 80% of the stabilized rate indicates that anesthesia should be lightened; heart rate is often the only reliable indicator of a reptile's level of anesthesia; it should be carefully monitored

C. Most reptiles (less than 500 g) can be induced by a mask or chamber at 2% to 4% isoflurane; use IV or IO propofol to induce anesthesia in larger reptiles; follow this with isoflurane gas anesthesia; nitrous oxide can be used for enhancing rate of induction and recovery and production of analgesia

  1. Watch for apnea

  2. Chelonians, aquatic squamates, and crocodilians can hold their breath for long periods of time; it can be difficult to extract a chelonian's head from its shell and open its beak; injectable sedatives are often required to allow intubation and positive-pressure respiration to maintain inhalant anesthesia; venomous or large, aggressive reptiles may require injectable anesthetics for safe restraint

    a. Propofol: 5 to 7 mg/kg in colubrid snakes; 10 to 12 mg/kg in birds; 12 to 15 mg/kg in chelonians; 5 to 14 mg/kg in lizards

    b. Ketamine: 20 to 60 mg/kg IM

    c. Ketamine: 5 to 15 mg/kg IV, IO

    d. Tiletamine/zolazepam: 10 to 40 mg/kg IM (squamates); 5 to 15 mg/kg IM (chelonians, crocodilians)

    e. Succinylcholine: *for intubation only*

      (1) No analgesia

      (2) Paralyzes muscles, including muscles of respiration

      (3) Intubate and assist respiration for approximately 1 hour after injection, sometimes longer

      (4) Do not repeat within 24 hours

      (5) 0.25 to 1.5 mg/kg IM (chelonians, crocodilians) in front half of animal

D. Intubation (similar to birds)

  1. The glottis is a slitlike opening between the arytenoids cartilages and located at the base of the tongue

  2. The glottis is harder to see in chelonians

  3. Crocodilians possess a pharyngeal membrane that allows them to breathe with a mouth full of food or water; this membrane must be pushed aside to see the glottis

  4. In some crocodilians the trachea is bent in on itself; therefore the endotracheal tube does not advance as far as expected

5. The tracheal rings are complete in chelonians and crocodilians; the trachea is short; to avoid intubation of only one bronchus, very short endotracheal tubes should be used
6. All reptiles attaining surgical levels of anesthesia must be intubated; exceptional care is needed for reptiles weighing less than 100 g to prevent tube-induced tracheitis

E. Maintenance
 1. Isoflurane (1% to 2%) or sevoflurane (2% to 4%) are the anesthetics of choice
 2. Oxygen flow rates: 1 L/0.3 to 1 kg; 1 L/5 to 10 kg for larger reptiles
 3. Ventilate the animal at least three to six times per minute
 4. Maintaining body temperature is essential
 5. Difficult to monitor anesthetic depth
  a. A surgical plane of anesthesia; decrease in muscle tone, obtunded palpebral and corneal reflexes, regular or even respiratory pattern

F. Analgesia (Table 25-5)

G. Recovery
 1. Recovery with isoflurane usually takes less than 20 minutes for procedures lasting less than 1 hour
 2. Recovery may take hours to days with injectable anesthetics
 3. Positive-pressure ventilation must be continued until the animal is breathing regularly on its own
  a. Some reptiles breathe when stimulated, but not on their own
  b. During recovery, reduce ventilation to two times per minute; room air or exhaled air may be used to increase the carbon dioxide concentration to stimulate respirations; be careful not to induce anoxia
 4. Heat and fluids accelerate recovery times

H. Emergencies
 1. Respiratory arrest
  a. Apnea is frequent; if the animal is stable, administer positive-pressure ventilation

  b. In turtles, extending and retracting the front legs can temporarily facilitate respirations while an endotracheal tube is being placed
  c. To reverse xylazine: yohimbine 1 mg/kg IV
  d. Doxapram: 5 mg/kg IV, IO, IM
 2. Cardiac arrest
  a. Administer 100% oxygen
  b. Use chest compressions in reptiles without shells
  c. Perform a laparotomy and manually compress the heart
  d. Epinephrine: 5 to 10 mg/kg IV, IO, IC, intratracheally
  e. See Chapters 28 and 29 for further information

AMPHIBIAN ANESTHESIA

 I. Indications
  A. Any painful procedure
  B. Diagnostic imaging
 II. Preanesthetic considerations
  A. See the general considerations section at the beginning of this chapter
  B. Amphibians are commonly grouped with reptiles in veterinary literature, it is more appropriate to include them with fish when discussing anesthesia
  C. If kept moist, amphibians can remain out of water for long periods
  D. Significant respiration occurs across moist skin
   1. Do not allow skin to completely dry out
   2. Handle the animal with wet latex gloves or wet hands
   3. Intubation may not be necessary unless surgical procedures require supplemental inhalant anesthesia
  E. The dermis of amphibians acts as a semipermeable membrane and allows not only for cutaneous respiration but also for absorption of other substances with which it comes in contact
  F. Some species of amphibians secrete a toxin from their skin; it is wise to wear gloves, although reports of toxicity in humans are rare

G. Withhold food from the animal 24 hours before anesthesia
H. Preanesthetic medications are not commonly used
I. Ectotherm
    1. Maintain adequate body temperature with external heat sources
    2. Hypothermia prolongs recovery and depresses the immune system
J. Animals weighing more than 100 g should be intubated (see avian anesthesia earlier in this chapter)

III. Stages of anesthesia
A. Similar to mammals
B. Erythema of ventral abdomen during induction
C. Abdominal respirations cease with heavy sedation, but pharyngeal (gular) respirations continue
    1. Cutaneous respiration in amphibians is adequate to prevent clinical hypoxia during anesthetic events
D. Corneal reflex is lost before loss of the withdrawal reflex
E. Normal values for heart rate and blood oxygen levels have not been published

IV. Anesthetic agents (Table 25-6)
A. Tricaine methanesulfonate, MS-222; Finquel MS-222

TABLE 25-6
ANESTHETIC AGENTS IN AMPHIBIANS

AGENTS	CONCENTRATION	COMMENTS
MS-222*	250-500 mg/L	Tadpoles and newts
	1-2 g/L	Frogs and salamanders
	2-3 g/L	Toads
Isoflurane†	3 ml/L	Topical bath
Isoflurane/KY-Jelly/ water††	0.025-0.0035 ml/g of body weight	Topical application to dorsum

*Solutions greater than 1 g/L should be buffered using sodium bicarbonate.
†Use a 25-gauge needle to spray isoflurane into water (beneath the surface).
††Mix 3 ml isoflurane, 1.5 ml water, and 3.5 ml KY-Jelly. Shake solution vigorously until uniform gel forms. Gel should be removed with moist gauze pad once anesthetic induction has occurred.

1. Routes
   a. Immersion baths; keep tank of untreated water for recovery tank
   b. Parenteral—IM or SQ; use sterile solution
2. Dose is species-dependent
   a. Immersion bath: 250 mg to 3 g/L
   b. 100 mg/kg SQ or IM (0.1 ml/10 g body weight with a 1% solution)
3. Induction takes 5 to 20 minutes
4. Pharmacology
   a. Rapidly absorbed through the gills
   b. Rapidly metabolized primarily by the liver but also in the kidneys, blood, and muscle
5. Recovery takes 10 to 30 minutes; keep skin moist with untreated water and maintain normal temperature
6. Wide margin of safety
7. Suppliers
   a. Argent Chemical Laboratories
      8702 152nd Ave NE
      Redmond, WA 98052
      1-800-426-6258
      http://www.argent-labs.com/
   b. Crescent Research Chemicals
      2810 S. 24th St. Suite #110
      Phoenix, AZ 85044
      1-480-893-9234
      http://www.aqualogy.com/crescent/

B. Isoflurane
   1. Use the unvaporized liquid form
      a. Inject directly into a water bath
      b. Mixed into a viscous solution with water-soluble lubricant (KY-Jelly, Johnson & Johnson) and water and then apply topically
   2. Intubate and ventilate after masking the animal
      a. Induce at 3% to 4% for 5 to 15 minutes
      b. Maintain at 1% to 2.5%
      c. Keep skin moist and maintain normal temperature
      d. Isoflurane is a respiratory depressant; use intermittent positive-pressure ventilation

      e. Recovery takes 10 to 30 minutes; keep the animal warm and moist

   3. Bubble the vaporized gas into water after induction with an induction chamber

   4. Isoflurane may be irritating to amphibian skin

  C. Ketamine

   1. Good for diagnostics, but not surgery

   2. 100 to 200 mg/kg SQ or IM

   3. Reflexes remain intact

   4. Induction takes 10 to 20 minutes

   5. Recovery takes 20 to 60 minutes

V. Recovery

  A. Recovery of amphibians from general anesthesia is relatively long when compared with fish

  B. It is not important not to raise their body temperatures for rapid recovery because they are poikilothermic

FISH ANESTHESIA

I. Indications

  A. Any painful procedure

  B. Sedation during shipping

  C. Diagnostic imaging

  D. Stripping milt (eggs)

II. Preanesthetic considerations

  A. See the General Considerations section at the beginning of this chapter

  B. Obligate water breathers

   1. Require oxygenated water moving over gills to oxygenate blood

   2. Normal water flow pattern is through the mouth, over the gills, and out the operculum

   3. Provide water flow during anesthesia by using frequent immersion or a small recirculating pump and airstone; a pump tube should be placed in the fish's mouth so that water flow is maintained across the gills

  C. Exterior mucus layer is an important part of the integument

   1. Use the least amount of restraint possible

2. Use wet latex gloves when handling the fish to minimize disruption to the mucus layer
D. Withhold food 12 to 24 hours before anesthesia
E. Have a recovery tank ready with water identical to the fish's preanesthetic conditions
F. Preanesthetic medications are not commonly used
G. Ectotherms
  1. Maintain adequate body temperature with external heat sources
  2. Hypothermia prolongs recovery and depresses the immune system

III. Stages of anesthesia

STAGES OF ANESTHESIA IN FISH			
STAGE	**PLANE**	**CATEGORY**	**FISH RESPONSES**
0		Normal	Normal
I	1	Light sedation	Decreased response to visual stimuli
I	2	Deep sedation	Voluntary swimming stopped, normal posture, no response to external stimuli
II	1	Light narcosis	Excitement, loss of balance
II	2	Deep narcosis	Equilibrium lost, normal respiratory rate responds to pain
III	1	Light anesthesia	Decreased respiratory rate, deep pain present
III	2	Surgical	Low respiratory rate, low anesthesia heart rate, no deep pain
IV		Medullary	Cardiac and respiratory collapse arrest

IV. Anesthetic agents (Table 25-7)
A. Tricaine methanesulfonate, MS-222; Finquel MS-222
  1. The only anesthetic licensed for use in fish

TABLE 25-7
ANESTHETIC AGENTS IN FISH

AGENTS	CONCENTRATION	COMMENTS
MS-222*	75-125 mg/L	Induction dose
	50-75 mg/L	Maintenance dose
Etomidate	2-4 mg/L	The minimum effective dose
	7-20 mg/L	The maximum safe dose
Clove oil	40-100 mg/L	Use 95% ethanol to create stock solution of 100 mg/ml
Isoflurane†	0.4-0.75 ml/L	Induction dose
	0.25-0.4 ml/L	Maintenance dose

*Solutions should be buffered using sodium bicarbonate. Lower dose are recommended for young fish and for medically compromised animals.
†Use a 25-gauge needle to spray isoflurane into water (beneath the surface).

2. Commonly used as an immersion bath; keep tank of untreated water for recovery bath
3. Dose is species-dependent; sedation is generally achieved at 20 to 50 mg/L, induction of anesthesia at 75 to 125 mg/L, maintenance of anesthesia at 50 to 75 mg/L; the depth of anesthesia is controlled by switching from a water bath that contains an anesthetic to an untreated water bath
4. Acidic solution: buffer with imidazole or sodium hydroxide to normal tank pH
5. Rapid induction—1 to 5 minutes
6. Rapid recovery—10 to 15 minutes; to prevent hypoxia, keep water moving over the fish's gills
7. Wide margin of safety
8. Suppliers (see amphibian section)

B. Etomidate
1. The minimum effective dose ranges from 2 to 4 mg/L; the maximum safe dose ranges from 7 to 20 mg/L
2. At 4 mg/L, fish typically enter anesthesia within 90 seconds and recover within 40 minutes
3. More effective in alkaline water and higher water temperature but is not affected by total hardness

C. Clove oil
1. Popular for koi and trout
2. The active ingredient is eugenol

      3. Add into the induction chamber water at 40 to 100 mg/L

  D. Isoflurane

      1. Not a preferred anesthetic agent

      2. Liquid isoflurane can be added to water

V. Treatment of anesthetic overdose

  A. Move the fish to untreated, oxygenated water

  B. Increase gentle water flow over the gills

  C. If spontaneous respirations do not occur in 2 minutes, assist respirations

      1. Move the fish gently through the water

      2. Slowly pump oxygenated water into the fish's mouth and across its gills

RABBIT AND RODENT ANESTHESIA

I. Generalities

  A. Rabbits, guinea pigs, and chinchillas frequently hold their breath and then take deep, rapid breaths when being masked down or induced in a chamber; this behavior can result in death if the concentration of anesthetic gases is high; to reduce risk, do the following:

      1. Use preanesthetics (diazepam or midazolam)

      2. Use nitrous oxide followed by an anesthetic agent

      3. Use a low induction setting

  B. Levels of anesthesia

      1. Excitement phase

      2. Loss of coordination

      3. Muscle relaxation

      4. Surgical anesthesia is attained when toe, ear, and tail pinches do not elicit a withdrawal (no or decreased reflexes)

      5. Loss of corneal reflexes varies significantly among individual animals and anesthetic agents; a loss of these reflexes in an animal that previously had them indicates that anesthesia should be lightened

      6. A decreasing respiratory or heart rate or abnormal breathing patterns are also indications to lighten anesthesia

II. Intubation (Table 25-8)
  A. It is difficult to intubate rodents and lagomorphs because of their small size and long, thin oral cavities; laryngeal masks may be easier
  B. Masks are effective for short procedures
  C. Intubation techniques and considerations
     1. Small endotracheal tubes clog and kink easily
        a. Check tube patency with positive-pressure ventilation at least every 2 minutes
        b. Have a replacement tube ready
        c. If a tube is clogged, try to reposition or suction it; if the tube does not become patent, maintain anesthesia by mask or injectables or place a new tube
     2. Be careful not to create iatrogenic tracheitis
     3. Prolonged, oral, or thoracic procedures require intubation
     4. Oxygen flow
        a. 500 ml/min minimum
        b. 0.5 to 2 L/min/kg; 3 to 4 L/min maximum
        c. 1 L every 5 to 10 kg
  D. Oral intubation: requires practice and luck (Fig. 25-1)
     1. Dorsal, lateral, or ventral recumbency
     2. Extend the head and neck
     3. Keep animal straight

TABLE 25-8
ENDOTRACHEAL INTUBATION: EQUIPMENT REQUIRED

SPECIES	BODY WEIGHT	ENDOTRACHEAL TUBE DIAMETER
Rabbit	1-3 kg	2-3 mm O/D*
	3-7 kg	3-6 mm O/D
Rat	200-400 g	18-12 gauge plastic cannula
Mouse	25-35 g	1.0 mm
Guinea pig	400-1000 g	16-12 gauge plastic cannula
Hamster	120 g	1.5 mm
Primate	<0.5 kg	Not reported
	0.5-20 kg	2-8 mm O/D
Pig	1-10 kg	2-6 mm O/D
	0.5-20 kg	6-15 mm O/D

*O/D, Outside diameter.

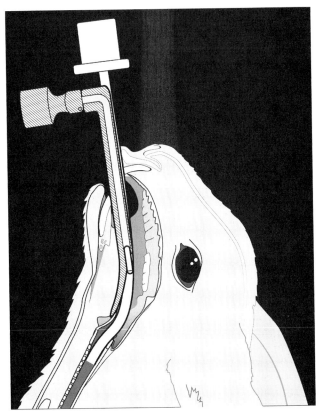

Fig. 25-1
A laryngoscope and a stylet to stiffen the endotracheal tube are frequently used to place an endotracheal tube in the trachea of larger rabbits.

4. Grasp the animal's tongue and pull it forward or around the incisors
5. Stylet or tube is inserted into the oral cavity, around the incisors, and positioned towards the larynx. Advance the tube when condensation is observed in the tube during exhalation

6. A laryngoscope is helpful in larger animals (Fig. 25-2)
7. In large rabbits, a small, rigid arthroscope can be introduced into the mouth to allow visualization of the glottis; however, damage to the instrument by the animal's molars is possible
8. Use of topical lidocaine can suppress laryngospasm
9. Repeated attempts at intubation can cause life-threatening hemorrhage and swelling

E. Retrograde technique
1. Aseptically prepare the ventral neck
2. Pass an over-the-needle catheter into the trachea
3. Retrograde it through the larynx

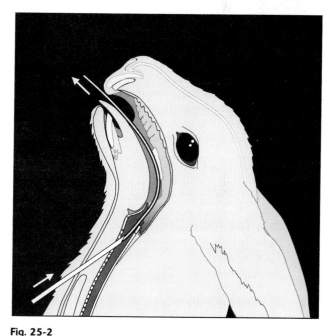

Fig. 25-2
A, A through-the-needle catheter can be placed into the trachea and passed retrogradely out the mouth to be used as a guide for endotracheal intubation. *Continued*

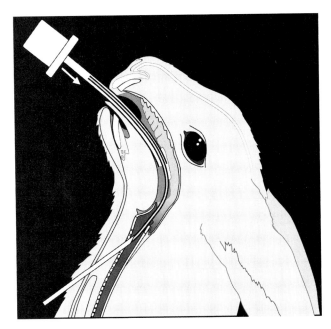

Fig. 25-2, cont'd
B, The endotracheal tube is passed over the catheter, which is used a guide for placement of the endotracheal tube in the trachea.

    4. Use the catheter as a stylet for the endotracheal tube
    5. Remove the catheter
    6. In animals with fat necks, a "cut down" to the trachea is required
  F. Induction
    1. Isoflurane: 2% to 3%
    2. Sevoflurane: 3% to 5%
  G. Maintenance
    1. Isoflurane: 0.25% to 2%
    2. Sevoflurane: 2% to 3%
    3. Use of nitrous oxide is similar to use in other domestic mammals

H. Recovery
1. Isoflurane or sevoflurane takes 5 to 15 minutes for surgeries that last less than one hour
2. Keep the animal warm
3. Monitor the animal's hydration and energy needs
I. Analgesia (Table 25-9)
J. Injectable anesthetics (Table 25-10)
1. Results vary significantly among individual animals
2. Poor muscle relaxation and poor analgesia are the most frequent problems
3. Injectable anesthetics are most useful for diagnostics or minor procedures
4. Dosages listed are only guidelines (Tables 25-9 and 25-10)
5. Barbiturates produce excellent muscle relaxation
   a. Their margin of safety is very low
   b. They are not recommended for use in pets
   c. Barbiturates are useful for euthanasia
   d. Pentobarbital: dilute to less than 10 mg/ml

BARBITURATE DOSES IN EXOTIC SPECIES		
SPECIES	**PENTOBARBITAL (mg/kg)**	**THIOPENTAL (mg/kg)**
Rat	25 to 40 IP, IV	20-40 IV
Mouse	40 to 80 IP, IV	20-50 IV
Guinea pig	30 to 40 IP, IV	
Chinchilla	35 to 40 IP	
Rabbit	25 to 40 IV	15-30 IV
Hamster	50 to 90 IP	
Gerbil	40 to 60 IP	

IP, Intraperitoneally.

K. Emergencies (see Chapters 28 and 29)

FERRET ANESTHESIA

I. Information in Chapters 7 and 20 is applicable to ferrets; ferret anesthesia is similar to that of domestic cats

TABLE 25-9
PREANESTHETICS AND ANALGESIC DRUGS FOR RABBITS AND RODENTS (mg/kg)

DRUG	RABBIT	RAT
Atropine	0.08 IV, IM, SQ	0.05 IM, SQ
Glycopyrrolate	0.01-0.1 IV, IM, SQ	0.01-0.02 IM, SQ
Acepromazine	0.2-0.75 IV, IM, SQ	0.5-2.5 IM, SQ
Diazepam	0.5-5 IV, SQ	3-5 SQ, IM
Midazolam	0.5-5 IV, IM	3-5 SQ, IM
Xylazine	1-5 IV, IM	5-10 IM, IP
Medetomidine	0.1-0.5 IV, IM	0.03-1 SQ
Aspirin	100 PO	100 PO
Carprofen	1.5 PO bid	5 SQ
Flunixin	1.1 SQ, IM q 12 hr	2.5 SQ, IM q 12 hr
Ketoprofen	3 IM	—
Buprenorphine	0.01-0.05 IV, IM, SQ, 8-12 hourly	0.01-0.05 SQ, IV or 0.1-0.25 PO 8-12 hourly
Butorphanol	0.1-0.5 IV, IM 4 hourly	2 SQ 4 hourly
Morphine	2-5 SQ, IM 2-4 hourly	2.5 SQ 2-4 hourly
Oxymorphone	0.1-0.2 IV, IM	
Meperidine	5-10 IM	
Fentanyl/fluanisone (Hypnorm)	0.5 ml/kg IM	0.4 ml/kg IM, IP
Fentanyl/droperidol	0.22 ml/kg IM	

SQ, Subcutaneous; *IM*, intramuscular; *IP*, intraperitoneal; *IV*, intravenous.
Note that considerable individual and strain variation in response may be encountered; therefore it is essential to assess the analgesic effect in each animal.

II. Introduction
   A. Because they lack substantial claws, ferrets are easier to hold in a towel and mask down with isoflurane than cats
   B. Mask induction is used for very ill ferrets to eliminate the side effects associated with many injectable anesthetics and for short procedures such as diagnostics; this allows the ferret to be returned to the owner quickly
   C. Monitoring the depth of anesthesia
      1. Loss of pedal withdrawal reflex and muscle tone provides an indication of plane of anesthesia

MOUSE	GERBIL	HAMSTER	GUINEA PIG
0.05 IM, SQ	0.05 IM, SQ	0.05 IM, SQ	0.05 IM, SQ
0.01-0.02 IM, SQ	0.01-0.02 IM, SQ	0.01-0.02 IM, SQ	
		5 IM, SQ	5 SQ, IP
3-5 SQ, IM	3-5 SQ, IM	3-5 SQ, IM	2-5 SQ, IP
3-5 SQ, IM	3-5 SQ, IM	3-5 SQ, IM	2-5 SQ, IP
5-10 IM, IP	5-10 IM, IP	5-10 IM, IP	5-10 SQ, IP
0.03-1 SQ	0.1-0.2 SQ	0.1 SQ	0.5 SQ
120 PO			87 PO
—			—
2.5 SQ, IM q 12 hr			—
—			—
0.05-0.1 SQ 12			0.05 SQ 8-12 hourly
1-5 SQ 4 hourly	—		
2.5 SQ 2-4 hourly		2-5 SQ, IM 4 hourly	
0.01 ml/30 g IP	0.5 ml/kg IM, IP	0.5 ml/kg IM, IP	1 ml/kg IM

    2. At a surgical plane of anesthesia, palpebral and corneal reflexes are lost

D. Because of their small size, ferrets require a non-rebreathing system; the oxygen flow must be two to three times the patient's minute ventilation (approximately 200 to 350 ml/kg/min)

E. Ferrets are easily intubated

    1. 2.0- to 3.5-mm internal diameter cuffed endotracheal tubes

    2. A laryngoscope is helpful

TABLE 25-10
RABBIT AND RODENT ANESTHESIA (mg/kg)

DRUG	RABBIT	RAT
Ketamine	15-30 IM	50-100 with sedatives
Ketamine/xylazine	35 + 5 IM	
Ketamine/xylazine/ butorphanol	35 + 5 + 0.2 IM	
Ketamine/medetomidine	15-25 + 0.25-0.5 IM, SQ	
Ketamine/acepromazine	15-30 + 0.2 IM	
Ketamine/diazepam	10-20 + 0.5 IV	
Ketamine/midazolem		
Tiletamine/zolazepam	5-25 IM	10-30 with sedatives
Fentanyl/droperidol		0.01-0.33 ml/kg SQ, IP
Fentanyl/fluanisone (Hypnorm®)/diazepam	0.3 ml/kg IM + 2 mg/kg IV, IP	0.3 ml/kg IM + 2.5 mg/kg IP
Fentanyl/fluanisone (Hypnorm)/midazolam*	0.3 ml/kg IM + 2 mg/kg IP	2.7 ml/kg IP
Alphaxalone/alphadolone	6-9 IV	10-12 IV
Propofol	8-10 IV	10 IV

*Mixture of midazolam 1.25 mg/ml, fentanyl 0.079 mg/ml, and fluanisone 2.5 mg/ml. Midazolam and hypnorm are each diluted with an equal volume of water before mixing. *SQ,* Subcutaneous; *IM,* intramuscular; *IP,* intraperitoneal; *IV,* intravenous.

   III. Inhalant anesthetics (Table 25-4)
      A. Isoflurane or sevoflurane
         1. Induce at 2.5% to 4%
         2. Maintain at 1% to 3%
         3. Recovery time is similar to that in cats
   V. Injectable anesthetics (Table 25-11)
  VI. Analgesia (Table 25-12)
 VII. Emergencies (see Chapters 28 and 29)

EXOTIC CAT ANESTHESIA

   I. Preanesthetic considerations
      A. See the general considerations section at the beginning of this chapter

MOUSE	GERBIL	HAMSTER	GUINEA PIG
50-200 with sedatives			
	50-70 + 2-3 SQ, IP	50-150 + 5-10 SQ, IP	40-80 + 5-10 SQ, IP
	40 + 0.5 SQ, IP		40 + 0.5 SQ, IP
			125 + 5 SQ, IP
		100 + 5 SQ, IP	
	10-30 with sedatives		40-60 IM
		0.5 ml/kg IM	
0.01 ml/30 g IP + 5 mg/kg IP			1 ml/kg IM + 2.5 mg/kg IP
10 ml/kg IP			8 ml/kg IP
10-15 IV 26 IV	80-120 SQ, IP	150 IP	40 IP

*Mixture of midazolam 1.25 mg/ml, fentanyl 0.079 mg/ml, and fluanisone 2.5 mg/ml. Midazolam and hypnorm are each diluted with an equal volume of water before mixing.
SQ, Subcutaneous; *IM*, intramuscular; *IP*, intraperitoneal; *IV*, intravenous.

      B. Withhold food from the animal for 24 hours; withhold water for 12 hours

      C. Respect the animal's strength

      D. Remote delivery (pole syringe, darting equipment) is often needed to ensure human safety

      E. Premedication is similar to that used in domestic cats but often is not needed

      F. Big cats usually require less anesthetics than smaller domestic cats

      G. Higher drug doses are needed for excited animals; create a calm and quiet environment for induction to anesthesia

   II. Stages of anesthesia

      A. Similar to other mammals

TABLE 25-11
ANESTHETIC DRUGS FOR FERRETS (mg/kg)

DRUG	DOSES
Alphaxalone/alphadolone	8-12 IV, 12-15 IM
Ketamine/acepromazine	25 + 0.25 IM
Ketamine/diazepam	5-25 + 0.5-2 IM
Ketamine/medetomidine	5-8 + 0.08-0.1 IM
Ketamine/xylazine	25 + 1-2 IM
Ketamine/butorphanol	15 + 0.2 IM
Ketamine/butorphanol/diazepam	15 + 0.2 + 3 IM
Ketamine/butorphanol/acepromazine	15 + 0.2 + 0.1 IM
Tiletamine/zolazepam	5-22 IM
Tiletamine/zolazepam/xylazine/ butorphanol	1.5-3 + 1.5-3 + 0.2 IM
Pentobarbitone	25-30 IV, 36 IP
Propofol	5-8 IV
Urethane	1500 IV

TABLE 25-12
PREMEDICANTS AND ANALGESIC DRUGS FOR FERRETS (mg/kg)

DRUG	DOSES
Atropine	0.02-0.05 IV, IM, SQ
Glycopyrrolate	0.01 IV, IM, SQ
Acepromazine	0.1-0.3 IV, IM
Diazepam	0.5-3 IM, SQ
Midazolam	0.5-3 IM SQ
Xylazine	1-2 IM. SQ
Medetomidine	0.08-0.2 IM, SQ
Ketamine	5-15 IM
Aspirin	200 PO
Flunixin	0.5-2 SQ; 12-24 hourly
Buprenorphine	0.01-0.03 IV, IM, SQ; 8-12 hourly
Butorphanol	0.4 IM; 4-6 hourly 0.1-0.5 IV, IM, SQ
Morphine	0.5 SQ, IM; 6 hourly 0.2-2 IM, SQ
Oxymorphone	0.05-0.2 IV, IM, SQ
Pethidine (meperidine)	5-10 SQ, IM; 2-4 hourly
Fentanyl/droperidol	0.15 ml/kg IM

Note that considerable individual and strain variation in response may be encountered; therefore it is essential to assess the analgesic effect in each animal.

    B. Sudden arousal of animals sedated with xylazine alone or medetomidine and ketamine is possible; supplementation may be needed

III. Anesthetic agents

    A. Xylazine

        1. Rarely used alone because of the possibility of sudden arousal

        2. Significant respiratory depressant

    B. Ketamine

        1. Used alone for short procedures in small cats; 5 to 20 mg/kg IM

        2. Sole use often causes salivation and muscle rigidity

        3. Seizures have been reported in some species of exotic cats recovering from ketamine or ketamine-combination anesthesia; control with diazepam

    C. Medetomidine/ketamine IM

        1. Medetomidine: 0.04 to 0.1 mg/kg

        2. Ketamine: 2 to 4 mg/kg

        3. Intubate and place on isoflurane or be prepared to supplement ketamine at 1 to 2 mg/kg IV if procedure is longer than 20 minutes

        4. At the conclusion of the procedure or after 20 minutes (whichever comes first), reverse medetomidine with atipamazole at five times the medetomidine dose IM or IV

        5. Bradycardia is common with medetomidine; this is rarely a clinical problem, but animals should be supplemented with O_2; this combination may not be appropriate for severely debilitated felines

    D. Ketamine/xylazine combination IV

        1. Ketamine: 8 to 10 mg/kg

        2. Xylazine: 0.6 to 1 mg/kg

        3. Intubate and place the animal on isoflurane inhalation anesthesia if the procedure takes longer than 20 minutes

    E. Ketamine/diazepam combination IV

        1. Ketamine: 5 to 8 mg/kg

        2. Diazepam: 0.1 mg/kg

        3. Intubate and place the animal on isoflurane inhalation anesthesia if the procedure takes longer than 20 minutes

F. Tiletamine/zolazepam (Telazol®)
   1. A 500-mg vial can be reconstituted to a final concentration of 100 to 500 mg/ml depending on the volume of diluent added for use in darting equipment
   2. Dose: 1.5 to 5 mg/kg IM for most species
      a. Sufficient for intubation
      b. Induces anesthesia in large felids in 2 to 5 minutes
      c. Intubate and place the animal on isoflurane inhalation anesthesia if the procedure takes longer than 20 minutes
      d. Snow leopards require a higher dose
      e. Excessive salivation is seen in some species; atropine can be combined to prevent this
      f. Recovery from anesthesia is smooth but prolonged compared with ketamine alone or ketamine combinations
      g. Delayed (3 to 10 days after immobilization) adverse drug reaction is seen in some Siberian and white tigers
G. Isoflurane or sevoflurane are the inhalation anesthetics of choice
   1. Small cats can be anesthetized in a chamber
   2. Face mask delivery can be used to supplement other anesthetics
   3. Dose
      a. Induce at 3% to 4%
      b. Maintain at 1% to 2% isoflurane; 2% to 3% sevoflurane
      c. Oxygen flow rate is 1 to 6 L/min
   4. Intubate the animal if the procedure takes longer than 20 minutes

IV. Treatment of anesthetic overdose
   A. Treat an overdose as an anesthetic emergency in domestic cats, but be prepared for arousal of the animal
   B. Xylazine can be reversed with yohimbine (0.125 mg/kg IM or IV), although results are not as dramatic as in other species
   C. Adverse tiletamine/zolazepam reactions in tigers have been treated with diazepam and dexamethasone
   D. Medetomidine can be reversed with atipamazole at one half the volume of medetomidine IM or IV

E. Telazol® can be partially antagonized with Romazicon (flumazenil)

CAMELID ANESTHESIA (LLAMAS, CAMELS, ALPACAS)

I. Preanesthetic considerations
   A. See the general considerations section at the beginning of this chapter
   B. Withhold food from the animal for 24 to 48 hours; withhold water for 24 hours, weather permitting
   C. Patient positioning is important to reduce regurgitation
      1. Keep the animal's head elevated above the rumen
      2. Do not roll an anesthetized animal dorsally
      3. If regurgitation occurs, position the animal's head with the muzzle below the level of the poll and ensure an open airway; rumen tubes can be placed to prevent aspiration
   D. Intubate animals if the procedure takes longer than 20 minutes
   E. Place a jugular catheter
II. Stages of anesthesia are similar to ruminants
III. Anesthetic agents
   A. Neonates: mask with isoflurane; intubate the animal if the procedure takes longer than 20 minutes
   B. Juveniles and adults
      1. Local anesthesia
         a. See Chapter 5
         b. A line block or an inverted L block using standard agents is common
         c. Regional nerve blocks are more difficult
         d. Dosage must be tailored to animal size
   C. Sedation
      1. Xylazine: 0.1 to 0.9 mg/kg IV or IM for large camelids, 0.1 to 0.3 mg/kg for llamas
      2. Medetomidine: 0.01 to 0.02 mg/kg IV, 0.02 to 0.04 mg/kg IM; can be reversed with atipamezole 0.125 mg/kg IV 0.02 to 0.04 mg/kg IM
      3. Acepromazine 0.1 mg/kg IM
      4. Butorphanol: 0.05 to 0.1 mg/kg IM
   D. IV anesthetics
      1. Ketamine/xylazine

a. Ketamine: 4 to 8 mg/kg IM
   3 to 5 mg/kg IV
b. Xylazine: 0.4 to 0.8 mg/kg IM
   0.25 mg/kg IV
c. Xylazine can be reversed with tolazoline 2 mg/kg IM

2. Medetomidine/ketamine
   a. Ketamine: 2 to 4 mg/kg IM or IV
   b. Medetomidine: 0.04 to 0.08 mg/kg IM or IV
3. Telazol®: 0.75 to 1.5 mg/kg IM
4. Thiopental: 8 to 10 mg/kg IV
5. Propofol: 1 to 3 mg/kg IV

E. Inhalation anesthetics (Table 25-10)

IV. Analgesics
A. Phenylbutazone: 2 to 4 mg/kg orally once a day (SID); may consider administration of cimetidine: 2.2 mg/kg concurrently
B. Flunixin meglumine: 1.1 mg/kg IV SID
   1. Avoid intraarterial injection
   2. Ulcerogenic: administer cimetidine concurrently
C. Aspirin: 25 to 50 mg/kg orally twice a day

V. Treatment of anesthetic overdose
A. Treat as anesthetic emergency as in other mammals
B. Xylazine can be reversed with yohimbine 0.25 mg/kg IV or tolazoline 2 mg/kg IM
C. Atipamezole is used to antagonize medetomidine at one half the volume of medetomidine IM or IV

POT-BELLIED PIG ANESTHESIA

I. Preanesthetic considerations
A. See the general considerations section at the beginning of this chapter
B. Withhold food from the animal for 24 hours
C. Warn the owner and the hospital staff that the pig may squeal when restrained—recommend wearing ear protection
D. Premedication is not generally needed
E. Endotracheal intubation can be challenging (see Chapter 23)

F. Watch for hyperthermia, although it is less of a problem in pot-bellied pigs than in other pigs

II. Stages of anesthesia are similar to other mammals

III. Anesthetic agents

A. Isoflurane or sevoflurane

1. Can be used as the sole anesthetic agent in small animals
2. Agents of choice for inhalation anesthesia
3. Deliver from a precision vaporizer with a face mask or an endotracheal tube
   a. Induction: 3% to 4% isoflurane; 3% to 5% sevoflurane
   b. Maintenance: 1% to 2% isoflurane; 2% to 4% sevoflurane
   c. Oxygen flow rate: 2 to 3 L/min

B. Tiletamine/zolazepam/ketamine/xylazine injectable combination

1. Reconstitute a 500-mg vial of Telazol® with 2.5 ml of 10% ketamine and 2.5 ml of 10% xylazine
2. Each milliliter of resultant mixture contains the following:
   a. 50 mg tiletamine
   b. 50 mg ketamine
   c. 50 mg zolazepam
   d. 50 mg xylazine
3. Dose
   a. Sedation: 0.006 to 0.012 ml/kg IM
   b. Surgical anesthesia and intubation: 0.018 to 0.024 ml/kg IM
   c. Requires 20 to 40 minutes to take effect
   d. Can be supplemented with 0.1- to 0.5-ml bolus in the auricular vein

C. Midazolam/medetomidine/butorphanol

1. Midazolam: 0.3 mg/kg IM
2. Medetomidine: 0.07 to 0.08 mg/kg IM
3. Butorphanol: 0.3 mg/kg IM
4. Supplementation
   a. Intubate and maintain on isoflurane
   b. Propofol: 1 mg/kg IV
   c. Ketamine: 1 mg/kg IV

5. Antagonists
   a. Atipamazole: 0.08 mg/kg IM or IV
   b. Naltrexone: 0.05 to 0.1 mg/kg IM or IV
   c. Restrain the animal until it is coordinated
D. Telazol®/medetomidine/butorphanol
   1. Telazol®: 0.5 mg/kg IM
   2. Medetomidine: 0.07 to 0.08 mg/kg IM
   3. Butorphanol: 0.3 mg/kg IM
   4. Supplementation (see section C4 above)
   5. Antagonists (see section C5 above)
E. Provide supplemental oxygen to all immobilized pigs with nasal tube at 5 L/min

VI. Treatment of anesthetic overdose
A. If using isoflurane, turn vaporizer off and flush system
B. Administer oxygen
C. If xylazine has been given, reverse with yohimbine 0.125 mg/kg IV
D. If medetomidine has been given, antagonize with atipamazole at one half the volume of medetomidine
E. If a narcotic has been given, antagonize with naltrexone 0.1 mg/kg IM or IV
F. Perform cardiopulmonary resuscitation as for other mammals

CHAPTER TWENTY-SIX

Fluid Administration During Anesthesia

"One can drink too much, but one never drinks enough."
GOTTHOLD EPHRAIM LESSING

OVERVIEW

Fluid therapy is a vital adjunct to any anesthetic plan. Almost all drugs used to produce chemical restraint and anesthesia decrease the force of cardiac contraction and relax blood vessels, increasing intravascular volume. These effects decrease cardiac output (blood flow) and arterial blood pressure. The routine administration of fluids during anesthesia helps to maintain an adequate and effective circulating blood volume and near-normal cardiac output. Choices for acute fluid therapy include balanced electrolyte solutions (crystalloids), colloids, cell-free blood substitutes, and blood.

GENERAL CONSIDERATIONS (TABLE 26-1)

I. Anesthesia, surgery, and many of the diseases for which surgical intervention is required disturb water and acid-base balance and decrease the effective circulating blood volume
   A. Disease produces changes in fluid, electrolyte, and acid-base balance (Table 26-2)
   B. Imbalances caused by anesthesia
      1. Inhalation and intravenous (IV) anesthetics
         a. Depress myocardial contractility, decreasing cardiac output and tissue perfusion; metabolic acidosis may ensue
         b. Produce vasodilation; relative hypovolemia; hypotension may occur

485

TABLE 26-1
NORMAL ELECTROLYTE COMPOSITION OF SERUM (mEq/L)

	NA^+	K^+	CA^{++}	MG^{++}	HPO_4	CL^-	HCO_3
Dog	143-153	4.2-5.4	5.0-6.1	0.43-0.60	3.2-8.1	109-120	18-25
Cat	146-156	3.2-5.5	4.9-5.5	0.43-0.70	3.2-6.5	114-126	18-22
Horse	132-142	2.4-4.6	6.0-7.2	0.46-0.66	1.2-4.8	97-105	23-31
Cow	133-143	3.9-5.2	8.9-5.4	0.47-0.65	3.8-7.7	98-108	23-31

TABLE 26-2

COMMON DISEASES AND EXPECTED ELECTROLYTE ABNORMALITIES

DISEASE SYNDROME	WATER	NA^+	K^+	CA^{++}	MG^{++}	HPO_4	CL^-	HCO_3
Gastric loss, vomiting	Loss	↓↓↓	↓↓↓↓		↓↓↓↓		↓↓↓	↑
Pancreatic or intestinal fluid loss	Loss	↓↓↓	↓↓↓		↓↓↓↓		↓↓↓	↓
Diarrhea	Loss		↕↓		↓↓		↓↓↓	↓
Starvation	Loss	↑	↑		↓↓		↓	
Acute hemorrhagic pancreatitis	Loss			↓↓↓↓	↓↓	↓↓	↓	↓
Malabsorption syndrome	Loss		↓	↑	↑	↑↓	↑	↓
Acute renal failure (oliguric)	Excess	↑↓	↓↕↑	↓	↓	↑↓		↑
Renal tubular dysfunction	Loss	↑↓	↓↕	↑	↑	↑	↑	↓
Chronic renal disease	Loss	↕↓↑	↓↕	↓	↓			↓
Diabetes insipidus	Loss	↓↓↓↑		↓↓↕↓↑↓	↑↓	↑↓		
Burns	Loss	↑↓	↓	↑↓	↓		↑	↑
Primary aldosteronism	Excess							
Stress, surgery, including antidiuretic hormone	Excess							
Hypoadrenocorticalism (Addison's disease)	Loss						↑↓	↓↕
Hypopituitarism	Excess							
Hyperadrenocorticalism (Cushing's disease)	Excess							
Excess citrated blood								
Hyperparathyroidism								
Excess lactation (milk fever)								
Acidosis (metabolic)								
Alkalosis (metabolic)								

↑, Increased serum concentration; ↓, decreased serum concentration; —, normal serum concentration.

        c. Depress minute ventilation; respiratory acidosis may occur

        d. Decrease urine formation and renal concentrating ability

        e. Promote hypothermia

        f. Depress autoregulatory compensation mechanisms

    2. General anesthesia usually depresses the sympathoadrenal response to hypercapnea and hypotension

  C. Imbalances caused by surgery

    1. Blood loss

    2. Evaporative fluid loss from exposed tissues

    3. Pain-induced redistribution of fluids

II. Fluid losses leading to a decrease in effective circulating blood volume usually cause metabolic acidosis

III. Blood loss is usually replaced with crystalloid fluids when the hematocrit is greater than 20% and total protein is above 3.5 g/dl

  A. Colloids, 6% dextran 70, or hetastarch can be administered as alternatives to crystalloids, especially when the total protein is less than 4 g/dl

  B. Blood substitutes or blood are indicated if the packed cell volume (PCV) is acutely decreased below 20% during surgery or in patients with a PCV <15% as a result of chronic anemia

IV. Fluid administration in young or small patients should be supplemented with a source of calories (dextrose) and monitored closely to prevent overhydration

V. The administration of large quantities of room-temperature fluids can produce hypothermia and hemodilution, producing coagulation abnormalities

VI. Fluid administration (Tables 26-3 and 26-4)

  A. Most fluid administration sets deliver 10 drops/ml (regular drip) or 60 drops/ml (mini-drip)

  B. Larger diameter needles or IV catheters offer less resistance to fluid flow and increase the rate of fluid administration

  C. Occasionally, fluids are administered at extremely rapid rates (>90 ml/kg/hr) with fluid pumps

  D. Infusion pumps and syringe infusion pumps facilitate delivery of accurate volumes of fluid (Figs. 26-1 and 26-2)

TABLE 26-3

CATEGORIES, DISTRIBUTION, AND CLINICAL INDICATIONS FOR COMMONLY AVAILABLE FLUIDS FOR INTRAVENOUS FLUID THERAPY

FLUID TYPE	EXAMPLES	VOLUME NEEDED TO INCREASE PLASMA VOLUME BY 1 LITER	DISTRIBUTION	EXAMPLES OF CLINICAL INDICATIONS
Colloid	Starch Gelatin Dextrans	1 L	Plasma volume	Hypovolemia, hypotension, normovolemic hemodilution, hypoalbuminemia
Hypertonic crystalloid	7.5% Saline (NaCl)	300 ml	Immediate plasma volume expansion causing ICFV reduction	Hypovolemic shock, cerebral edema
Hypotonic crystalloid	5% Dextrose	14 L	Total body water	Free water deficit, hypernatremia
Isotonic crystalloid	0.9% NaCl lactated Ringer's solution	4 L or more	ECFV (plasma volume and ISFV expansion)	Dehydration, hypovolemia, hypotension, normovolemia, hemoconcentration

ICFV, Intracellular fluid volume; *ECFV*, extracellular fluid volume; *ISFV*, interstitial fluid volume.

TABLE 26-4
GUIDELINES FOR CRYSTALLOID FLUIDS FOR SURGICAL PATIENTS

Step 1

Start IV fluids, replace insensible (feces, saliva, skin, respiratory tract $\cong$ 20 ml/kg/day) loss with maintenance-type solutions, 2-5 ml/kg/hr, during interval since last oral intake

Step 2

Change to replacement-type solution for intraoperative losses. Administer LRS, Normosol-R, or in some cases 0.9% NaCl, 2 ml/kg/hr

Step 3

Estimate surgical trauma and add appropriate volume of replacement-type solution to that given in Step 2:
Minimal trauma, add 5 ml/kg/hr
Moderate trauma, add 10 ml/kg/hr
Extreme trauma, add 15 ml/kg/hr
Replace 1 ml of blood loss with 3 ml of crystalloid
Administer appropriate fluid; when in doubt give balanced electrolyte solution

Step 4

Give appropriate colloid solution for each volume of blood lost over 15%-20% of the patient's estimated blood volume

Step 5

Monitor vital signs and urine output. Adjust fluids to keep urine output at 1 ml/kg/hr

Modified from Glesecke AH, Egbert LD: Perioperative fluid therapy—crystalloids. In Miller RD, editor: *Anesthesia*, ed 2, New York, 1986, Churchill Livingstone, p. 1315.

NORMAL BODY WATER DISTRIBUTION (FIG. 26-3)

I. Total body water represents 55% to 75% of body weight (use 60%), primarily depending on age and body fat

II. Extracellular water constitutes 23% to 33% of body weight (use 30%); the percentage is greater in very young animals

III. Interstitial water constitutes 15% to 25% of body weight

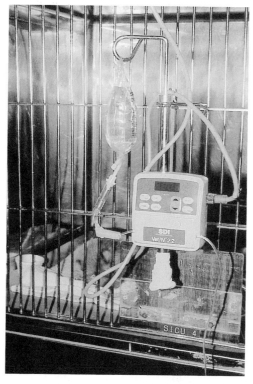

Fig. 26-1
Volumetric infusion pump that uses a fluid administration set.

IV. Plasma water constitutes approximately 5% of body weight
V. Extracellular water equals plasma water plus interstitial water
VI. Intracellular water constitutes 35% to 45% of body weight
VII. Blood volume constitutes 8% to 10% of body weight (approximately 90 ml/kg), depending on the hematocrit level; blood volume equals plasma water plus red blood cell (RBC) volume

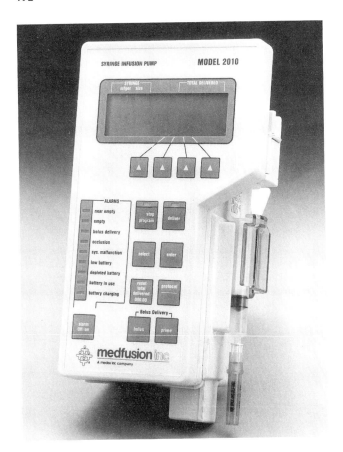

Fig. 26-2
Syringe infusion pump.

ELECTROLYTE DISTRIBUTION

I. Extracellular water contains large quantities of sodium and chloride ions

II. Intracellular water contains large quantities of potassium ions

III. Table 26-1 shows the normal electrolyte composition of serum

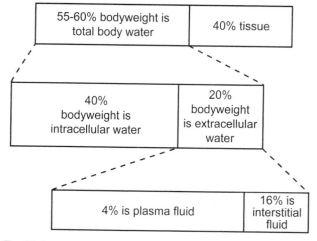

Fig. 26-3

The body fluids are distributed among the intravascular, interstitial (extracellular), and intracellular fluid compartments. Approximately 55% to 60% of the body is water.

PRINCIPLES OF FLUID ADMINISTRATION

I. Correct dehydration and electrolyte and acid-base imbalances before anesthesia when possible

II. Do not attempt to replace chronic fluid losses acutely; severe dilution of plasma proteins, RBCs, and electrolytes may be produced (Table 26-2)

III. Monitor pulmonary, renal, and cardiac function when administering fluids rapidly (e.g., for shock)

    A. Pulmonary function—overhydration can lead to pulmonary edema

    B. Renal function

        1. Improve or reestablish glomerular perfusion rate (renal perfusion) before anesthesia

        2. Administer mannitol at 1 to 2g/kg over a 30-minute period after hydration has been restored

        3. Monitor urine output: 1 to 2 ml/kg/hr

C. Cardiac function
1. Monitor central venous pressure; normally 0.5 to 5 cm H_2O
2. Auscultate the chest; if the total protein (TP) drops below 3.5 g/dl from fluid administration, pulmonary edema may occur
3. In cases of left-sided heart failure, monitor pulmonary capillary wedge pressure, if possible

FLUID ADMINISTRATION DURING ANESTHESIA (TABLES 26-3 THROUGH 26-5)

I. Fluids administered during anesthesia are usually polyionic isotonic crystalloid solutions (Table 26-6)
II. Rate of initial crystalloid fluid administration depends on fluid loss during surgery
   A. Initial minimal rates of fluid administration:

MAINTENANCE RATES FOR CRYSTALLOIDS	
Small animals	3 to 10 ml/kg/hr
Large animals	3 to 5 ml/kg/hr

TABLE 26-5
GUIDE TO MONITORING FLUID THERAPY IN SURGICAL PATIENTS

1. Auscultation: normal bronchovesicular lung sounds
2. Packed cell volume >20%
3. Total protein >3.5 g/dl
4. Electrolytes
   a. Sodium 145-155 mEq/L
   b. Chloride 95-110 mEq/L
   c. Potassium 4.0-5.0 mEq/L
   d. Calcium 8.0-10.0 mg/dl
5. Blood pH 7.3-7.45; $PaCO_2$ 35-45 mm Hg
6. Urine output >1 ml/kg/hr
7. Hemodynamics
   a. Central venous pressure 0-5 cm H_2O
   b. Pulmonary capillary wedge pressure 5-10 mm Hg
   c. Mean arterial blood pressure 70-90 mm Hg

    B. Increase this rate if blood loss occurs

    C. Monitor PCV and TP for hemodilution

III. Estimate blood loss and administer at least 3 ml of crystalloid solution for each milliliter of blood loss (unless blood transfusion is indicated; PCV <20%) over and above the basic fluid rate provided during anesthesia

    A. Crystalloids are rapidly redistributed from the blood into the extracellular fluid, which is approximately three times larger than the blood volume

IV. Maximum volume and rate of safe administration of fluids during shock therapy varies considerably; the rule of thumb is 20 to 90 ml/kg/hr

V. Colloids (Tables 26-3, 26-7, and 26-8)

    A. Restore and maintain intravascular volume

    B. Duration of effect ($t_{1/2}$) determined by molecular size; larger size, longer duration

    C. Colloids produce acute and lasting increases in the following:

        1. Intravascular volume

        2. Arterial blood pressure

        3. Cardiac output

        4. Tissue perfusion and oxygen delivery

    D. Small volumes (5 to 10 ml/kg IV) produce immediate increases in arterial blood pressure and cardiac output

        1. Helps to maintain plasma oncotic value and delay fluid extravasation

        2. May cause an autotransfusion when plasma colloid osmotic pressure is increased

    E. May prolong bleeding time

VI. Hypertonic saline solution (Tables 26-3 and 26-6)

    A. Normal saline solution contains 0.9% NaCl

        1. Commonly used hypertonic saline solutions contain 3%, 5%, and 7% NaCl

    B. Hypertonic fluids increase vascular volume by pulling water from the extracellular fluid space into the vascular space

    C. Hypertonic fluids produce acute increases in the following:

        1. Arterial blood pressure

        2. Cardiac output

        3. Renal perfusion and diuresis

TABLE 26-6

CHARACTERISTICS AND CONTENTS OF COMMONLY USED CRYSTALLOIDS AND NATURAL COLLOIDS

NAME	FLUID COMPARTMENT	OSMOLARITY (mOsm/L)	pH	Na^+ (mEq/L)
Crystalloids				
Maintenance				
2.5% Dextrose in half-strength Lactated Ringer's solution	Extra-cellular	264 (isotonic)	4.5-7.5	65.5
ProcalAmine[*]	Extra-cellular	735 (hypertonic)	6-7	35
3% Freamine III[*]	Extra-cellular	405 (hypertonic)	6-7	35
Replacement				
0.9% Saline	Extra-cellular	308 (isotonic)	5.0	154
Lactated Ringer's solution	Extra-cellular	275 (isotonic)	6.5	130
Plasmalyte-A pH 7.4†	Extra-cellular	294 (isotonic)	7.4	140
7.0% saline	Extra-cellular	2396 (hypertonic)	—	1197
Normosol-R‡	Extra-cellular	295 (isotonic)	5.5-7	140
5% Dextrose in H_2O	Intra-cellular	252 (hypotonic)	4.0	0
Natural				
Whole blood	Extra-cellular	300 (isotonic)	Variable	140
Frozen plasma	Extra-cellular	300 (isotonic)	Variable	140
Albumin	Extra-cellular	309 (5%; isotonic) 312 (25%; hypertonic)	6.4-7.4	130-160

COP, Colloid oncotic pressure.
*McGaw Inc.
†Baxter Healthcare, Corp.
‡Abbott Laboratories.

Cl^- (mEq/L)	K^+ (mEq/L)	Mg^{++} (mEq/L)	Ca^{++} (mEq/L)	DEXTROSE (q/L)	BUFFER	COP (mm Hg)
55	2	0	1.5	25	Lactate	0
41	24	5	0	30	Acetate, Phosphate	0
41	24	5	0	0	Acetate, Phosphate	0
154	0	0	0	0	None	0
109	4	0	3	0	Lactate	0
98	5	3	0	0	Acetate, Gluconate	0
98	5	3	0	0	Acetate, Gluconate	0
1197	0	0	0	0	None	0
0	0	0	0	50	None	0
100	4	0	0	0-4	None	20
110	4	0	0	0-4	None	22
130-160	<1	0	0	0	None	19

TABLE 26-7
CHARACTERISTICS AND CONTENTS OF COMMONLY USED SYNTHETIC COLLOIDS AND BLOOD SUBSTITUTE

NAME	FLUID COMPARTMENT	OSMOLARITY (mOsm/L)	pH	Na^+ (mEq/L)
Synthetic colloids				
6% Hetastarch	Extra-cellular	310 (isotonic)	5.5	154
6% Hetastarch in lactated electrolyte (Hextend)	Extra-cellular	307 (isotonic)	5.9	143
10% Pentastarch	Extra-cellular	326 (isotonic)	5.0	154
Dextran 40	Extra-cellular	311 (isotonic)	3.5-7.0	154
Dextran 70	Extra-cellular	310 (isotonic)	3-7	154
Oxypolygelatin	Extra-cellular	200 (hypotonic)	7.4	155
Blood substitute (O_2 carriers)				
Oxyglobin	Extra-cellular	300 (isotonic)	7.7	150

D. 7% NaCl is used as acute fluid therapy for hypotension or shock; 4 to 7 ml/kg IV

E. Overdose produces hypernatremia, hyperchloremia, and nonrespiratory acidosis; cardiac arrhythmias are also a possibility

VII. Blood substitutes (Table 26-7)

A. Oxygen-carrying solutions that are ultrapurified and hemoglobin-based can be used to replace volume and improve tissue oxygen delivery after trauma and hemorrhage

B. Uses

1. Improve oxygen delivery by increasing oxygen content of the blood and expanding vascular volume

2. Replace hemoglobin in anemic animals

C. Polymerized bovine hemoglobin (Oxyglobin; hemoglobin = 13 g/dl) in modified lactated Ringer's solution is a colloid solution that carries oxygen

1. Immediate availability and ready to use

2. Not 2,3-diphosphoglycerate (DPG)-dependent; chloride-ion dependent

Cl^- (mEq/L)	K^+ (mEq/L)	Mg^{++} (mEq/L)	Ca^{++} (mEq/L)	DEXTROSE (g/L)	BUFFER	COP (mm Hg)
154	0	0	0	0	None	32
124	3	0.9	5	0	Lactate	36
154	0	0	0	0	None	25
154	0	0	0	0	None	82
154	0	0	0	0	None	62
100	0	0	1	0	None	45-47
110	4.0	—	1.0	—	None	43

      3. Stored at room temperature (2-year shelf life)

      4. No typing and cross-matching (no transfusion reactions)

      5. No disease transmission

      6. Saves time, labor, and materials (no need for donor dog)

      7. Dose: 30 ml/kg at 10 ml/kg/hr

   D. Clinical issues

      1. Temporary interference with some serum chemistries

      2. Transient discoloration of urine, sclera, and mucous membranes

      3. Potential for overexpansion of vascular volume in normovolemic patients

   E. Contraindications

      1. Plasma volume expanders, such as colloids and Oxyglobin, are contraindicated in dogs with advanced cardiac disease (i.e., congestive heart failure) or otherwise severely impaired cardiac function or renal impairment with oliguria or anuria

      2. Use during sepsis and endotoxemia has been questioned

TABLE 26-8

CHARACTERISTICS OF COMMON COLLOID SOLUTIONS

COLLOID	MOLECULAR WEIGHT (RANGE)	MOLECULAR WEIGHT (AVERAGE)	NUMBER AVERAGED MOLECULAR WEIGHT	COP (mm Hg)	OSMOLARITY (mOsm/L)
Saline	0	0	0	0	310
Albumin	66,000-69,000	68,000	68,000	19	309 (5%) 312 (25%)
Plasma	66,000-400,000	119,000	88,000	22	285
10% Dextran 40	10,000-90,000	40,000	26,000	82	310
6% Dextran 70	10,000-1,000,000	450,000	69,000	62	310
6% Hetastarch	15,000-3,400,000	70,000	41,000	32	310
6% Hetastarch in lactated electrolyte (Hextend)	15,000-3,400,000	70,000	41,000	36	307
10% Pentastarch	10,000-2,000,000	268,000	110,000	25	326
Pentafraction	10,000-1,000,000	280,000	120,000	—	—
4% Gelatins	5,000-100,000	30,000	22,600	—	—

TABLE 26-9

DRUG DOSES AND ROUTE OF ADMINISTRATION FOR USE IN TRANSFUSION REACTIONS

---

1. STOP TRANSFUSION
2. Drugs

Short-acting glucocorticoids
    Methylpredonisolone succinate 30 mg/kg IV once
    Dexamethasone sodium phosphate 4-6 mg/kg IV once
Diphenhydramine 2 mg/kg IV as required
Regular insulin 0.5 U/kg IV given with 50% dextrose 2 g per unit of insulin as required
Calcium gluconate (10% solution) 50-150 mg/kg IV over 20-30 min; discontinue if bradycardia occurs
    Repeat if hypocalcemia persists
Calcium chloride (10% solution) 50-150 mg/kg IV over 20-30 min; discontinue if bradycardia occurs
    Repeat if hypocalcemia persists
Furosemide 2-4 mg/kg IV
Nitroglycerin paste (2%) $\frac{1}{4}$-1 inch applied to skin; monitor blood pressure, may cause hypotension
Aspirin 10 mg/kg orally once

Modified from Hohenhaus AE, Blood transfusions and blood substitutes. In DiBartola SP: *Fluid, electrolyte, and acid-base disorders in small animal practice,* ed 3, Philadelphia, 2006, W.B. Saunders, p. 577.

    3. Warnings
        a. Overdose or an excessively rapid administration rate (more than 10 ml/kg/hr) may result in circulatory overload; see the product's package insert for complete information

PERIOPERATIVE FLUID THERAPY

    I. Normal daily fluid maintenance rates vary as follows:
        A. 30 to 60 ml/kg/day (mature animal)
        B. 40 to 80 ml/kg/day (young animal)
    II. Calculation of replacement fluid volume in dehydrated animals
        A. Body weight (kg) × % dehydration (figured as a decimal) = fluid deficit (L) (e.g., 20 kg × 10% dehydration = 2 L fluid deficit); reassess periodically to determine the response to volumes administered

B. Fluid administration to correct dehydration can be administered over a 6- to 12-hour period or added to the maintenance fluid volume and administered over a 24-hour period

CLINICAL ASSESSMENT OF HYDRATION			
	MINIMAL (4%)	**MODERATE (6% TO 8%)**	**SEVERE (10% TO 12%)**
Skin resiliency	Pliable	Leathery	Absolutely no pliability
Skin tenting	Tented skin immediately disappears and tent persists up to 2 sec	Tented skin slowly disappears and tent persists up to 3 sec or more	Twist and tent persists indefinitely
Eye	Bright	Duller than normal	Cornea dry
	Slightly sunken	Obviously sunken	Deeply sunken, 2- to 4-mm space between eyeball and bony orbit
Mouth	Moist, warm	Sticky to dry, warm	Dry, cyanotic, warm to cold

BLOOD TRANSFUSION—MAJOR BLOOD GROUPS

I. Dogs
  A. At least eight specific antigens have been identified on the dog erythrocyte
    1. Dogs that are 1.1 negative and 1.2 negative are universal donors
    2. Dog erythrocyte antigen $(DEA)_1$, DEA_2, and DEA_7 have the greatest potential to induce hemolytic antibody production in recipients; dogs negative for these RBC antigens are desirable as donors

       3. Transfusion reactions related to the remaining blood-group antigens are usually clinically insignificant

       4. Donor dogs should test negative for heartworms and other blood-borne diseases

II. Cats

    A. Three major antigens have been identified on the cat erythrocyte

       1. Transfusion reactions are rare in cats; blood typing is rarely performed

       2. RBC survival time may decrease after multiple transfusions

III. Horses

    A. At least nine specific blood group antigens have been identified

       1. Compatibility testing should be done before transfusion

         a. Blood typing

         b. Major and minor antigen agglutination

         c. Lysis cross-matching test

       2. When compatibility cannot be tested, a healthy male that has never had a transfusion is the most suitable donor

IV. Cows: at least 11 antigenic blood groups

V. Swine: at least 15 antigenic blood groups

VI. Sheep: at least 8 antigenic blood groups

INDICATIONS FOR BLOOD OR BLOOD SUBSTITUTES

  I. Restoration of oxygen-carrying capacity

    A. Anemia

       1. PCV <15% to 20%; hemoglobin is <5 to 7 g/dl in a normally hydrated patient being prepared for surgery

       2. Nonsurgical, chronically anemic patients may not require transfusion unless PCV is <15 in dogs or <10 in cats

    B. Hemorrhage (Table 27-2)

       1. Crystalloid infusions adequately treat 15% to 30% total blood volume loss

2. Colloids should be considered when blood loss exceeds 20% of blood volume (>15 ml/kg)
3. Whole blood or blood substitutes are necessary for replacement of more than 50% total blood volume loss
   a. Stored blood is a poor carrier of oxygen because the hemoglobin cannot off-load oxygen efficiently
   b. Fresh whole blood or blood substitutes should be administered to replace acute blood loss and improve oxygen delivery to tissues

II. Restoration of blood volume after severe (>20 ml/kg) blood loss

III. Coagulation factor replacement
   A. Poor viability of platelets and coagulation factors in stored blood
   B. Choose fresh blood (stored for <12 hours) when treating coagulopathies

COLLECTING AND STORING BLOOD FOR TRANSFUSION

I. Obtain blood from the jugular vein or with a cardiac puncture

II. Anticoagulant solutions used
   A. Acid citrate dextrose
   B. Citrate phosphate dextrose maintains higher pH, adenosine triphosphate, and 2,3-DPG content during storage
   C. Heparin
      1. Heparin activates platelet aggregation and inhibits thrombin formation by inhibiting factor IX activation
      2. Do not use blood collected with heparin as the anticoagulant if it has been stored longer than 48 hours

III. Plastic containers are recommended for blood collection; they are less likely to activate platelet and coagulation factors

IV. Suggested guidelines for blood storage
   A. Maintain temperature between 1° and 6° C for the following storage times:
      1. Acid citrate dextrose anticoagulant: 21 days
      2. Citrate phosphate dextrose anticoagulant: 28 days
      3. Feline blood: 30 days
   B. 70% to 75% RBCs are viable at the end of the storage times listed above

MODIFICATIONS OF STORED BLOOD

I. RBCs become less deformable because of the following conditions:
   A. Hypertonicity of anticoagulant solution
   B. Decreasing erythrocyte adenosine triphosphate content
   C. Hypoxemia and metabolic acidosis
II. Erythrocyte 2,3-DPG content is decreased
   A. The oxygen dissociation curve shifts to the left; decreased oxygen is released at the tissue level
      1. Stored blood is a poor choice when increased oxygen delivery to tissues is required; blood substitutes (Oxyglobin) are recommended in these circumstances
   B. 2,3-DPG content in RBCs is restored within hours of transfusion
III. pH decreases (less than 6.5 after 3 weeks of storage); citrate anticoagulants are converted to bicarbonate within minutes by the liver; bicarbonate therapy with blood transfusion is not necessary unless inadequate liver blood flow or altered liver metabolism is suspected
IV. Platelet numbers decrease; functional platelets are nonexistent after 2 to 3 days of storage
V. Ammonia content increases; this may be detrimental for patients with impaired hepatic function
VI. Plasma potassium concentration increases because of progressive hemolysis during storage
VII. Metabolic transformations in stored blood are largely reversed during the first 24 hours after transfusion

ADVERSE, IMMUNE-MEDIATED EFFECTS OF BLOOD TRANSFUSION

I. Nonhemolytic hypersensitivity reactions
   A. Activation of kallikrein-kinin system or immunoglobulin E
   B. Release of biogenic amines
   C. Clinical signs are muscle tremor, vomiting, pyrexia, hypotension, tachycardia, and urticaria
II. Hemolytic reactions
   A. Hemolysis results from the following:

1. Recipient antibodies interacting with incompatible antigen of donor
2. Antibodies of a previously sensitized donor interacting with recipient antigen

B. Immediate transfusion reactions are unlikely during a first transfusion

C. Clinical signs usually develop within an hour after a transfusion and include hypotension, pyrexia, muscle tremor, emesis, convulsions, hemoglobinemia or hemoglobinuria, and bilirubinemia or bilirubinuria

D. Shock, renal failure, and disseminated intravascular coagulation may ensue

E. Delayed transfusion reactions can occur up to 2 weeks after a transfusion
   1. The recipient mounts an immune response to incompatible erythrocytes
   2. Clinical signs include pyrexia, anorexia, jaundice, and bilirubinuria

F. Hemolysis in neonates resulting from previous sensitization of the mother (neonatal isoerythrolysis) can be avoided by preventing colostrum absorption; withhold mother's milk from the neonate in the first 48 hours of life

NONIMMUNOLOGIC ADVERSE TRANSFUSION REACTIONS

I. Sepsis: improper collection, storage, or handling may result in bacterial contamination and overgrowth

II. Transmission of infectious or parasitic diseases

III. Circulatory overload

IV. Citrate toxicity
   A. Citrate toxicity is rarely seen because of the rapid metabolism of citrate by the liver; it is more likely in animals with liver dysfunction or excessively rapid blood administration
   B. Excessive circulating citrate causes chelation of serum ionized calcium

PLASMA TRANSFUSION

I. Indications
  A. Hypoproteinemia: total protein ≤ 4 g/dl; albumin ≤ 1.5 g/dl
  B. Failure of passive transfer; inadequate colostral antibody absorption
  C. Thrombocytopenia: use fresh plasma
  D. Coagulopathies: use fresh plasma
II. Plasma can be stored in a conventional freezer for up to 1 year

---

PLASMA REPLACEMENT

Milliliters of plasma to administer =
$$\frac{(\text{Desired TP} - \text{Existing TP}) \times (\text{ml/kg PV} \times \text{Recipient BW [kg]})}{\text{Donor TP}}$$

TP, Total protein; *PV*, plasma volume.

ROUTES AND VOLUME OF FLUID ADMINISTRATION

I. A peripheral or jugular vein
II. Intraperitoneal administration
  A. Administer slowly
  B. RBCs are poorly recovered into the system; approximately 40% of blood is absorbed in 24 hours
III. Medullary cavity of femur, tibia, or humerus
  A. Adequate for neonatal small animals
  B. Use a 20-gauge needle or a bone-marrow aspiration needle
  C. 95% of the blood is absorbed within 5 minutes
IV. Rewarm stored blood to decrease viscosity and prevent hypothermia in recipients; immerse transfusion tubing in water that is maintained at a temperature below 40° C; auto-agglutination occurs at higher temperatures
V. Volume of colloid or blood to be administered
  A. General rule: 1 ml of colloid or blood per milliliter of blood lost
  B. General rule: 2 ml of whole blood per kilogram raises the PCV by 1% (assuming there is a donor PCV of 40%)

C. The amount of blood lost in aspirated fluids

Volume of blood in suction fluid =
$$\frac{PCV \text{ of fluid} \times \text{Volume of fluid}}{PCV \text{ of animal}}$$

D. Plasma volume needed to attain a target TP

Amount of donor plasma needed (ml) =
Desired TP – Actual TP × Recipient plasma volume

VI. Blood administration
  A. Use an administrative set with a filter to remove aggregated debris
    1. Micropore filter with pore size 20 to 40 μm
    2. Cloth filter of administration set with pore size 170 μm
  B. Flush tubing before introducing blood
    1. This reduces resistance to blood flow
    2. Isotonic saline solution is the recommended fluid
    3. Lactated Ringer's or other calcium-containing solutions may recalcify blood and trigger coagulation
    4. Dextrose solutions may cause agglutination and/or hemolysis
VII. Blood administration rate depends on clinical circumstances
  A. Administer rapidly after massive hemorrhage
  B. Blood replacement

BLOOD REPLACEMENT

Milliliters of blood to administer =
$$\frac{(\text{Desired HP} - \text{Existing HP}) \times (\text{ml/kg BV} \times \text{Recipient BW [kg]})}{\text{Donor HP}}$$

Hb, Hemoglobin; *BV*, blood volume.

C. In other cases
    1. Transfuse blood slowly at 0.25 ml/kg during the first 30 minutes; observe for adverse reactions
    2. Afterward, the rule of thumb is 10 ml/kg/hr, until the desired PCV is achieved
    3. Monitor for signs of fluid overload (e.g., central venous pressure, thoracic auscultation)
VIII. Intravenous fluid supplement (Table 26-10)

TABLE 26-10
FLUID INTRAVENOUS SUPPLEMENTS

SUPPLEMENT	EMERGENCY DOSE	OSMOLARITY (mOsm/L)	pH	COMPOSITION (mmol/L)
Calcium chloride (10%)	0.05-0.1 ml/kg slowly	2040	5.5-7.5	34 Calcium 68 Chloride
Calcium gluconate (10%)	0.5-3 ml/kg slowly or 60-90 mg/kg/day	680	6.0-8.2	465 Calcium gluconate (no data)
Dextrose (50%)	500 mg/kg diluted, for immediate bolus	2530	4.2	No data
Magnesium sulphate (1 g/2 ml)	0.15-0.3 mmol/kg over 5 min	4060	5.5-7.0	4.06 Magnesium sulphate (no data)
Mannitol (25%)	0.25-3 g/kg diluted and slowly over 30 min	1373	4.5-7.0	No data
Potassium chloride (2 mmol/ml)	0.5-1 mmol/kg/hr	4000	4-8	2000 Potassium 2000 Chloride
Sodium bicarbonate (8.4%), (1 mmol/ml)	0.3 × body weight (kg) × base deficit (mmol/L) or 1 mmol/L immediately	2000	7.8	1000 Sodium 1000 Bicarbonate
Tromethamine	Milliliter needed = body weight (kg) × base deficit (mmol/L) × 1.1	380	8.6	300 Tromethamine

CHAPTER TWENTY-SEVEN

Shock

"I'm late, I'm late for a very important date" (early recognition and treatment is essential to prevent death).

LEWIS CARROLL

OVERVIEW

Traditional approaches to the classification of shock emphasize the importance of various potential causes (hemorrhage, trauma, sepsis, allergies, and drug reactions) or the functional relationship between the effective circulating volume, the heart, and peripheral vasculature. These approaches ascribe shock to hypovolemia, cardiac failure, obstruction (high resistance) to blood flow, or the abnormal distribution (low resistance) of blood flow. Although instructive, only the functional categorization provides the necessary knowledge required for a rational approach to therapy. The temporal pathophysiologic processes responsible for the circulatory changes that occur are vitally important. Shock activates the immune system and white blood cells, leading to systemic inflammatory response syndrome (SIRS). The development of SIRS can also result from opportunistic infections in depressed, debilitated, or severely stressed animals. Sustained shock with or without hyperthermia predisposes animals to multiple organ failure and coagulopathies, including disseminated intravascular coagulopathy. This chapter defines shock and discusses current thoughts regarding the pathophysiology of shock, circulatory compensation and decompensation, signs and symptoms, the value of monitored physiologic variables, and the treatment of shock syndromes.

DEFINITION OF SHOCK

I. Definition: shock is a disease syndrome best characterized by impaired tissue perfusion and oxygenation

    A. Importantly, the success of therapy is more closely linked to microhemodynamic events (functional capillary density) and tissue PO_2 (PtO_2) than heart rate, respiratory rate, and arterial blood pressure (macrohemodynamic events)

II. Etiology (Table 27-1)

    A. Hypovolemic

    B. Cardiogenic

    C. Distributive

    D. Obstructive

III. Pathophysiology (Fig. 27-1)

    A. Poor tissue perfusion can result from the following

        1. Trauma, hemorrhage (Table 27-2)

            a. Blood loss

                (1) 20% loss: mild signs of shock

                (2) 30% loss: obvious signs of shock

            b. Release of catecholamines

            c. Vasoconstriction

            d. Hypovolemia

        2. Heart failure

            a. Forward failure

                (1) Cardiomyopathy

                (2) Aortic and pulmonic stenosis

                (3) Ventricular septal defect

            b. Backward failure

                (1) Mitral insufficiency

                (2) Aortic insufficiency

            c. Cardiac arrhythmias

                (1) Multiform ventricular tachycardia

        3. Endotoxin

            a. Endotoxin-induced extravasation of fluids (third space loss)

            b. Release of vasoactive substances (histamine, catecholamines, serotonin, bradykinins, prostaglandins, tumor necrosis factor, interleukins)

TABLE 27-1
CAUSES OF SHOCK

CATEGORY	CAUSE
HYPOVOLEMIC SHOCK	
Exogenous	Blood loss caused by hemorrhage
	Plasma loss caused by thermal or chemical burns and inflammation
	Fluid and electrolyte loss caused by dehydration, vomiting, diarrhea, renal disease, severe exercise, heat stress, or excessive diuresis
Endogenous	Extravasation of fluids, plasma, or blood into a body cavity or tissues (third-space losses) caused by trauma, endotoxins, hypoproteinemia, anaphylaxis, or burns
CARDIAC SHOCK	
	Myocardial mechanical problems caused by regurgitant or obstructive defects
	Myopathic defects caused by inheritable traits, chemicals, or toxins
	Cardiac arrhythmias (rapid or multiform wide QRS tachycardias, bradycardia)
DISTRIBUTIVE SHOCK	
High resistance	Abnormal distribution of blood volume and flow to vital organs caused by endotoxins, anesthetic drug overdose, CNS trauma, anaphylaxis
Low resistance	Distribution of blood away from vital organs caused by severe infections, abscesses, or arteriovenous fistulas
OBSTRUCTIVE SHOCK	
	Obstruction to blood flow through the heart (pericardial tamponade, neoplasia, embolism), aorta (embolism, aneurysm), vena cava (gastric bloat, heartworm, neoplasia), lungs (embolism, heartworm, positive-pressure ventilation)

CNS, Central nervous system.

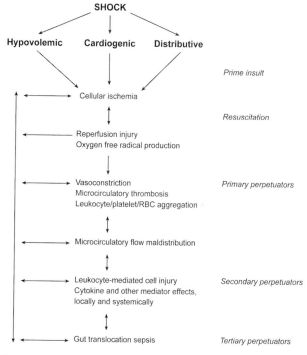

Fig. 27-1
Progressive pathophysiologic processes in shock.

       c. Generalized vasoconstriction (occurs early in septic shock)
       d. Capillary damage with loss of volume
       e. Selective capillary dilatation
       f. Relative hypovolemia
       g. The opening of arteriovenous shunts may result in blood flow bypassing capillary beds, regardless of cardiac output

B. Traumatic, hemorrhagic, or cardiogenic shock eventually leads to the following
    1. Ischemic anoxia: can be caused by decreased effective circulatory volume, decreased venous return, reduced

TABLE 27-2
THE FOUR CLASSES OF HEMORRHAGE

Class 1	Loss of up to 15% (approximately 10-12 ml/kg)* of the circulating blood volume	Clinical symptoms are minimal as suggested by mild tachycardia, no changes in arterial blood pressure, pulse pressure, or respiratory rate
Class 2	Loss of 15%-30% (approximately 23-25 ml/kg)* of the circulating blood volume	Clinical signs include tachycardia, tachypnea, and a decrease in pulse pressure
Class 3	Loss of 30%-40% (approximately 30-32 ml/kg)* of the circulating blood volume	Clinical signs include pale mucous membranes, prolonged capillary refill time, tachycardia, tachypnea, depression, and a decrease in arterial blood pressure
Class 4	Loss of greater than 40% of the circulating blood volume	Clinical signs include very pale or white mucous membranes, prolonged capillary refill time, cold extremities, tachycardia, tachypnea, rapid thready pulse, markedly decreased arterial blood pressure, delirium, and depression

Reproduced with permission from American College of Surgeons' Committee on Trauma. *Advanced Trauma Life Support for Doctors (ATLS) Student Manual 7th Edition.* Chicago: American College of Surgeons, 2004.
*Assumes a total blood volume of 80 ml/kg.

cardiac output, increased total peripheral resistance, decreased tissue perfusion, and increased catecholamines
2. Hypoxia, ischemia, and acidosis leading to the activation of monocytes, macrophages, and leukocytes, which trigger the release of cellular reactant substances
   a. Various interleukins (1, 6, 8, and others) are products of activated monocytes and macrophages:
      (1) Stimulate fever by initiating prostaglandin synthesis
      (2) Stimulate activation and release of neutrophils
      (3) Initiate proteolysis in skeletal muscles
      (4) Stimulate insulin and glucagon production
      (5) Activate the immune system
   b. Activated leukocytes release lytic enzymes (proteases, lipases) and oxygen free radicals, resulting in SIRS:
      (1) Initiation of the complement cascade
      (2) Damage to cell membranes by lysosomal enzymes
      (3) Production of autocoids (histamine, bradykinin, and serotonin)
      (4) Increased capillary membrane permeability
   c. Arachidonic acid metabolism is activated, producing a number of biologically active cyclooxygenase and lipoxygenase products (prostaglandins)
      (1) Prostacyclin relaxes vascular smooth muscle and inhibits platelet aggregation
      (2) Thromboxane A_2 constricts vascular smooth muscle, releases lysosomes, and causes platelet and leukocyte activation and aggregation
      (3) Leukotrienes (e.g., the slow-reacting substance of anaphylaxis) produce many detrimental effects such as vasoconstriction, bronchoconstriction, and increased capillary membrane permeability
   d. Cellular damage causes the production of cardiac depressant substances and vasoactive peptides; factor XII is produced, which converts kallikreinogen to kallikrein, bradykinin, and other active peptides, resulting in vasodilation and increased capillary membrane permeability

(1) Factor XII initiates the intrinsic system in the coagulation cascade

(a) Fibrin thrombi are formed, perpetuating hypoxia, acidosis, and tissue damage; fibrin split products are formed, thrombocytopenia develops, culminating in disseminated intravascular coagulopathy

3. Stagnant anoxia can be caused by anoxia, stagnation, acidosis, microthrombosis, and arteriovenous shunting (venous admixture): bacteria-tissue interaction and/or atelectasis in the lungs may contribute to shunting

4. Time: ischemic anoxia to stagnant anoxia may take hours to occur in hemorrhagic shock; it occurs in seconds to minutes in anaphylactic or septic shock

5. The ultimate outcome is cell damage and death

C. Cellular events
1. Reduced oxygen and nutrient supply
2. Anaerobic metabolism
3. Decreased adenosine triphosphate and energy
4. Increased membrane permeability
5. Influx of sodium and water
6. Efflux of intracellular potassium
7. Cellular edema
8. Mitochondrial damage (swelling)
9. Intracellular acidosis
10. Lysosomal membrane rupture
11. Extracellular lytic enzymes
12. Extracellular acidemia
13. Cell damage and death

IV. Compensation and decompensation
A. Most compensatory changes are initiated in an attempt to sustain tissue oxygen (PtO_2) and preserve cellular metabolic functions (Table 27-3; Fig. 27-2)

1. Hemorrhage decreases blood volume, cardiac output, arterial blood pressure, and oxygen delivery; activating the sympathetic nervous system

a. Compensatory mechanisms include tachycardia, systemic and pulmonary vasoconstriction, and increased myocardial contractility

TABLE 27-3

COMPENSATORY AND CORRECTIVE RESPONSES TO A DECREASE IN THE EFFECTIVE CIRCULATING BLOOD VOLUME

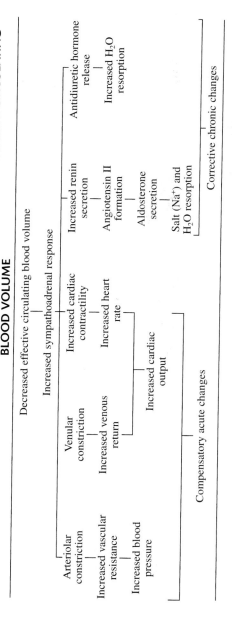

Decreased effective circulating blood volume

Increased sympathoadrenal response

Arteriolar constriction → Increased vascular resistance → Increased blood pressure

Venular constriction → Increased venous return → Increased cardiac output

Increased cardiac contractility → Increased cardiac output

Increased heart rate → Increased cardiac output

Compensatory acute changes

Increased renin secretion → Angiotensin II formation → Aldosterone secretion → Salt (Na^+) and H_2O resorption

Antidiuretic hormone release → Increased H_2O resorption

Corrective chronic changes

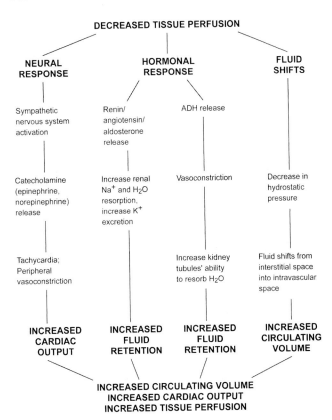

Fig. 27-2
Compensatory mechanisms activated in shock.

b. Blood flow is preferentially redistributed to the heart, brain, lungs, and liver at the expense of the kidneys, gut, skin, and muscle
c. Continued or severe untreated hemorrhage (more than 50% blood volume) causes cardiac output and arterial blood pressure to decrease until death

     d. Prolonged intense vasoconstriction predisposes the patient to tissue ischemia, hypoxia, and cellular acidosis

2. Trauma (blunt force, surgery), with or without major blood loss, increases sympathetic neural activity; this stimulates the cardiorespiratory centers

     a. Compensatory mechanisms include tachycardia, increased force of cardiac contraction, and increased arterial blood pressure and peripheral vascular resistance

     b. When hypovolemia is severe (>25% blood volume), cardiac output decreases

     c. Respiratory alkalosis occurs as a result of increased ventilation

     d. The duration and magnitude of the traumatic event determine the onset of various decompensatory events

        (1) Persistent tachycardia

        (2) Decreased cardiac output (<90 ml/kg/min)

        (3) Decreased arterial pressure (mean <60 mm Hg; systolic <80 mm Hg)

        (4) Activation of neuroendocrine, immune complement, and arachidonic acid systems

3. Heart failure and severe cardiac arrhythmias (ventricular tachycardia) decrease cardiac output, which activate the sympathetic nervous system and various neuroendocrine and renal mechanisms designed to restore blood volume and flow

     a. Compensatory mechanisms include tachycardia, vasoconstriction, and increased total blood volume

     b. Peripheral vascular resistance increases

     c. Cardiac decompensation produced by progressive heart failure results in reduced cardiac output, tachycardia, arterial hypotension, elevated venous pressures, pulmonary edema, and ascites

4. Sepsis activates neuroendocrine, immune, arachidonic acid (prostaglandin), and complement systems

     a. Compensatory responses include fever, chills, leukocytosis with or without hypotension, and tachycardia; cardiac output and alveolar ventilation are initially increased

b. Cardiac output is increased and systemic vascular resistance is decreased early during sepsis to meet the increased metabolic demands for oxygen and the production of nitric oxide

c. Hyperthermia increases metabolic (oxygen) and circulatory demands

d. Endotoxins damage endothelial cells and cause the release of vasoactive peptides, which result in the following:

(1) Activation of the complement cascade

(2) Activation of the coagulation system

(3) Activation of factor XII, which produces bradykinin and the release of other autocoids

(4) Activation of the fibrinolytic system

(a) Formation of fibrin split products

(b) Consumption of coagulation factors

(c) Thrombocytopenia

5. Extreme dehydration, hemorrhage, or trauma can cause redistribution of body water from plasma, interstitial, and intracellular compartments

a. Body fluid shifts occur after hemorrhage in an attempt to refill the plasma compartment and result in a gradual reduction in hemoglobin concentration (packed cell volume [PCV])

b. Inappropriate fluid shifts after trauma, surgery, and hemorrhage lead to hypovolemia, excessive interstitial water, reduced intracellular water, and increased total body water

(1) Peripheral edema may occur

(2) Pulmonary edema may occur

B. Decompensation, which can take hours or minutes, is an extension of the hyperdynamic state; progressive increases in tissue oxygen demand and maldistribution of blood flow eventually lead to tissue ischemia, hypoxia, and acidosis

V. Clinical signs of shock (Tables 27-4 and 27-5)

A. The signs of shock are indicative of exaggerated adrenergic responses and the products of tissue ischemia, hypoxia, and acidosis

TABLE 27-4
STAGES OF SHOCK

CHARACTERISTIC	EARLY STAGE	LATE STAGE
Cardiovascular		
Heart rate	Moderately increased	Markedly increased
Heart rhythm	Regular, rapid, normal	Regular or irregular
Pulse pressure	Normal	Reduced (weak, thready pulse)
Capillary refill time	Minimally prolonged	Markedly prolonged (>3 sec)
Mucous membrane color	Pale pink (injected in septic shock)	White (red or blue in septic shock)
CVP	Minimally reduced	Markedly reduced (<1 cm H_2O)
Arterial blood pressure	Normal or decreased (elevated in septic shock)	Decreased (mean pressure <60 mm Hg)
ECG	Normal, tachycardia	Tachycardia, arrhythmic, S-T segment deviation
Respiratory		
Respiratory rate	Increased	Rapid, shallow breathing
Pattern of respiration	Regular	Normal, intermittent dyspnea
Auscultation	Normal, increased tracheal sounds	Increased bronchovesicular sounds, crackles
Tidal volume	Increased	Decreased
Arterial oxygen tension	Normal	Normal or decreased
Arterial carbon dioxide	Decreased	Normal, decreased or increased

CVP, Central venous pressure; *ECG,* electrocardiogram; *BUN,* blood urea nitrogen.

Continued

TABLE 27-4
STAGES OF SHOCK—cont'd

CHARACTERISTIC	EARLY STAGE	LATE STAGE
Central nervous system		
Level of consciousness	Alert, anxious, minimally depressed	Depressed, semiconscious, coma
Laboratory evaluation		
Packed cell volume	Normal or increased	Normal or decreased
Total protein	Normal or increased	Decreased
Blood lactate	Normal	Increased
Serum K^+	Normal or decreased	Increased
BUN and creatinine	Normal	Normal or increased
Urine volume and Na^+	Decreased	Markedly decreased
White blood cell count	Increased (left shift)	Decreased (left shift)

CVP, Central venous pressure; *ECG,* electrocardiogram; *BUN,* blood urea nitrogen.

TABLE 27-5
CLINICALLY USEFUL VARIABLES FOR ASSESSING SHOCK

	UNIT	NORMAL VALUE OR CONDITION
Mucous membrane color	—	Pink
Capillary refill time	Sec	<2
Respiratory rate	Breaths/min	
Dog		<20
Cat		<30
Arterial oxygen tension, PaO_2	mm Hg	100-120
Arterial oxygen saturation	%	>85
Central venous oxygen saturation, SvO_2	%	>70
Heart rate	Beats/min	
Dog		70-180
Cat		150-210
Urine output	ml/kg/hr	2-5
Blood glucose concentration	mg/dl	70-150
Potassium	mEq/L	4-5
Packed cell volume	%	30-45
Hemoglobin	g/dl	12-16
Temperature	°F	100-102
Lactic acid concentration	mmol/L	<1.0
Central venous pressure	mm Hg	<1.0
Arterial blood pressure	mm Hg	
Systolic		80-150
Diastolic		50-90
Mean		60-110

1. Hemorrhage causes activation of the autonomic nervous system; redistribution of blood to the heart, brain, and lungs; and a shift of body fluids to the plasma volume
   a. Depression, unconsciousness
   b. Pale or white mucous membranes
   c. Decreased skin temperature
   d. Prolonged capillary refill time
   e. Tachycardia
   f. Oliguria
   g. Delayed reduction in PCV

2. Severe physical or surgical injury increases autonomic neural activity, which stimulates central cardiac and respiratory centers and activates humoral mechanisms
   a. History of trauma or surgery
   b. Physical evidence of injury (fractures, lacerations)
   c. Depression, collapse
   d. Signs of hemorrhage (see above)
   e. Tachypnea, respiratory distress
3. Heart failure reduces cardiac output, which activates the autonomic and neuroendocrine systems; this results in retention of electrolytes (Na^+, Cl^-) and water
   a. Reduced exercise tolerance, depression, or fainting
   b. Pale and cold mucous membranes
   c. Prolonged capillary refill time
   d. Cardiac arrhythmias
   e. Weak peripheral pulses
   f. Cardiac murmurs
   g. Oliguria
   h. Pulmonary edema and ascites
4. Localized or systemic infection (SIRS), with or without bacteremia and endotoxemia, is associated with sympathetic activation of the cardiorespiratory centers and the immune, coagulation, complement, and kinin systems and the release of various hormones, prostaglandins, and vasoactive peptides
   a. Depression
   b. Fever, chills
   c. Warm skin and mucous membranes
   d. Normal or red mucous membranes
   e. Tachycardia
   f. Strong or weak pulse
   g. Tachypnea
   h. Oliguria
   i. Leukocytosis or leukopenia
   j. Thrombocytopenia

CLINICAL AND LABORATORY FEATURES

I. Shock is divided into early (reversible) and late (irreversible) stages (Table 27-4)

II. Laboratory findings: laboratory data vary greatly and in many instances depend on the cause of the shock syndrome and the stage of shock (refer to Fig. 15-10)

A. PCV

    1. In hemorrhagic shock

        a. Normal early, then below normal in hypovolemic and progressive phases of oligemic shock; plasma volume increases as interstitial fluid moves into the vascular system during the first 30 to 45 minutes during hemorrhage (0.25 ml/kg/min); in many species (dogs, horses), the spleen serves as a blood reservoir and buffers the effects of acute blood loss on PCV; because of the ability of splenic contraction to restore blood volume, hemorrhage must be severe to produce PCV decreases

        b. With traumatic burns, endotoxic shock, and colic, PCV increases and hemoconcentration occurs

    2. Blood glucose is elevated; epinephrine is released

    3. Blood serum protein concentration may be normal or increased at first, but it is generally reduced during later stages of shock

    4. Platelet count is usually decreased

    5. Blood urea nitrogen and creatinine are elevated, and creatinine clearance is reduced

    6. Urinalysis generally shows no specific abnormalities

    7. Electrolyte patterns vary considerably, but there is a tendency toward a low serum sodium level and a low serum chloride level

    8. Serum potassium may be high, low, or normal

    9. Plasma bicarbonate is usually low, and blood lactate is elevated

    10. Respiratory alkalosis occurs early in shock and is manifested by a low $PaCO_2$

    11. Hypoxia and metabolic acidosis develop as shock progresses; PaO_2 values are below 70 mm Hg (normal values are 75 to 100 mm Hg)

B. The lungs in shock: respiratory failure is the most frequent cause of death in patients with shock, particularly after the hemodynamic alterations have been corrected; this syndrome is characterized by pulmonary congestion, hemorrhage, atelectasis, edema, and the formation of thrombi; pulmonary surfactant decreases, and pulmonary compliance becomes progressively compromised

MONITORING

Monitoring provides vital information for evaluating patient trends and guiding the course of therapy. A global monitoring approach is necessary, including a detailed medical history and physical examination supplemented by physiologic, laboratory (pH, PO_2, lactate), and radiographic or other imaging information (e.g., ultrasound). Serial measurements are mandatory (Table 27-5).

I. Hemodynamic monitoring should stress tissue perfusion and emphasize variables reflecting oxygen transport
   A. Heart rate
   B. Heart and lung sounds
   C. Pulse pressure measurement
   D. Mucous membrane capillary refill time (less than 2 seconds)
   E. Mucous membrane color (pink)
   F. Temperature (more than 37.8° C [100° F]; less than 38.6° C [101.5° F])
   G. PCV and hemoglobin concentration (PCV >20%; hemoglobin >7 g/dl)
   H. Arterial blood pressure measurement (mean >60 mm Hg; systolic >80 mm Hg)
      1. Direct arterial catheters
      2. Indirect blood pressure cuffs (oscillometric or Doppler blood pressure monitors)
   I. Electrocardiogram
   J. Pulse oximetry for noninvasive assessment of tissue oxygenation and heart rate
   K. Blood gas (PO_2, PCO_2) and pH measurements
      1. Arterial blood gases are indicative of oxygenation and ventilation

2. Venous blood gases and pH indicate tissue metabolic status and adequacy of blood flow (cardiac output)

II. Respiratory system monitoring should evaluate ventilation and must stress arterial oxygenation

A. Mucous membrane color: cyanotic (blue) mucous membrane color suggests at least 5 g/dl of reduced (desaturated) hemoglobin

B. Respiratory rate

C. Thoracic radiographs

D. Effort of breathing (dyspnea)

E. Tidal volume

1. Subjectively assessed by rebreathing from a bag (anesthetic machine)

2. Ventilometer: measures V_T (mls)

F. End-tidal CO_2 determination noninvasively assesses the adequacy of ventilation

G. Blood gases and pH

1. Arterial blood gases are used to assess oxygenation (PO_2) and ventilation (PCO_2)

III. Hydration should be assessed to ensure adequate tissue perfusion and to prevent dehydration

A. Skin turgor

B. Mucous membrane color and capillary refill time

C. Urinary output

D. Urine sodium concentration

E. Urine and plasma osmolality

F. Responses of central venous pressure to a fluid challenge

1. Sudden increases in central venous pressure (more than 5 cm H_2O) with small fluid infusions indicate poor cardiac function, an infusion rate that is too rapid, or a transfusion volume that is too large

IV. Laboratory evaluation may provide insights regarding blood loss, infection, and prognosis

A. Hemogram (hematocrit, total protein, platelets)

B. White cell counts

C. Electrolytes (Na^+, K^+, Cl^-, Ca^{2+}), anion gap, strong ion difference

D. Blood urea nitrogen and creatinine to evaluate renal function

E. Tests of visceral organ damage
   1. Possible liver damage: alanine transaminase and alkaline phosphatase measurements
   2. Possible general tissue damage: aspartate transaminase and lactic dehydrogenase measurements
   3. Possible pancreatic damage: lipase or amylase measurements
F. Lactate
   1. Excellent indicator of the severity of tissue acidosis and prognosis (normal value less than 15 mmol/L)
G. Blood gases and pH
H. Coagulation screening tests
   1. Clotting time
   2. Fibrin split products

THERAPY (TABLES 27-6 THROUGH 27-8)

I. Support of respiration: in many patients with shock, ventilation and arterial PO_2 are significantly depressed; oxygen may be administered nasally or by mask; endotracheal intubation and the use of an Ambu bag or positive-pressure respirator if appropriate

II. Fluid replacement: blood volume should be replaced with appropriate fluids; oliguria in the presence of hypotension is not a contraindication for fluid therapy (crystalloids, colloids)

III. In addition to fluids, inotropes, antiarrhythmics, antibiotics, and glucocorticosteroids may be indicated; small volume (3 to 4 ml/kg) hypertonic (7%) saline solution in 6% of hetastarch may help to rapidly restore and maintain cardiovascular function
   A. Hypertonic (7%) saline solutions mixed with colloidal solutions can be used to treat hemorrhagic, traumatic, and endotoxic shock with remarkably good response
      1. This can be made by adding 2 ml of hetastarch to 1 ml of 23.4% Na^+Cl^-

IV. Antibiotics: blood cultures and cultures of relevant body fluids or exudates are ideally taken before the administration of antimicrobial therapy, but they do not usually provide substantial information (Table 27-7)

TABLE 27-6

THERAPEUTIC MANAGEMENT OF PROBLEMS ASSOCIATED WITH SHOCK

PROBLEM	TREATMENT	TRADE NAME	DOSAGE	SIDE EFFECTS OR CONTRAINDICATIONS
Hypovolemia				
Fluid loss	Crystalloid	Lactated Ringer's	50-100 ml/kg/hr IV	Hypervolemia, pulmonary edema, hypoproteinemia
Plasma loss	Colloid expander			Hypervolemia, pulmonary edema, allergic reactions (rare)
	6% Dextran 70	Reomacrodex	10-20 ml/kg IV	
	6% Hetastarch	Hespan	5-10 ml/kg IV	
		Hextend	5-10 ml/kg IV	
Blood loss	Whole blood	—	10-40 ml/kg IV	Hypervolemia, allergic reactions
	Blood substitute	Oxyglobin	10-30 mg/kg	Hypervolemia
			3-4 ml/kg/hr	
	Hypertonic saline	7% crystalloid	3-4 mg/kg IV until effective	Hypernatremia, hypokalemia, hyperosmolality

Continued

TABLE 27-6

THERAPEUTIC MANAGEMENT OF PROBLEMS ASSOCIATED WITH SHOCK—cont'd

PROBLEM	TREATMENT	TRADE NAME	DOSAGE	SIDE EFFECTS OR CONTRAINDICATIONS
Hypovolemia—cont'd				
Hypotension	Correct hypovolemia first			
	Dopamine	Intropin (Armar-Stone)	3-10 µg/kg/min IV	Hypertension, tachycardia
	Dobutamine	Dobutrex (Lilly)	3-10 µg/kg/min IV	Hypertension, tachycardia
	Ephedrine	Ephedrine sulfate	5 mg IV	Hypertension, tachycardia
	Epinephrine	Adrenaline (Parke-Davis)	3-5 µg/kg IV	Hypertension, tachycardia, arrhythmias
Cardiac arrhythmias				
Bradycardia	Atropine	—	0.01-0.02 mg/kg IV	Tachycardia
	Glycopyrrolate	Robinul (Robins)	0.005-0.01 mg/kg IV	Tachycardia
	Digoxin	Lanoxin (Burroughs-Wellcome)	0.01-0.02 mg/kg IV slowly	Bradycardia, cardiac arrhythmias
Tachycardia	Propranolol	Inderal (Ayerst)	0.05-0.1 mg/kg IV	Bradycardia, cardiac failure
	Esmolol	Brevibloc	10-50 µg/kg/min IV	Bradycardia, hypotension
Atrial arrhythmias	Quinidine	Quinidine gluconate (Lilly)	4-8 mg/kg/10 min IV	Hypotension
Ventricular arrhythmias	Lidocaine	Xylocaine (Astra)	2-4 mg/kg IV	CNS excitement; may require K+ (0.5 mEq/kg/hr) supplementation

Acute heart failure

	Dopamine	Intropin (Amar-Stone)	3-10 µg/kg/min IV
	Dobutamine	Dobutrex (Lilly)	3-10 µg/kg/min IV
	Epinephrine	Adrenaline (Parke-Davis)	3-5 µg/kg IV

Hypertension, tachycardia, cardiac arrhythmias

Respiratory failure

Hypoxia	O_2 nasal catheter; oxygen cage		2-4 L/min	Decreased venous return, respiratory alkalosis
Hypercarbia	Doxapram	Dopram V (Robins)	1-2 mg/kg	CNS excitement
	Ventilation		$V_T = 14$ ml/kg	Decreased venous return, respiratory alkalosis
Dyspnea	Tracheostomy			
	Chest tubes	Heimlich valve		
	Ventilation		$V_T = 14$ ml/kg	Decreased venous return, respiratory alkalosis
Sepsis	Surgery			
	Gentamicin	Gentocin (Schering)	4 mg/kg four times daily IM	Muscle weakness, renal toxicity

Continued

*Questionable efficacy during severe low-flow states.
IV, Intravenously; *CNS,* central nervous system; *IM,* intramuscularly; *CSF,* cerebrospinal fluid; *SQ,* subcutaneously.

TABLE 27-6
THERAPEUTIC MANAGEMENT OF PROBLEMS ASSOCIATED WITH SHOCK–cont'd

PROBLEM	TREATMENT	TRADE NAME	DOSAGE	SIDE EFFECTS OR CONTRAINDICATIONS
Metabolic acidosis				
	Sodium lactate*		Bicarbonate dose = Base deficit × 0.3 × wt (kg) or 0.5 mEq/kg 10min IV, give to effect	Metabolic alkalosis, hyperosmolarity, CSF acidosis, hyperkalemia, hypocalcemia
	Sodium acetate* Sodium bicarbonate			
Hyperkalemia	Sodium bicarbonate 0.9% NaCl solution		0.5-1 mg/kg IV 10-40 ml/kg/hr IV	As above Hypervolemia, hypoproteinemia Tachycardia
	Calcium gluconate		0.5 ml/kg of 10% solution IV	
	Hyperventilation		V_T = 14 ml/kg	Decreased venous return, respiratory alkalosis
Hypoglycemia	50% dextrose		1-2 ml/kg IV 0.5-1 g/kg/hr 10% glucose	Hyperosmolarity

Renal ischemia	Fluids	Lactated Ringer's	10-40 ml/kg/hr IV	Hypervolemia, hypoproteinemia, pulmonary edema
				Hyperosmolality
	Mannitol (20%)	Osmitrol (Travenol)	0.5-2 mg/kg IV	Decreased cardiac output
	Furosemide	Lasix (National)	1-2 mg/kg IM, IV	Hypervolemia,
	Fluids	Lactated Ringer's	10-40 ml/kg/hr IV warmed to 37° C	hypoproteinemia, pulmonary edema
Hypothermia	H₂O-filled heating pad		Warmed slowly to 38° C	
Disseminated intravascular coagulation	Correct hypotension	Lactated Ringer's	10-40 mg/kg/hr IV	Hypervolemia, hypoproteinemia, pulmonary edema
	Correct hypoxemia	Nasal catheter Ventilation	2-4 L/min V_T = 14 ml/kg	Decreased venous return, respiratory alkalosis
	Correct acidosis	Sodium bicarbonate	0.5-1 mg/kg IV	Metabolic alkalosis, hyperosmolarity, CSF acidosis, hyperkalemia, hypocalcemia
	Heparin		Dog: 500 IU/kg three times daily SQ Cat: 250-400 IU/kg three times daily SQ	

*Questionable efficacy during severe low-flow states.

IV, Intravenously; CNS, central nervous system; IM, intramuscularly; CSF, cerebrospinal fluid; SQ, subcutaneously.

Continued

TABLE 27-6
THERAPEUTIC MANAGEMENT OF PROBLEMS ASSOCIATED WITH SHOCK—cont'd

PROBLEM	TREATMENT	TRADE NAME	DOSAGE	SIDE EFFECTS OR CONTRAINDICATIONS
Metabolic acidosis—cont'd				
Cellular ischemia	Fluids	Lactated Ringer's	10-40 ml/kg/hr IV	Hypervolemia, hypoproteinemia, pulmonary edema
	Oxygen	Nasal catheter	2-4 L/min	
	Dexamethasone sodium phosphate	Azium SP (Schering)	4-6 mg/kg IV	
	Prednisolone sodium succinate	Solu-Delta-Cortef (Upjohn)	>10 mg/kg	

IV, Intravenously; *CNS,* central nervous system; *IM,* intramuscularly; *CSF,* cerebrospinal fluid; *SQ,* subcutaneously.

TABLE 27-7
ANTIBIOTICS USED TO TREAT SEVERE BACTERIAL
INFECTIONS

DRUG IV	DOSAGE
Gentamicin	6 mg/kg/24 hr
Amikacin	10 mg/kg/8 hr
Ampicillin	20-40 mg/kg/8 hr
Metronidazole	10 mg/kg/8 hr
Cefazolin	20 mg/kg/8 hr

V. Surgical intervention: many patients with shock may have an abscess or internal hemorrhage that requires surgical drainage and excision or control, respectively; immediate surgical intervention may be of paramount importance; some patients will continue to deteriorate unless surgical intervention is undertaken

VI. Temperature control: hypothermic shock patients usually do not survive. Every effort should be made to maintain a body temperature above 36° C

VII. Nutritional support should be considered for chronically debilitated patients and those that do not respond well to initial therapies (Table 27-8)

TABLE 27-8
ENTERAL FEEDING ALTERNATIVES FOR PATIENTS WITH SEPSIS

SPECIES	CONDITION	PROTEIN REQUIREMENT (g/100 kcal)	EXAMPLE DIETS	CALORIES (kcal/ml)	PROTEIN (g/100 kcal)
Dog	Normal protein	4.0–8.0	312 g Prescription Diet a/d* + 50 ml water CliniCare Canine†	1.0 0.9	9 5.5
	Protein loss	>8.0	312 g Prescription Diet a/d* + 50 ml water 237 ml Sustacal‡ + 24 g ProBalance Max Stress Feline§	1.0 1.2	9 8.8
Cat	Normal protein	6.0–9.0	Blenderized 224 g Prescription Diet Feline p/d* + 170 ml water 50 ml Sustacal‡ + 50 ml Pulmocare§ + 4.8 g ProBalance Max Stress Feline§	0.9 1.3	9.3 6.4
	Protein loss	>9.0	312 g Prescription Diet a/d* + 50 ml water 237 ml Sustacal‡ + 24 g ProBalance Max Stress Feline§	1.0 1.2	9 8.8

Choose a diet that meets the protein requirement of the animal.
Calculate the volume of diet required: (kcal/day)/(kcal/ml) = ml of formula/day.
Calculate the volume of each feeding: (ml of formula/day)/(number of feedings/day).
*Hills Pet Nutrition, Inc., Topeka, Kansas.
†PetAg, Hampshire, Illinois.
‡Bristol-Meyers Squibb, Princeton, New Jersey.
§Pfizer Animal Health, Exton, Pennsylvania.

CHAPTER TWENTY-EIGHT

Respiratory Emergencies

"Each person is born to one possession which out values all his others–his last breath."

MARK TWAIN

OVERVIEW

Respiratory depression occurs during every anesthetic episode. Respiratory depression can lead to hypoventilation ($\uparrow PaCO_2$), hypoxemia ($\downarrow PaO_2$), and apnea. Hypoventilation ($\uparrow PaCO_2$) cannot always be determined by visual inspection but can be assessed by arterial blood gas analysis or capnography. Although potentially devastating, respiratory emergencies and depression, if recognized early, are easily treated by establishing a patent airway and providing adequate inflation of the lungs to ensure appropriate gas exchange.

GENERAL CONSIDERATIONS

I. Definition: a respiratory emergency is the inability to maintain adequate ventilation such that tissue oxygenation and acid-base status become compromised

II. Clinical causes
   A. Major causes
      1. Hypoventilation caused by drug-induced respiratory depression
      2. Improper placement (e.g., esophageal) of the endotracheal tube
      3. Parenchymal pulmonary disease (diffusion impairment)
      4. Pleural cavity disease (pneumothorax, fractured ribs)
      5. Airway obstruction

      a. Laryngeal disease

         (1) Laryngeal paralysis (Labradors and horses)

         (2) Laryngeal spasm with intubation

      b. Small or obstructed endotracheal tubes. Do not overinflate the cuff

      c. Restricted chest wall movement; improper physical restraint or positioning for surgery, improper bandaging

      d. Nasal obstruction or edema

      e. Displacement of the palate

    6. Low inspired O_2 (FiO_2)

      a. Oxygen flow turned off on anesthetic machine

III. Patient age and size determine respiratory frequency, rate of lung inflation, inflation pressure, and tidal volume delivered; large adults generally require slower inflation rates, lower frequencies of breathing, and larger volumes

  A. Pneumothorax should be corrected immediately to ensure adequate lung expansion and prevent development of tension pneumothorax

  B. Intrathoracic air or fluid should be removed

IV. Treating apnea

  A. If the animal is breathing slowly or is apneic, establish an airway and institute artificial ventilation with room air or oxygen; oxygen is preferred

    1. Deliver oxygen to endotracheal or tracheotomy tube

    2. Nasal intubation with oxygen administration

    3. Face mask and oxygen

    4. Mouth-to-nose

    5. Mouth-to-mouth

  B. Control breathing rate if apneic; assist ventilation if breathing

    1. Rate: 6 to 15 breaths/min

    2. Inspiratory time: 1 to 3 seconds, depending on size of the patient

    3. Maintain proper inspiratory/expiratory ratio of 1:2,1:3, or 1:4

    4. Inflate lungs to 15 to 20 cm H_2O if chest is closed (up to 20 to 30 cm H_2O in large animals)

    5. Inflate lungs to 20 to 30 cm H_2O if chest is open or atelectasis of lungs has occurred (up to 40 cm H_2O in large animals)

6. Tidal volume
   a. Approximately 10 to 15 ml/kg
   b. 12 to 20 ml/kg if mechanical ventilator is used

PRINCIPAL POINTS

Establish a patent airway!
Administer O_2

V. Support of ventilation (assisted or controlled ventilation) should be continued until the patient can maintain consciousness, normal mucous membrane color, and normal blood gases
   A. Familiarity with the use of a ventilator is valuable (see chapter 14)

CLINICAL SIGNS OF RESPIRATORY DISTRESS

I. Apnea or dyspnea
II. Increased frequency of breathing; respiratory rate, depth, and effort are generally increased in animals with respiratory disease
III. Stridor or sonorous breathing sounds are associated with airway obstruction
IV. Cyanosis: bluish discoloration of the mucous membranes
   A. Cyanosis may be absent in severely anemic animals (hemoglobin less than 5 g/dl)
V. Abnormal postures
   A. Open mouth breathing
   B. Extension of the head and neck
   C. Abduction of the forelimbs

TREATMENT OF RESPIRATORY DISTRESS

I. Treat the cause and administer oxygen (O_2)
II. Control or assist breathing when necessary
   A. Ambu bag
   B. Use a volume-cycled ventilator with a standing bellows (see Chapter 14)

III. Use respiratory stimulants when necessary
  A. Doxapram: 1 to 4 mg/kg IV; repeat if necessary; or 5 to 10 μg/kg/min IV infusion
  B. Antagonize respiratory depressant drugs if indicated

AIRWAY OBSTRUCTION

  I. Partial airway obstruction may be associated with respiratory disease or obstruction/kinking of the endotracheal tube
  II. Conditions that predispose animals to airway collapse
  A. Stenotic nares in brachycephalic breeds
  B. Edema of the nasal turbinates in horses
  C. Elongated or displaced soft palate
    1. Brachycephalic breeds
    2. Beagles and cocker spaniels
    3. Horses
  D. Collapsing arytenoid cartilages
    1. Congenital in Bouvier des Flandres, Bull terriers, and Siberian huskies
    2. Acquired in giant-breed dogs (e.g., St. Bernards)
  E. Everting laryngeal ventricles
    1. Brachycephalic breeds
    2. English bulldogs
    3. May be associated with hypothyroidism
  F. Collapsing trachea
    1. Middle-aged to older, obese toy-breed dogs, especially miniature Poodles, Yorkshire terriers, and Chihuahuas
    2. Calves
  G. Laryngeal paresis or paralysis
    1. Horses
      a. Naturally occurring
      b. Postsurgical paralysis
    2. Congenital, especially in Bouvier des Flandres, Bull terriers, and Siberian huskies
    3. Acquired in giant-breed dogs, especially St. Bernards
  H. Hypoplasia of the trachea
    1. Congenital in brachycephalic breeds
    2. English bulldog
  III. Other causes of airway obstruction
  A. Foreign bodies
  B. Nasal disease (e.g., tumor, fungal)

C. Mucus or blood in airway or endotracheal tube

D. Other causes
1. Tumors of the nasal passages, pharynx, or larynx
2. Horse: displaced soft palate, guttural pouch infections or tympany, ethmoidal hematoma, tumors
3. Cat: asthma
4. Sheep: nasal parasites
5. Pig: atrophic rhinitis
6. Llamas, alpacas: congenital choanal atresia

E. Clinical signs
1. Noisy, stridorous, or labored breathing (snoring)
   a. Loudest at larynx and pharynx during upper airway obstruction
   b. Low-pitched honking sound during tracheal collapse
2. History of exercise intolerance, cyanosis, and/or collapse
3. Choking, retching, and vomiting
4. Severely distressed animals may paw or claw at the face and throat
5. Abnormal body positions
6. Diagnosis (consider establishing a patent airway before attempting a diagnosis)
7. History of facial injuries, epistaxis, or wounds to the neck
8. The presence of stenotic nares, foreign bodies or tumors, and soft tissue swelling
9. Radiography
   a. Survey
   b. Contrast
   c. Fluoroscopy
   d. Bronchoscopy or endoscopy to confirm airway obstruction

F. Electromyography to confirm denervation of laryngeal muscles

IV. Treatment of airway obstruction
A. Establish patent airway
1. Intubate
2. Remove oral, nasal, or tracheal foreign material or blood using forceps, suction, and postural drainage
3. Perform nasotracheal intubation or tracheotomy, if necessary, to relieve or bypass obstruction (Fig. 28-1)

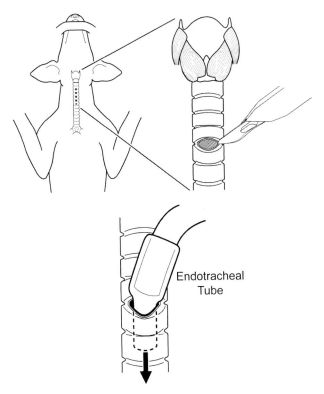

Fig. 28-1
A tracheotomy can be easily performed in most species.

    4. Apply local anesthetic creams (lidocaine) to prevent laryngospasm
B. Provide oxygen
C. Avoid stress
D. Supportive care
    1. Oxygen
    2. Intravenous fluid therapy
    3. Bronchodilators (albuterol, clenbuterol)
    4. Respiratory stimulants, if necessary
    5. Sedation

6. Antibiotics
7. Corticosteroids
8. Maintain normal body temperature

E. Treat coexisting problems; prepare for surgery
   1. Remove foreign bodies or tumors
   2. Repair fractures and wounds of the respiratory system
   3. Drain fluid or air from the thorax
   4. Correct anatomic defects if possible

F. Care of tracheotomy tube
   1. Apply suction every 2 hours using aseptic technique
   2. Nebulize with saline solution or acetylcysteine diluted with saline solution to prevent drying of the airway
   3. Maintain normal hydration
   4. Monitor body temperature
   5. Take periodic chest radiographs

RESPIRATORY DISEASES

I. Classification
   A. Life-threatening pneumonia
      1. Acute, fulminating bronchopneumonia
      2. Smoke inhalation
      3. Aspiration pneumonia
   B. Pulmonary contusion
   C. Pulmonary edema
   D. Pulmonary embolism

II. Diagnosis
   A. Physical signs, including lethargy
   B. Radiographs of the chest
   C. Laboratory tests
      1. Complete blood count
      2. Transtracheal aspirate, bronchoalveolar lavage
      3. Bronchoscopy
      4. Blood gas determination
      5. $PaCO_2$, end-tidal CO_2

III. Treatment
   A. Remove aspirated material, if present
   B. Maintain the patency and function of the airways
   C. Supply O_2 and apply positive end-expiratory pressure
   D. Treat infection

E. Enhance removal of secretions (suction, acetylcysteine, guaifenesin)
F. Supportive care
   1. Administer oxygen (40% or more) using the following methods:
      a. Face mask
      b. Nasal catheter
      c. Pediatric incubator
      d. Oxygen cage
      e. Tracheotomy and positive-pressure ventilation (if laryngeal spasm or airway obstruction with secretions persist)
   2. Humidify the air by nebulization with normal saline solution to improve removal of secretions
   3. Maintain normal body hydration with fluids intravenously or subcutaneously to prevent drying and thickening of secretions
   4. Perform periodic coupage (percussion of the chest)
   5. Provide physiotherapy with deep breathing; this aids in removal of secretions, increases lymphatic drainage of the lungs, and activates surfactant
   6. The use of diuretics, corticosteroids, and antiprostaglandins in pneumonia is controversial
   7. Bronchodilators are helpful in reversing bronchial spasm and constriction (e.g., aminophylline, clenbuterol)
   8. Anticoagulants and oxygen in patients with pulmonary embolism
   9. Pneumonia with viscous secretions may require expectorants (e.g., guaifenesin)
   10. Analgesics may be used for pain and apprehension in selected patients
      a. Monitor blood gases to detect respiratory depression
   11. Medical therapy of pulmonary edema
      a. Confine the animal to a cage to decrease the workload of its heart; administer oxygen and sedation (low-dose opioids)
      b. Improve ventilation by endotracheal suctioning
      c. Nebulize with 40% alcohol
      d. Eliminate excessive fluids with diuretics and vasodilators

PLEURAL CAVITY DISEASE

I. Definition: pleural cavity disease includes problems that decrease the functional capacity of the lungs because of fluid, masses, or inflammation in the thoracic cavity, or damage to the integrity of the thoracic wall

II. Classification

    A. Pneumothorax

        1. Open

        2. Closed

        3. Spontaneous

        4. Tension

    B. Pleural effusion

        1. Chylothorax

        2. Pyothorax

        3. Hydrothorax

        4. Hemothorax

        5. Neoplastic effusion

        6. Infectious, inflammatory effusion

    C. Diaphragmatic hernia

    D. Flail chest

III. Causes

    A. Pneumothorax: accumulation of free air in the pleural cavity

        1. Trauma, resulting in pleural or parenchymal lacerations or tracheobronchial ruptures, is the most common cause of pneumothorax

        2. Pneumothorax—occurs spontaneously in Afghan hounds (Fig. 28-2, *A*)

        3. Tension pneumothorax: air accumulates in pleural space during inspiration and is not expelled during expiration; intrapleural pressure increases, collapsing the lungs and great vessels (Fig. 28-2, *B*)

        4. Other causes

            a. Penetrating injuries from bite wounds and projectiles

            b. Rupture of congenital bullous emphysematous or granulomatous lung lesions (blebs or bullae)

            c. Rupture of parasitic cysts (*Paragonimus*); neoplasia

            d. Hardware disease in cattle

            e. Pleuritis

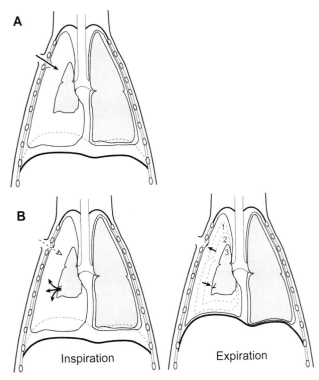

A Inspiration

B Inspiration Expiration

Fig. 28-2
A, Open pneumothorax. Air moves into the chest. The lung collapses as a result of loss of negative pressure. **B,** Tension pneumothorax. During inspiration, air moves one way into the chest, gradually increasing intrathoracic pressure and collapsing the lung. Note: because the mediastinum is incomplete in most species, the effects discussed are usually bilateral.

    f. Iatrogenic causes
       (1) Overzealous intermittent positive-pressure ventilation (particularly in cats) can result in pulmonary barotrauma
       (2) After pneumomediastinum from trauma, air migrates from the trachea or esophagus to the chest

(3) Intrathoracic surgical procedures

(4) Cardiopulmonary resuscitation

B. Pleural effusion: abnormal fluid accumulation within the pleural cavity

1. Hemothorax

   a. Rupture of cardiac and intrathoracic blood vessels from trauma

   b. Clotting disorders

   c. Bleeding neoplasms (e.g., hemangiosarcoma)

   d. Lung-lobe torsion

   e. Pleuritis

2. Chylothorax

   a. Accumulation of lymphatic fluid in the pleural space

      (1) Rupture of the thoracic duct

      (2) Idiopathic lymphatic obstruction

3. Hydrothorax

   a. Hypoproteinemia

   b. Heart failure and cardiomyopathy

4. Pyothorax (pleuritis)

   a. Penetrating wounds of the thorax or esophagus

   b. Migrating foreign bodies

   c. Spread of pulmonary infection and pleuritis

   d. Organisms: *Escherichia coli, Staphylococcus, β-Streptococcus, Pasteurella, Nocardia*

C. Chest wall abnormalities

   a. Diaphragmatic hernias displace the lungs with abdominal viscera

   b. Flail chest is caused by proximal and distal fractures of several consecutive ribs

      (1) Chest wall is drawn inward with expiration and blown outward with inspiration (paradoxic movement [Fig. 28-2, *B*])

      (2) Lung contusion and hemopneumothorax may be present, precipitating acute respiratory distress

IV. Diagnosis

A. Auscultation and percussion

B. Thoracic radiography

C. Ultrasound examination

D. Thoracocentesis

V. Treatment
   A. Establish a patent airway
   B. Oxygen therapy
   C. Intravenous fluid therapy for shock
   D. Bandage penetrating wounds
   E. Chest tube
   F. Remove the cause
      1. Needle aspiration (air or liquid)
      2. Tube thoracostomy (Fig. 28-3)
         a. Indications
            (1) Acute severe pneumothorax
            (2) Tension pneumothorax
            (3) Pneumothorax associated with rib fractures, emphysema, or hemothorax

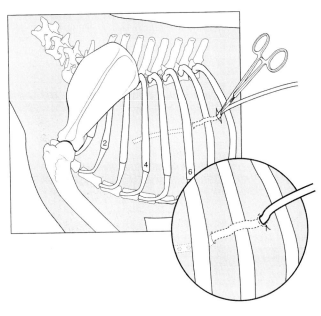

Fig. 28-3
A chest tube is placed to restore negative intrathoracic pressure by connecting it to a Heimlich valve (Fig. 28-4) or a three-bottle negative pressure system (Fig. 28-5).

(4) Fluid accumulation

(5) In situations where repeated needle evacuations are necessary

b. Methods of drainage

(1) Intermittent aspiration using a syringe and three-way stopcock

(2) Unidirectional flutter (Heimlich) valves (Fig. 28-4)

(3) Intermittent connection of the chest tube to a suction pump (10 to 15 cm H_2O negative pressure)

(4) Connection of the chest tube to underwater seal units (Fig. 28-5). Thoracic drainage units are commercially available

3. Complications

a. Chest tube attaches to an underwater seal and requires constant monitoring (disconnection causes pneumothorax)

b. Accumulation of fibrin and blood

c. Displacement of tube

d. Kinking of tube

e. Subcutaneous emphysema

f. Lung tissue entrapment and infarction after vigorous suction

g. Infection

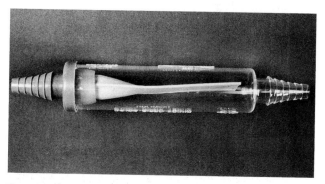

Fig. 28-4
Heimlich (one-way) valve.

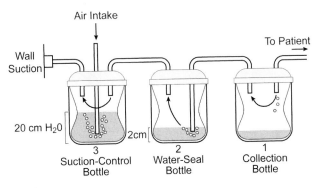

Fig. 28-5
Underwater seal system (three-bottle) for connection to a chest tube and creating negative intrathoracic pressure.

IATROGENIC CAUSES OF RESPIRATORY EMERGENCIES

I. Inadequate patient evaluation
II. Poor anesthetic techniques
    A. Anesthetic overdose (e.g., barbiturates)
    B. Excessive dead space in anesthetic equipment, incompetent nonrebreathing valves
    C. Lack of oxygen delivery
        1. Nitrous oxide on; oxygen off
        2. Excessive use of N_2O (more than 70%)
        3. Oxygen supply depleted
        4. Anesthetic system not connected properly
        5. Endotracheal tube too small
        6. Overdistended endotracheal tube cuff
            a. Collapse of tracheal tube within cuff
            b. Postsurgical stenosis of trachea
        7. Inappropriately placed endotracheal tube
            a. In esophagus
            b. In pharynx
            c. At or caudal to bifurcation of trachea
    D. Kinked or obstructed anesthetic delivery hoses and tubes

E. Overdistention of lungs during mechanical ventilation

F. Neuromuscular paralysis of diaphragm and intercostal muscles without ventilatory support

III. Restrictive bandages around the chest

IV. Inadequate monitoring of the patient

A. Patterns of respiration

1. Eupnea: normal rate and rhythm
2. Tachypnea: increased respiratory rate; caused by fever, hypoxia, hypercapnea, pneumonia, or lesions of the central nervous system respiratory centers
3. Bradypnea: slow but regular respirations; caused by sleep, anesthesia, opiates, hypothermia, neoplasia, or respiratory decompensation
4. Apnea: absence of respiration; may be periodic; caused by drug depression, muscle paralysis, overventilation, obstruction, shock, increased intracranial pressure, or surgical manipulation of vagus and splanchnic nerves
5. Hyperpnea: large respirations (increased tidal volume); rate normal; caused by excitement, pain, surgical stimulation, hypoxia, hypercarbia, heat, or cold
6. Cheyne-Stokes respiration: respirations become faster and larger, then slower, followed by an apneic pause; caused by increased intracranial pressure from head trauma or neoplasia, meningitis, renal failure, severe hypoxia, anesthetic drug overdose, or high altitude
7. Biot's respiration: respirations that are faster and deeper than normal, with abrupt pauses between them; each breath has approximately the same tidal volume; caused by anesthesia in normal, athletic horses and greyhounds; spinal meningitis; or drugs that cause generalized central nervous system depression
8. Kussmaul's respiration: regular and deep respirations without pauses; patient's breathing usually sounds labored, with breaths that resemble sighs; caused by renal failure, metabolic acidosis, or diabetic ketoacidosis
9. Apneustic: prolonged gasping inspiration, followed by extremely short, inefficient expirations; caused by high doses of drugs (e.g., ketamine in cats and horses or excessive doses of guaifenesin in horses) or lesions in the pons and thalamus

OTHER CAUSES OF PULMONARY INSUFFICIENCY

I. Ventilation-perfusion inequalities
  A. Hypoventilation
  B. Decreased cardiac output
  C. Atelectasis
    1. Absorption: absorption of oxygen from behind blocked small airways
    2. Compression: compression of lungs by distended abdominal viscera pressing against the diaphragm (colic in horses; rumen in cattle, sheep, and goats; bloat in dogs)
    3. Gravitational effects
II. Increased venous admixture (shunts)
  A. Pulmonary arteriovenous shunts
  B. Bronchial vessel shunts
  C. Atelectasis (physiologic shunt)
  D. Pulmonary neoplasia
  E. Congenital cardiac disease (tetralogy of Fallot)

RESPIRATORY ARREST

I. Cessation of breathing from any of the previously discussed causes
II. Correct immediately (within 1 to 3 minutes)
III. Treatment
  A. Establish a patent airway
    1. Remove the obstruction or foreign material
    2. Intubate
    3. Consider a tracheostomy if unable to orotracheally intubate (Fig. 28-1)
  B. Provide artificial ventilation
    1. Room air delivered through Ambu-bag (Fig. 28-6)
    2. 100% oxygen delivered through anesthetic system
    3. Transtracheal insufflation of O_2; 3 to 6 L/min in dogs
  C. Proceed with cardiopulmonary resuscitation, if necessary (see Chapter 29)
  D. Acupuncture resuscitative techniques have been used successfully in emergency situations

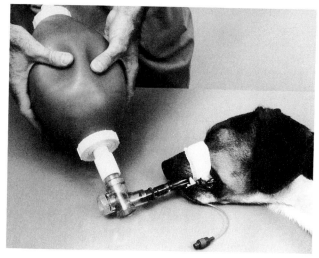

Fig. 28-6
Ventilation with an Ambu-Bag.

1. Use 25- to 28-gauge hypodermic needle, 25 to 50 mm long
2. Insert the needle 10 to 20 mm into the nasal septum at point GV 26, along the midline of the nasolabial cleft at the left of the lower canthi of the nostril
3. Twirl the needle strongly and move it up and down
4. Use this technique as an adjunct to, but not a replacement for, conventional techniques

PREVENTION OF RESPIRATORY EMERGENCIES

I. Proper preanesthetic evaluation
   A. Clinical signs
   B. Auscultation
   C. Radiography
   D. Blood gas analysis (i-STAT; IRMA)
II. Use of proper anesthetic and monitoring equipment (see Chapter 15)

III. Adequate inspection of anesthetic equipment
IV. Administer oxygen with a face mask for 3 to 5 minutes before induction of anesthesia (preoxygenate)
V. Proper administration of preanesthetic and anesthetic agents
VI. Careful and continuous monitoring during anesthesia
VII. Awareness of possible problems

USE OF RESPIRATORY STIMULANTS, BICARBONATE, AND BRONCHODILATOR DRUGS

I. Doxapram hydrochloride (1 to 4 mg/kg IV in small animals; 0.2 to 0.6 mg/kg IV in large animals) is a general central nervous system and respiratory center stimulant and can be administered by infusion (5 to 10 μg/kg/min) until effective; a centrally acting respiratory stimulant; increases tidal volume and, in larger doses, respiratory rate; causes small elevations in arterial blood pressure and heart rate and may cause arousal from anesthetic depression, increases cerebral metabolic rate

II. Sodium bicarbonate (1 to 4 mEq/kg IV); used to correct metabolic (nonrespiratory) acidosis, which may occur during hypoxia, or complete respiratory and cardiac arrest; excessive administration may produce hypokalemic metabolic alkalosis or paradoxic cerebrospinal fluid acidosis. Use is controversial

III. Aminophylline: up to 4 mg/kg IV slowly over 30 minutes, 2 to 4 mg/kg intramuscularly; dilates bronchial smooth muscle and may be useful in asthmatics and bronchospasm; has inotropic action on the heart

IV. Specific antagonists (see Chapter 3)
  A. Narcotic antagonists (naloxone, nalorphine, levallorphan); act by competitively displacing narcotic analgesics from opiate and nonopiate receptors
  B. Neostigmine, edrophonium: reversal of nondepolarizing neuromuscular blocking drugs (see Chapter 11)
  C. α_2-Antagonists (yohimbine, tolazoline, atipamazole); reversal of xylazine, medetomidine, or detomidine (see Chapter 3)

TREATMENT OF PULMONARY EDEMA

I. Measures to improve ventilation-gas exchange
  A. Oxygen (FiO_2 40% to 50%)
  B. Reduction of activity (cage rest): to decrease oxygen demand
  C. Sedation, relief of anxiety
    1. Morphine (dogs): 0.2 to 0.5 mg/kg subcutaneously, intramuscularly, intravenously
    2. Acepromazine: 0.1 to 0.2 mg/kg subcutaneously, intramuscularly (maximum of 4 mg)
    3. Xylazine (horses): 0.2 mg/kg intravenously, intramuscularly
  D. Endotracheal suctioning in severe cases to clear foam from airways
  E. Ethyl alcohol nebulization (40%) into O_2 (prevents foaming in airways)
  F. Positive-pressure ventilation through an endotracheal tube
    1. Manual or mechanical
      a. Criteria for ventilation: PaO_2 less than 60 mm Hg, $PaCO_2$ more than 60 to 70 mm Hg, persistent cyanosis, dyspnea, or tachypnea (all while breathing 60% O_2)
    2. Positive end-expiratory pressure, 5 to 10 cm H_2O, is used to ventilate stiff lungs (e.g., pulmonary edema, pneumonia)
II. Measures to reduce capillary hydrostatic pressure and pulmonary edema
  A. Oxygen
  B. Decrease circulating blood volume
    1. Diuretics: furosemide 2 to 4 mg/kg intravenously, intramuscularly, subcutaneously, by mouth every 6 to 8 hours
    2. Phlebotomy: remove 6 to 10 ml/kg; rarely used
  C. Redistribute pulmonary blood flow to other circulatory beds
    1. Morphine: in addition to sedative effects, increases systemic venous capacitance

2. Furosemide (Lasix): in addition to diuresis, redistributes pulmonary blood flow by increasing systemic venous capacitance
3. Vasodilators carefully
   a. Sodium nitroprusside, nitroglycerine
   b. Peripheral vasodilation redistributes circulation away from pulmonary beds (noncardiogenic) and decreases resistance to left ventricular outflow (afterload; cardiogenic)
D. Improve cardiac function (cardiac output); mostly used in cardiogenic edema
   1. Positive inotropes (dopamine, dobutamine)
   2. Antiarrhythmics to control arrhythmias, if present

III. Other therapy
   A. Corticosteroids (e.g., prednisolone sodium succinate: 20 to 30 mg/kg intravenously)

IV. Monitoring the response to therapy
   A. Physical examination (including rate and depth of breathing, auscultation, mucous membrane color)
   B. Sequential arterial blood gas analyses (see Chapter 15)
   C. Thoracic radiography
   D. Pulmonary capillary wedge pressure

CHAPTER TWENTY-NINE

Cardiovascular Emergencies

"It is by presence of mind in untried emergencies that the native metal of a man is tested."

JAMES RUSSELL LOWELL

OVERVIEW

Most drugs used for anesthesia can produce hypotension. Cardiac arrhythmias (bradycardia), hypotension, and decreased peripheral perfusion (low cardiac output) leading to shock can occur after the administration of sedatives and anesthetics. The potential for cardiac emergencies is increased in severely debilitated or traumatized patients. A variety of physical and pharmacologic approaches have been developed to prevent or reverse deterioration of the circulation and reestablish normal hemodynamics. It is imperative to have a physical, technical, and working knowledge of the various pharmacologic approaches to cardiopulmonary resuscitation. Successful resuscitation should be followed by continuous intensive nursing care and close patient monitoring for at least 3 to 7 days.

GENERAL CONSIDERATIONS

I. Definition: a cardiovascular emergency is any condition involving the heart or vasculature that results in the inability to maintain adequate tissue perfusion and oxygenation

II. Common causes
   A. Respiratory failure (hypoxia)
      1. Hypoventilation (hypercarbia, $PaCO_2$)
      2. Hypoxemia
      3. Ventilation-perfusion abnormalities
      4. Shunt
      5. Diffusion abnormalities

557

B. Acid-base imbalance
   1. Respiratory acidosis ($PaCO_2$)
   2. Metabolic acidosis (usually lactic) leading to myocardial depression
   3. Respiratory alkalosis ($PaCO_2$)
   4. Mixed metabolic and respiratory alkalosis or acidosis
C. Electrolyte imbalance
   1. Hyperkalemia (bradycardia; poor contractility, vasodilation)
   2. Hypokalemia (tachycardia)
   3. Hypocalcemia (hypocontractility, hypotension)
D. Autonomic imbalance
   1. Increased sympathetic tone; increased myocardial automaticity and irritability
   2. Increased parasympathetic tone; predisposition to bradycardia and various forms of heart block; predisposition to atrial arrhythmias, including atrial fibrillation
   3. Increased sympathetic and parasympathetic tone, predisposition to ventricular arrhythmias
E. Hypothermia (35° C, 95° F)
F. Air embolism
G. Excessive or inappropriate drug administration
   1. Any hypersensitivity or drug overdose such as a hypotensive crisis caused byrate or amount of drug administered
      a. Most commonly observed after intravenous drug administration
      b. Treatment includes fluids, steroids, and occasionally vasopressors
      c. Administration of catecholamines during inhalation anesthesia (ventricular arrhythmias, tachycardia)
   2. Accidental intraarterial drug administration (e.g., accidental intracarotid administration of preanesthetic drugs [phenothiazines, xylazine] in horses and cattle); treatment should include adequate padding, anticonvulsants (diazepam), fluids, and steroids
   3. Myocardial depressant factors produced by ischemic organs (e.g., pancreas)
H. Cardiac disease and/or arrhythmias (Table 29-1)

TABLE 29-1

DISTINGUISHING CHARACTERISTICS OF SEVERAL TYPES OF CARDIAC FAILURE OR ARREST

CAUSE	PERIPHERAL PULSE	AUSCULTATION OF HEART SOUNDS	ELECTROCARDIOGRAM	VISUAL OBSERVATIONS
Bradycardia	Slow; may be irregular	Slow	Infrequent or irregular QRS complexes	Infrequent coordinated ventricular contractions
Ventricular tachycardia	Rapid, irregular Pulse deficits	Muffled; may be variable intensity	May have wide bizarre looking QRS complexes; absence of P-QRS relationship	Disorganized, rapidly beating heart
Ventricular fibrillation	None	None	Absence of QRST complexes; Fibrillation waves	Fine-to-coarse rippling of the ventricular myocardium
Ventricular asystole	None	None	Absence of QRST complexes; straight-line ECG	No cardiac movement
Pulseless electrical activity	None	None	Normal PQRST complexes (Systolic arterial blood pressure <50 mm Hg)	Feeble or absent cardiac contractions

ECG, Electrocardiogram.

1. Cardiovascular collapse: cardiac failure that is unresponsive to therapy
   a. Occurs primarily in patients who have heart disease or are inadvertently administered too much drug too fast
2. Bradycardia: lower than acceptable heart rate
   a. Increased parasympathetic tone
   b. Hypothermia
   c. Hyperkalemia
   d. Specific medications (opioids, α_2-agonists)
   e. Cardiac disease (e.g., sick sinus syndrome, atrioventricular fibrosis)
   f. Drug overdose
3. Tachycardia: higher than acceptable heart rate
   a. Increased sympathetic tone
      (1) Not adequately anesthetized
      (2) Pain, stress
      (3) Hypotension
      (4) Hypoxia
      (5) Hypokalemia
   b. Specific drug administration (catecholamines, atropine, ketamine)
4. Atrial or ventricular arrhythmias (atrial tachycardia, ventricular tachycardia); associated with conditions that cause ischemia, hypoxia, hypotension, hypercarbia, metabolic acidosis or alkalosis, hyperkalemia, hypothermia, hypotension. Cardiac arrhythmias are also caused by surgical manipulation, anesthetic drugs, and cardiac catheterization
   a. Atrial fibrillation
      (1) Variable-intensity heart sounds
      (2) Variable-strength pulses and "dropped" (missing) pulses
      (3) Regularly irregular heart rates
   b. Ventricular fibrillation
      (1) Most likely to occur during hypoxia because of the instability of autonomic reflexes and endogenous release of catecholamines
      (2) Rarely associated with too rapid infusion of thiobarbiturates or high initial concentrations of inhalation anesthetics

(3) May follow severe hypercarbia, hypoxia, hypovolemia, acidosis, and/or hyperkalemia
c. Ventricular asystole (lack of ventricular contraction)
  (1) Usually associated with anesthetic overdose
  (2) Seen during shock or in toxic animals
d. Pulseless electrical activity; electrocardiogram is present, but poor cardiac contraction produces low arterial blood pressure. Electromechanical dissociation is a special type of pulseless electrical activity wherein ventricular contraction is uncoupled from electrical activation
  (1) Hypoxia and ischemia
  (2) Drug overdose

INDICATORS OF POOR CARDIAC FUNCTION

    I. Weak or absent peripheral pulses
       A. Weak cardiac apex beat
   II. Irregular pulses or heart sounds
  III. Cyanosis (not seen in anemic patients)
  IV. Poor perfusion; prolonged capillary refill time (>2 seconds)
   V. Cardiac arrhythmias
  VI. Abnormal breathing pattern or apnea
 VII. Dilated pupils
VIII. Depression, weight loss, or edema
  IX. No bleeding from cut surfaces
   X. Signs of shock (see Chapter 27)

EQUIPMENT NEEDED FOR CARDIAC EMERGENCIES

I. Equipment should be readily accessible in the event of cardiovascular collapse, timing is critical
   A. Cuffed endotracheal tubes and stylet (for small dogs and cats)
      1. Small
      2. Medium
      3. Large
   B. Lighted laryngoscope with blades
   C. Ambu-bag, demand valve, or anesthetic machine (Fig. 29-1)

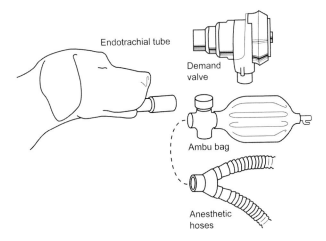

Endotrachial tube

Demand valve

Ambu bag

Anesthetic hoses

Fig. 29-1
Methods to provide breathing to an apneic animal.

D. Tongue depressors
E. Syringes
   1. Five 1-ml
   2. Five 3-ml
   3. Five 6-ml
   4. Five 12-ml
   5. Five 35-ml
F. Three-way stopcocks
G. One roll of 2.5-cm adhesive tape
H. One roll of 5-cm gauze
I. One pack of sterile 10×10 cm gauze pads
J. One roll of elastic bandage
K. Blood administration set
L. Needles
   1. Five 20-gauge
   2. Five 18-gauge
   3. Two 16-gauge
M. Butterfly administration needles
   1. Two 21-gauge
   2. Two 19-gauge

N. Intravenous fluid administration set and syringe infusion pump
O. Sterile emergency surgery pack
   1. Scalpel handle
   2. Blades: two no.10, two no. 15
   3. Two small hemostats
   4. Thumb forceps
   5. One pair of Metzenbaum scissors
   6. One pair of curved forceps
   7. Several packages of suture
   8. Needle holders
   9. One set of medium-sized rib retractors
P. Intravenous catheters: 16-gauge to 22-gauge
Q. Chest tube: Heimlich valve
R. Defibrillator/electrocardiogram

TREATMENT (TABLES 29-2 THROUGH 29-4; FIG. 29-2)

PRINCIPAL POINTS

Begin chest compression immediately if the arrest is witnessed

---

I. Airway (see Chapter 28)
II. Breathing (Table 29-3)
III. Circulation (Tables 29-4 and 29-5)
IV. Drugs (Table 29-6)
V. Electrocardiogram
VI. Defibrillation (Table 29-5)

TABLE 29-2
TREATMENT OF CARDIOPULMONARY ARREST

Unwitnessed CPA $\rightarrow$ Witnessed CPA $\rightarrow$

Patient evaluation: $\leftarrow$ 1. External cardiac massage
1. Ventilation   2. Ventilation (with oxygen)
2. Pupillary reflexes   3. IV fluids
3. Color/refill
4. Heartbeats
5. Arterial pulses
$\downarrow$

Yes $\leftarrow$ Pulse or heartbeats present? $\longrightarrow$ No $\rightarrow$

1. Intubate and ventilate   1. Begin chest compression
2. IV fluids   2. Intubate and ventilate
3. Sodium bicarbonate (if necessary)   3. IV fluids/emergency drugs
4. Inotropes, if necessary
5. Reevaluate

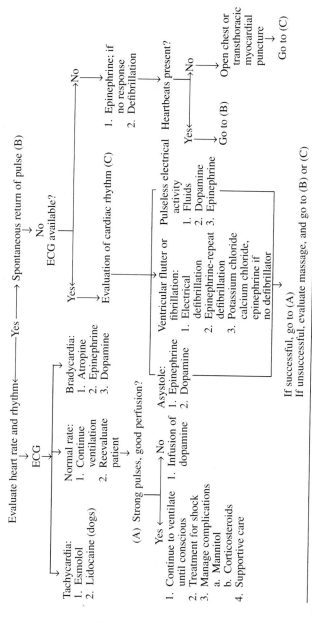

Evaluate heart rate and rhythm ← Yes ⟶ Spontaneous return of pulse (B)

↓ No

ECG available?

→ No

1. Epinephrine; if no response
2. Defibrillation

Heartbeats present?

→ No

Open chest or transthoracic myocardial puncture

Go to (C)

Yes ← Go to (B)

Yes ←

Evaluation of cardiac rhythm (C)

Pulseless electrical activity
1. Fluids
2. Dopamine
3. Epinephrine

Ventricular flutter or fibrillation:
1. Electrical defibrillation
2. Epinephrine-repeat defibrillation
3. Potassium chloride calcium chloride, epinephrine if no defibrillator

Asystole:
1. Epinephrine
2. Dopamine

ECG

Tachycardia:
1. Esmolol
2. Lidocaine (dogs)

Normal rate:
1. Continue ventilation
2. Reevaluate patient

Bradycardia:
1. Atropine
2. Epinephrine
3. Dopamine

(A) Strong pulses, good perfusion?

Yes ←
1. Continue to ventilate until conscious
2. Treatment for shock
3. Manage complications
   a. Mannitol
   b. Corticosteroids
4. Supportive care

→ No
1. Infusion of dopamine

If successful, go to (A)
If unsuccessful, evaluate massage, and go to (B) or (C)

CPA, Cardiopulmonary arrest; *IV*, intravenous.

TABLE 29-3
GUIDELINES FOR VENTILATING PATIENTS

PARAMETER	GUIDELINES
Respiratory rate	6-18/min
Tidal volume	15-20 ml/kg
Inspiratory time	<1.5 sec.
Inspiratory/expiratory ratio	1: 2–1: 3
Peak inspiratory pressure	20-25 cm H_2O
Positive-end expiratory pressure	3-5 cm H_2O
Sigh (every 5-10 min.)	30 cm H_2O
Assessment of ventilatory adequacy	1. Observe chest wall excursions 2. Monitor blood gases; preferred method (maintain $PaCO_2$ at 40 mm Hg)

TABLE 29-4
RECEPTOR ACTIVITY OF INOTROPIC AND VASOACTIVE AGENTS

	ALPHA$_1$	ALPHA$_2$	BETA$_1$	BETA$_2$	DOPAMINERGIC
Isoproterenol	0	0	++++	++++	0
Dobutamine	++/+++	?	++++	++	0
Dopamine	+	+	++++	++	++++
Ephedrine	+	?	++	+	
Epinephrine	++++	++++	++++	+++	0
Norepinephrine	+++	+++	+/++	+/++	0
Phenylephrine	++/+++	+	?	0	0

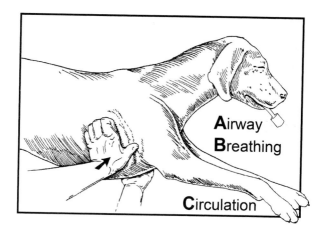

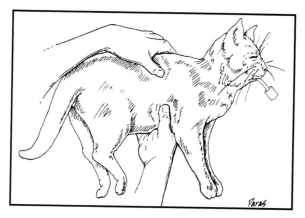

Fig. 29-2

Chest compression (approximately 100 compressions per minute) in dogs and cats.

TABLE 29-5

TREATMENTS FOR VENTRICULAR FIBRILLATION

DIRECT-CURRENT DEFIBRILLATORS	CHEMICAL DEFIBRILLATION
<ul><li>0.5 to 2 Ws/kg internal</li><li>5 to 10 Ws/kg external</li></ul> <ul><li>Small patient (<7 kg) 5 to 15 Ws internal 50 to 100 Ws external</li><li>Large patient (>10 kg) 20 to 80 Ws internal 100 to 400 Ws external</li></ul> Alternating-current defibrillators Small patient <ul><li>30 to 50 V internal</li><li>50 to 100 V external</li></ul>	1 mg potassium chloride and 6 mg acetylcholine/kg followed by 1ml/10 kg of 10% calcium chloride Unresponsive ventricular fibrillation <ul><li>Evaluate ventilation</li><li>Evaluate chest or cardiac compression</li><li>Repeat epinephrine and consider calcium chloride administration</li><li>Administer sodium bicarbonate</li><li>Administer lidocaine</li><li>Repeat electrical defibrillation</li></ul>

TABLE 29-6

ESSENTIAL DRUGS USED IN THE MANAGEMENT OF CARDIOPULMONARY ARREST

GENERIC NAME	TRADE NAME	BENEFICIAL EFFECTS (RECOMMENDED USE)	ADVERSE OR SIDE EFFECTS	DOSE AND ROUTE OF ADMINISTRATION
Vasoactive and cardiostimulatory agents				
Epinephrine HCl	Adrenaline	Positive inotrope; initiates heartbeats; increases heart rate and cardiac output; initially increases, then decreases mean arterial blood pressure and coronary blood flow	Intense vasoconstriction of renal and splanchnic vasculature; causes decreased perfusion of these tissues; increases myocardial oxygen consumption and cardiac work; arrhythmogenic, may cause ventricular fibrillation	6-10 µg/kg IC 10-30 µg/kg IV 0.1-0.2 ml/20 kg, small animals 1-3 ml/450 kg, large animals
Dopamine HCl	Inotropin	Positive inotrope; increases heart rate, cardiac output, and mean arterial blood pressure; improves blood flow to coronary, renal, and mesenteric circulation	May produce severe tachycardia if given rapidly; arrhythmogenic; vasoconstriction at higher doses	Give to effect, add 6 mg to 250 ml 5% dextrose; drip slowly at rate of 2-10 µg/kg/min

IC, Intracardiac; *IV,* intravenously; *PEA,* pulseless electric activity; *CPA,* cardiopulmonary arrest; *IM,* intramuscularly.

Continued

TABLE 29-6
ESSENTIAL DRUGS USED IN THE MANAGEMENT OF CARDIOPULMONARY ARREST—cont'd

GENERIC NAME	TRADE NAME	BENEFICIAL EFFECTS (RECOMMENDED USE)	ADVERSE OR SIDE EFFECTS	DOSE AND ROUTE OF ADMINISTRATION
Vasoactive and cardiostimulatory agents—cont'd				
Dobutamine HCl	Dobutrex	Positive inotrope; has lower chronotropic and vasopressor effect than dopamine	Tachyarrhythmias, vasoconstriction, and arrhythmias at higher doses	Give to effect, 1-10 μg/kg/min
Ephedrine sulphate	Ephedrine	Vasopressor; positive inotrope, chronotrope, vasoconstrictor	Tachycardia, hypertension	5-10 μg/kg
Drugs used specifically to increase contractility				
Calcium chloride		Positive inotrope; used to treat inhalant anesthetic overdose, hyperkalemia, and PEA	May cause asystole; myocardial calcium overload; "stone" heart	0.05-0.1 ml/kg of the 10% solution IV, IC
Digoxin	Lanoxin	Positive inotrope; increased vagal tone; used in cases of CPA caused by congestive heart failure; treat supraventricular tachycardia	Arrhythmogenic; increases oxygen consumption; causes vasoconstriction when given IV	0.01-0.02 mg/kg IV; given in four divided doses; dosed every hour give to effect; monitor ECG

Drugs used to combat acidosis

Sodium bicarbonate	Buffer acidosis; allows more effective defibrillation	Excessive administration may produce alkalosis, hyperosmolarity, paradoxical cerebrospinal fluid acidosis	1-2 mEq/kg IV, give to effect

Drugs used to treat acute cardiac arrhythmias

Atropine sulfate		Parasympatholytic effects; may correct supraventricular bradycardia or a slow ventricular rhythm by stimulating supraventricular pacemakers	May cause excessive tachycardia; increases myocardial oxygen consumption; lowers ventricular fibrillatory threshold; may predispose to sympathetic-induced arrhythmias	0.1-0.2 mg/kg IV
Glycopyrrolate	Robinul-V	Parasympatholytic (anticholinergic); may correct supraventricular bradycardia	May cause excessive tachycardia	0.005-0.01 mg/kg IV

Continued

TABLE 29-6
ESSENTIAL DRUGS USED IN THE MANAGEMENT OF CARDIOPULMONARY ARREST—cont'd

GENERIC NAME	TRADE NAME	BENEFICIAL EFFECTS (RECOMMENDED USE)	ADVERSE OR SIDE EFFECTS	DOSE AND ROUTE OF ADMINISTRATION
Drugs used to treat acute cardiac arrhythmias—cont'd				
Esmolol	Brevebloc	β_1-adrenergic blocker; treat supraventricular and ventricular tachycardia	Hypertension, bradycardia, heart failure	10-50 µg/kg/min IV
Propranolol HCl	Inderal	β-adrenergic blocker; antiarrhythmic; may correct supraventricular and ventricular tachycardia	Decreases contractility, an important adverse effect; may increase airway resistance	1 mg diluted in 1 ml saline solution; this dilution is given as 0.05-0.1 ml boluses IV give to effect
Lidocaine	Xylocaine	Ventricular antiarrhythmic	Dosage must be considerably decreased when used in cats	2-6 mg/kg dogs IV 0.5-1 mg/kg cats IV
Diltiazem	Cardiazem	Calcium channel blocker; treat supraventricular arrhythmias	Bradycardia hypotension	1-2 mg/kg PO
Sotalol	Betapase	Ventricular arrhythmias	Hypotension, proarrhythmia	5 mg/kg IV
Acetylcholine KCl cocktail		Chemical defibrillator?	Parasympathomimetic side effects	6 mg/kg ACh + 1 mEq/kg KCl, IC

Drugs used to stimulate ventilation

| Doxapram HCl | Dopram | Direct action on centers in the medulla | Respiratory alkalosis, hyperkalemia | 1-4 mg/kg IV
10 μg/kg/min give to effect |

Drugs used to combat cerebral edema

Oxygen		Prevents vasodilation	May cause pulmonary edema with prolonged administration; may suppress ventilatory drive	2-4 L/min (small animal) 15 L/min (large animal)
Mannitol	20% Osmitrol	Osmotic diuretic; reduces cerebral edema	May overload the volume of the circulatory system, causing edema	1-2 g/kg IV
Dexamethasone	Azium	(See section on shock)		

Drugs used to combat acute pulmonary edema

| Furosemide | Lasix | Potent loop diuretic promoting loss of Na^+, Cl^-, and H_2O | May cause dehydration or lead to hypokalemic metabolic alkalosis if used excessively | 1-2 mg/kg IV, 2-4 mg/kg IM |

Continued

TABLE 29-6
ESSENTIAL DRUGS USED IN THE MANAGEMENT OF CARDIOPULMONARY ARREST—cont'd

GENERIC NAME	TRADE NAME	BENEFICIAL EFFECTS (RECOMMENDED USE)	ADVERSE OR SIDE EFFECTS	DOSE AND ROUTE OF ADMINISTRATION
Steroids				
Prednisolone sodium	Solu-Delta-Cortef	Stabilizes lysosomal membranes; induces vasodilation; regulated fluid and electrolyte homeostasis		30 mg/kg IV
Dexamethasone Isotonic IV fluids Lactated Ringer's 0.9% saline solution	Azium SP	Increases cardiac output Expand the blood volume; hypotension; increase tissue perfusion	May increase edema in cats with congestive heart failure; fluid administration rate generally should not exceed 90 ml/kg/hr; administer at high rates initially to improve venous return	8 mg/kg IV 20-40 mg/kg/hr until effective

Specific drug antagonists

Naloxone	Narcan	Narcotic antagonist	None	50 µg/kg
Neostigmine	Prostigmine Stiglyn	Cholinesterase inhibitor; used to reverse nondepolarizing neuromuscular blocking agents	Cholinergic effects; a parasympatholytic must be given before drug administration (e.g., atropine, glycopyrrolate)	0.02 mg/kg
Pyridostigmine	Regonol	Cholinesterase inhibitor; used to reverse nondepolarizing neuromuscular blocking agents	Cholinergic effects; a parasympatholytic must be given before drug administration (e.g., atropine, glycopyrrolate)	0.1 mg/kg
Edrophonium	Tensilon	Cholinesterase inhibitor; used to reverse nondepolarizing neuromuscular blocking drugs	Same as neostigmine	0.2-1 mg/kg IV
Yohimbine	Yobine	α_2-Antagonist; used to reverse α_2-agonists	Excitement, disorientation	0.2-0.4 mg/kg IV
Tolazoline	Tolazine Antisedan	Same as yohimbine but more selective for α_2- receptors	Excitement	2-4 mg/kg IV 0.1-0.2 mg/kg IV
Flumazenil	Romazicon	Benzodiazepine antagonist	—	0.1 mg/kg IV

CHAPTER THIRTY

Euthanasia

"Sweet is true love though given in vain, and sweet is death
that puts an end to pain."
ALFRED LORD TENNYSON

OVERVIEW

Euthanasia is a personal and emotional decision often made in the face of incurable disease or uncontrollable pain. Almost all drugs used for chemical restraint and anesthesia have the capability of producing death, as long as a sufficient amount of the drug is administered. Anesthetic drugs used for euthanasia offer the advantage of producing total unconsciousness before cardiopulmonary arrest and the elimination of brain electrical activity. This chapter does not presume to identify what technique of anesthesia is the best but describes the various techniques applied to produce euthanasia.

GENERAL CONSIDERATIONS

I. Euthanasia is the act of inducing loss of consciousness and death without causing pain, distress, anxiety, or apprehension. It should result in cardiac and respiratory arrest and the ultimate loss of brain function; death may be defined as permanent abolition of central nervous system function
   A. Euthanasia often requires the animal to be physically restrained
   B. Methods of euthanasia
      1. Acceptable methods consistently produce a humane death when used as the sole means of euthanasia
      2. Conditionally acceptable methods are those techniques that by the nature of the technique or because of greater potential for operator error or safety hazards

576

might not consistently produce humane death or are methods not well documented in the scientific literature
   3. Unacceptable methods are those techniques deemed inhumane under any conditions or that pose a substantial risk to the human applying the technique
C. In many species, capturing and immobilizing the animal for euthanasia may cause a variety of aesthetically unpleasant responses
   1. Vocalization
   2. Avoidance or aggressive behavior
   3. Immobility (the animal may be "frozen with fear")
   4. Urination and defecation, evacuation of anal sacs
   5. Sweating, salivation
   6. Skeletal muscle tremors, spasms, or shivering
   7. Pupillary dilation
   8. Tachycardia
   9. "Playing dead" in certain species, particularly rabbits and chickens
D. Selection of a method of euthanasia depends on the following factors:
   1. Species and breeds of animal
   2. Size and weight
   3. The animal's behavior
   4. Type of physical restraint necessary; anesthetized or unconscious animals need less critical methods
   5. Owner preference
   6. Skill of personnel and risk involved
   7. Number of animals to be euthanatized
   8. Economics
   9. Facilities available
E. Tranquilizers or other depressant drugs (e.g., α_2-agonists, opioids) are recommended before the administration of euthanatizing drugs in excitable or vicious animals
F. Pain perception requires a functional cerebral cortex and subcortical structures; an unconscious animal does not experience pain, but pain-provoking stimuli in an unconscious animal may evoke a reflex motor or sympathetic response
G. Stress is defined as the effects of physical, physiologic, or emotional factors (stressors) that induce an alteration in an animal's homeostasis or adaptive state

H. Personnel who perform euthanasia must have appropriate certification, training, and experience in the humane restraint of the species of animal to be euthanatized, in order to ensure that animal pain and distress are minimized during euthanasia

AVAILABLE METHODS

I. Euthanatizing agents include gaseous, chemical, and physical (e.g., mechanical, electrical) methods of producing death (Table 30-1)
II. Euthanatizing agents produce death by three mechanisms
   A. Hypoxia; direct or indirect
   B. Direct depression of neurons necessary for life function
   C. Physical disruption of brain activity and destruction of neurons necessary for life
III. The most common drug used for euthanasia of dogs, cats, horses, and cattle is pentobarbital sodium, 100 mg/kg intravenously

EVALUATION CRITERIA

I. Criteria for evaluation of acceptable methods of euthanasia
   A. Ability to induce loss of consciousness and death without causing pain, distress, anxiety, or apprehension
   B. Time required to induce loss of consciousness
   C. Reliability
   D. Safety to personnel
   E. Irreversibility
   F. Compatibility with requirement and purpose
   G. Emotional effect on observers or operators
   H. Compatibility with subsequent evaluation, examination, or use of tissue
   I. Drug availability and human abuse potential
   J. Compatibility with species, age, and health status
   K. Ability to maintain equipment in proper working order
   L. Safety for predators/scavengers should the carcass be consumed

TABLE 30-1
ACCEPTABLE AGENTS AND METHODS OF EUTHANASIA BY SPECIES

SPECIES	AGENTS AND METHODS	DOSE
Dogs	Barbiturates*	
	Inhalant anesthetics†	
Cats	Barbiturates*	
	Inhalant anesthetics†	
Horses	Barbiturates*	
	Potassium chloride in conjunction with general anesthesia	1-2 mmol/kg rapid IV or intracardiac administration
Ruminants	Barbiturates*	
	Potassium chloride in conjunction with general anesthesia	1-2 mmol/kg rapid IV or intracardiac administration
Swine	Barbiturates*	
	CO_2	30%

*Sodium pentobarbital best fits euthanasia and is most widely used. Dose 100 mg/kg IV.
†Inhalant agents should not be used alone in animals less than 16 weeks old except to induce loss of consciousness, followed by the use of some other method to kill the animal.
‡Many reptiles and amphibians, including chelonians, are capable of holding their breath and converting to anaerobic metabolism and can survive long periods of anoxia; death in these species may not occur even after prolonged inhalant exposure.
IP, Intraperitoneal; IV, intravenous.

Continued

TABLE 30-1

ACCEPTABLE AGENTS AND METHODS OF EUTHANASIA BY SPECIES—cont'd

SPECIES	AGENTS AND METHODS	DOSE
Camelids	Barbiturates*	
Rabbits	Barbiturates*	
	Inhalant anesthetics†	
Rodents and other small mammals	Barbiturates*	
	Inhalant anesthetics†	
Birds	Barbiturates*	
	Inhalant anesthetics†	
Mink, fox, and other mammals	Barbiturates*	
produced for fur	Inhalant anesthetics†	
Reptiles	Barbiturates*	Sodium pentobarbital 60-100 mg/kg
	Inhalant anesthetics† (in appropriate	IV, IP
	species‡)	
Amphibians	Barbiturates*	Sodium pentobarbital 60-100 mg/kg
	Inhalant anesthetics† (in appropriate	IV, IP
	species‡)	
Zoo animals	Barbiturates*	
	Inhalant anesthetics†	
Fish	Barbiturates*	Sodium pentobarbital 60-100 mg/kg
	Inhalant anesthetics†	IV, IP
Free-ranging wildlife	Barbiturates* IV or IP	
	Inhalant anesthetics†	

UNACCEPTABLE DRUGS AND TECHNIQUES

I. Unacceptable drugs: depolarizing and nondepolarizing muscle relaxants, strychnine, magnesium sulfate, and nicotine are intravenous drugs that were commonly used for euthanasia in the past; their individual use as the sole euthanatizing agent is absolutely unwarranted; with other techniques that induce hypoxia, some animals may have motor activity after loss of consciousness, but this is reflex activity and is not perceived by the animal

  A. Strychnine produces violent muscular contractions associated with extreme pain

  B. Magnesium sulfate causes death from asphyxia

  C. Nicotine produces convulsions before death and is extremely hazardous to personnel

  D. Neuromuscular blocking drugs (e.g., succinylcholine, atracurium) cause paralysis without anesthesia

  E. Do not use drugs that exhibit the following characteristics:

    1. Do not produce unconsciousness

    2. Do not produce analgesia

    3. Have no anesthetic effect

    4. Lead to specific problems

    5. Produce death by hypoxia

II. Unacceptable techniques (used alone)

  A. Exsanguination

  B. Rapid freezing

  C. Air embolism

  D. Decompression

  E. Drowning

  F. Electrocution (stunning)

NOTE

Techniques A, B, C, and F have been used in anesthetized animals under special circumstances

Reference: "2000 Report of the AVMA Panels on Euthanasia" which is available on the AVMA website or from the Journal of the American Veterinary Medical Association:

http://www.avma.org/issues/animal_welfare/euthanasia.pdf

2000 Report of the AVMA Panel on Euthanasia. *J Am Vet Med Assoc* 218:669-96, 2001. (Erratum in: *J Am Vet Med Assoc* 218:1884, 2001.)

Partial Listing of Commonly Used Drugs, Anesthetic and Monitoring Equipment, and Their Manufacturers

ANTICHOLINERGICS

Atropine (*atropine*)
American Pharmaceutical Partners, Inc.
Schaumburg, Illinois
http://www.appdrugs.com

Robinul-V (*glycopyrrolate*)
Fort Dodge Animal Health, Division of Wyeth Holdings Corp.
Madison, New Jersey
http://www.wyeth.com

TRANQUILIZERS/ SEDATIVES

Domitor (*medetomidine*)
Pfizer, Inc.
New York, New York
http://www.pfizer.com

Dormosedan (*detomidine*)
Pfizer, Inc.
New York, New York
http://www.pfizer.com

PromAce (*acepromazine maleate*)
Fort Dodge Animal Health, Division of Wyeth Holdings Corp.
Madison, New Jersey
http://www.wyeth.com

TranquiVed Inject Injectable 20 mg/ml (*xylazine*)
Vedco, Inc.
St. Joseph, Missouri
http://www.vedco.com

Xylazine 100 mg/ml (*xylazine*)
Butler Animal Health Supply Co.
Dublin, Ohio
https://www.accessbutler.com

OPIOID ANALGESICS

Astramorph/PS Injection (*preservative-free morphine sulfate*)
AstraZeneca Pharmaceuticals LP, Inc.
Wilmington, Delaware
http://www.astrazeneca-us.com

**Buprenorphine HCl
   Injection** (*buprenorphine*)
Bedford Laboratories
Bedford, Ohio
http://www.bedfordlabs.com

ButorPhanol 10 mg/ml
   (*butorphanol*)
Butler Animal Health Supply
   Co.
Dublin, Ohio
https://www.accessbutler.com

Demerol (*meperidine*)
Abbott Laboratories
Chicago, Illinois
http://www.abbott.com

Fentanyl (*fentanyl*)
Abbott Laboratories
North Chicago, Illinois
http://www.abbott.com

Methadone HCl Injection
   (*methadone*)
AAIPharma, Inc.
Wilmington, North Carolina
http://www.aaipharma.com

Morphine Sulfate Injection
   (*morphine*)
Baxter Healthcare Corp.
Deerfield, Illinois
http://www.baxter.com

Nubain (*nalbuphine*)
DuPont Pharmaceuticals Co.
Wilmington, Delaware
http://www2.dupont.com

Numorphan (*oxymorphone*)
Endo Pharmaceuticals, Co.
Chadds Ford, Pennsylvania
http://www.endo.com

Sufenta (*sufentanil*)
Janssen Pharmaceutica, Inc.
Titusville, New Jersey
http://www.janssenpharmaceu-
   tica.com

Talwin (*pentazocine*)
Sanofi-Synthelabo, Inc.
Bridgewater, New Jersey
http://www.sanofi-aventis.us

Torbugesic 2 mg/ml
   (*butorphanol*)
Fort Dodge Animal Health,
   Division of Wyeth Holdings
   Corp.
Madison, New Jersey
http://www.wyeth.com

LOCAL ANESTHETICS

Carbocaine-V (*mepivacaine*)
Fort Dodge Animal Health,
   Division of Wyeth Holdings
   Corp.
New York, New York
http://www.pfizer.com

Lidocaine HCl 2%
Butler Animal Health Supply
   Co.
Dublin, Ohio
https://www.accessbutler.com

Naropin (*ropivacaine*)
AstraZeneca Pharmaceuticals
   LP, Inc.
Wilmington, Delaware
http://www.astrazeneca-us.com

Sensorcaine (*bupivacaine*)
AstraZeneca Pharmaceuticals
   LP, Inc.
Wilmington, Delaware
http://www.astrazeneca-us.com

Xylocaine MPF (*lidocaine*)
AstraZeneca Pharmaceuticals
   LP, Inc.
Wilmington, Delaware
http://www.astrazeneca-us.com

INJECTABLE ANESTHETICS

Amidate (*etomidate*)
Abbott Laboratories
North Chicago, Illinois
http://www.abbott.com

Brevital (*methohexital*)
King Pharmaceuticals, Inc.
Bristol, Tennessee
http://www.kingpharm.com

Chloral Hydrate Solution
   (*chloral hydrate*)
Sigma-Aldrich Corp.
St. Louis, Missouri
http://www.sigmaaldrich.com

Etomidate
Bedford Laboratories
Bedford, Ohio
http://www.bedfordlabs.com

Ketaset/Vetalar (*ketamine*)
Fort Dodge Animal Health,
   Division of Wyeth Holdings
   Corp.
Madison, New Jersey
http://www.wyeth.com

Nembutal (*pentobarbital*)
Abbott Laboratories
North Chicago, Illinois
http://www.abbott.com

Pentothal (*thiopental*)
Abbott Laboratories
North Chicago, Illinois
http://www.abbott.com

PropoFlo (*propofol*)
Abbott Laboratories
North Chicago, Illinois
http://www.abbott.com

Rapinovet (*propofol*)
Schering-Plough Animal
   Health Corp.
Kenilworth, New Jersey
http://www.spah.com

Telazol® (*tiletamine-zolazepam*)
Fort Dodge Animal Health, Division of Wyeth Holdings Corp.
Madison, New Jersey
http://www.wyeth.com

INHALANT ANESTHETICS

AErrane (*isoflurane*)
Baxter Healthcare Corp.
Deerfield, Illinois
http://www.baxter.com

Isoflo (*isoflurane*)
Abbott Laboratories
North Chicago, Illinois
http://www.abbott.com

Sevoflo (*sevoflurane*)
Abbott Laboratories
North Chicago, Illinois
http://www.abbott.com

Suprane (*desflurane*)
Baxter Healthcare Corp.
Deerfield, Illinois
http://www.baxter.com

MUSCLE RELAXANTS

Central

Guaifenesin Injection (*guaifenesin*)
Vedco, Inc.
St. Joseph, Missouri
http://www.vedco.com

Guaifenesin Injection 50 mg/ml (*guaifenesin*)
Phoenix Scientific, Division of IVAX Corp.
St. Joseph, Missouri
http://www.psiqv.com

Guailaxin (*guaifenesin sterile powder*)
Fort Dodge Animal Health, Division of Wyeth Holdings Corp.
Madison, New Jersey
http://www.wyeth.com

Midazolam 5 mg/ml (*midazolam*)
Bedford Laboratories
Bedford, Ohio
http://www.bedfordlabs.com

Valium (*diazepam*)
Roche Laboratories, Inc.
Nutley, New Jersey
http://www.rocheusa.com

Peripheral

Atracurium Novaplus (*atracurium*)
Boehringer Ingelheim Ben Venue Laboratories, Inc.
Bedford, Ohio
http://www.benvenue.com

Norcuron (*vecuronium*)
Organon, Inc.
Roseland, New Jersey
http://www.organon-usa.com

Pavulon (*pancuronium*)
Organon, Inc.
Roseland, New Jersey
http://www.organon-usa.com

Succinylcholine
    (*succinylcholine chloride*)
Abbott Laboratories
North Chicago, Illinois
http://www.abbott.com

ANTAGONISTS

Alpha-2

Antisedan (*atipamazole*)
Pfizer, Inc.
New York, New York
http://www.pfizer.com

Tolazine (*tolazoline HCl*)
Lloyd, Inc.
Shenandoah, Iowa
http://www.lloydinc.com

Yobine (*yohimbine*)
Lloyd, Inc.
Shenandoah, Iowa
http://www.lloydinc.com

Benzodiazepine

Romazicon (*flumazenil*)
Hoffman-La Roche, Inc.
Nutley, New Jersey
http://www.rocheusa.com

Opioid

Naloxone 4 mg/ml (*naloxone*)
Abbott Laboratories
North Chicago, Illinois
http://www.abbott.com

Revex (*nalmefene*)
Baxter Healthcare Corp.
Deerfield, Illinois
http://www.baxter.com

Peripheral Acting Muscle Relaxants

Enlon (*edrophonium*)
Baxter Healthcare Corp.
Deerfield, Illinois
http://www.baxter.com

Neostigmin (*neostigmine*)
American Pharmaceutical
    Partners, Inc.
Schaumburg, Illinois
http://www.appdrugs.com

Regonol (*pyridostigmine*)
Organon, Inc.
Roseland, New Jersey
http://www.organon-usa.com

RESPIRATORY STIMULANTS

Dopram-V (*doxapram*)
Fort Dodge Animal Health,
    Division of Wyeth Holdings
    Corp.
Madison, New Jersey
http://www.wyeth.com

CARDIAC STIMULANTS

Calcium Chloride Injection
10% *(calcium chloride)*
American Pharmaceutical
   Partners, Inc.
Schaumburg, Illinois
http://www.appdrugs.com

Calcium Gluconate Injection
   (calcium gluconate)
American Regent, Inc.
Shirley, New York
http://www.americanregent.com

Dobutamine *(dobutamine)*
Bedford Laboratories
Bedford, Ohio
http://www.bedfordlabs.com

Ephedrine *(ephedrine)*
Bedford Laboratories
Bedford, Ohio
http://www.bedfordlabs.com

Epinephrine (1:1000)
   (ephedrine)
Vedco, Inc.
St. Joseph, Missouri
http://www.vedco.com

Inotropin *(dopamine)*
Abbott Laboratories
North Chicago, Illinois
http://www.abbott.com

Magnesium Chloride
   Injection *(magnesium*
   chloride)
American Regent, Inc.
Shirley, New York
http://www.americanregent.com

Magnesium Sulfate Injection
   (magnesium sulfate)
American Regent, Inc.
Shirley, New York
http://www.americanregent.com

Procainamide *(procainamide)*
Abbott Laboratories
North Chicago, Illinois
http://www.abbott.com

EUTHANASIA SOLUTION

Euthasol *(pentobarbital)*
Virbac Corp.
Fort Worth, Texas
http://www.virbaccorp.com

OTHER PRODUCTS

Benadryl *(diphenhydramine)*
Parkedale Pharmaceuticals,
   Inc.
Rochester, Michigan
http://www.kingpharm.com

Dexamethasone Sodium
   Phosphate *(dexamethasone*
   sodium phosphate)
Vedco, Inc.
St. Joseph, Missouri
http://www.vedco.com

Dextrose Injection
Abbott Laboratories
North Chicago, Illinois
http://www.abbott.com

EMLA Anesthetic Cream
*(lidocaine 2.5% and
prilocaine 2.5%)*
AstraZeneca Pharmaceuticals,
Inc.
Wilmington, Delaware
http://www.astrazeneca-us.com

**Equi-Phar Furosemido
Injection 5%** *(furosemide)*
Vedco, Inc.
St. Joseph, Missouri
http://www.vedco.com

Mannitol Injection 25%
(mannitol)
Abbott Laboratories
North Chicago, Illinois
http://www.abbott.com

Metacam *(meloxicam)*
Boehringer Ingelheim
Vetmedica, Inc.
St. Joseph, Missouri
http://www.vetmedica.com

Nitropress *(sodium
nitroprusside)*
Abbott Laboratories
North Chicago, Illinois
http://www.abbott.com

Potassium Chloride
American Reagent
Shirley, New York
http://www.americanregent.com

Rimadyl *(carprofen)*
Pfizer, Inc.
New York, New York.
http://www.pfizer.com

**Sodium Bicarbonate Inj.
8.4%** *(sodium bicarbonate)*
Abbott Laboratories
North Chicago, Illinois
http://www.abbott.com

Solu-Delta-Cortef
*(prednisolone sodium
succinate)*
Pfizer, Inc.
New York, New York
http://www.pfizer.com

**Tears Renewed Ointment 3.5
GM** *(lubricant ophthalmic
ointment)*
Akorn, Inc.
Buffalo Grove, Illinois
http://www.akorn.com

ANESTHETIC AND RELATED EQUIPMENT

**Allied Health Care Products,
Inc.**
St. Louis, Missouri
http://www.alliedhpi.com

Bivona, Inc.
a Smiths Medical Co.
Keene, New Hampshire
http://www.smiths-
medical.com

Engler Engineering Corp.
Hialeah, Florida
http://www.engler-
engineering.com

Hallowell EMC Engineering and Manufacturing Corp.
Pittsfield, Massachusetts
http://www.hallowell.com

Henry Schein, Inc.
Melville, New York
http://www.henryschein.com

Hudson RCI
Research Triangle Park, North Carolina
http://www.hudsonrci.com

Mallard Medical
Redding, California
http://www.mallardmedical.net

Matrix Medical, Inc.
Minneapolis, Minnesota
http://www.matrixmedical.net

North American Drager
Telford, Pennsylvania
http://www.draeger.com

Ohio Medical Corporation
Madison, Wisconsin
http://ohmeda.ohiomedical.com

Parks Medical Electronics, Inc.
Aloha, Oregon
http://www.parksmed.com

Respironics, Inc.
Carlsbad, California
http://www.respironics.com

SurgiVet, Inc.
Waukesha, Wisconsin
http://www.surgivet.com

ANESTHETIC MONITORING AND RELATED EQUIPMENT

Anesthetic Agent Monitoring and Respiratory Monitors

Criticare Systems, Inc.
Waukesha, Wisconsin
http://www.csiusa.com

Datex-Ohmeda
Madison, Wisconsin
http://www.us.datex-ohmeda.com

Novametrix Medical Systems, Inc.
Carlsbad, California
http://www.respironics.com

Handheld Electrocardiogram Monitors

Vet/Ox Plus 4800
Heska
Loveland, Colorado
http://www.heska.com

PAM Cardiac Monitor
Technology Transfer, Inc.
Lafayette, Indiana
http://www.ttic.com

Blood Pressure/Electrocardiogram Monitors

Datascope Corp.
Montvale, New Jersey
http://www.datascope.com

Gould Life Science
Valley View, Ohio
http://www.lds-group.com

Space Labs Medical
Issaquah, Washington
http://www.spacelabs.com

Indirect Blood Pressure Monitors

General Electric Medical Systems
Waukesha, Wisconsin
http://www.gehealthcare.com

Heska
Loveland, Colorado
http://www.heska.com

Nellcor, Inc.
Pleasanton, California
http://www.nellcor.com

Parks Medical Equipment, Inc.
Aloha, Oregon
http://www.parksmed.com

Ramsey Medical, Inc.
Tampa, Florida
http://www.cardiocommand.com

Sharn Veterinary, Inc.
Tampa, Florida
http://www.sharnvet.com

Pulse Oximetry

Heska
Loveland, Colorado
http://www.heska.com

Nellcor, Inc.
Pleasanton, California
http://www.nellcor.com

Nonin Medical, Inc.
Plymouth, Minnesota
http://www.nonin.com

SurgiVet, Inc.
Waukesha, Wisconsin
http://www.surgivet.com

Noninvasive Cardiac Output Monitors

NICO
Novametrix Medical Systems, Inc.
Wallingford, Connecticut
http://www.novametrix.com

LiDCOplus
LiDCO Ltd.
Coppell. Texas
http://www.lidco.com

USCOM
USCOM Pty. Ltd.
Sydney, Australia
http://www.uscom.com.au

Syringe/Fluid Infusion Pumps

Autosyringe
Baxter International, Inc.
Deerfield, Illinois

Baxter
Deerfield, Illinois
http://www.baxter.com

Heska
Loveland, Colorado
http://www.heska.com

Medex, Inc.
Smiths Medical (Formerly
  Medex)
Duluth, Georgia
http://www.smiths-
  medical.com

Stat Electrolytes

IRMA
ITC
Edison, New Jersey
http://www.itcmed.com

i-STAT
Heska
Loveland, Colorado
http://www.heska.com

Stat Blood Gases and pH

IRMA
ITC
Edison, New Jersey
http://www.itcmed.com

i-STAT
Heska
Loveland, Colorado
http://www.heska.com

ABL 700/800
Radiometer America
Cleveland, Ohio
http://www.radiometeramerica.
  com

**Stat Profile Critical Care
  XPress**
Nova Biomedical Corp.
Waltham, Massachusetts
http://www.novabiomedical.
  com

Defibrillators

Datascope Corp.
Montvale, New Jersey
http://www.datascope.com

Temperature Monitors

Yellow Springs Instruments
Dayton, Ohio
http://www.ysi.com

Oxygen Cages

**Isolette: North American
  Drager**
Telford, Pennsylvania
http://www.draeger.com

Heating Devices

Thermadrape
Vital Signs, Inc.
Totowa, New Jersey
http://www.vital-signs.com

Bair Hugger
Arizant, Inc.
Eden Prairie, Minnesota
http://www.augustinemedical.
  com

Hotline (fluid warmer)
Smiths Level-1
Rockland, Massachusetts
http://www.smiths-level1.com

**Hallowell EMC Heated Hard
  Pad**
Hallowell EMC
Pittsfield, Massachusetts
http://www.hallowell.com

APPENDIX II

Physical Principles of Anesthesia

I. Laws
   A. *Boyle's law*

   $$\text{Volume} = \frac{k}{\text{Pressure}}; \; V \times P = k$$
   $$P_1V_1 = P_2V_2$$

   B. *Charles' law*

   $$V = k + T \qquad T = {}^\circ\text{Kelvin (K)}$$
   $$\frac{V_1}{V_2} = \frac{T_1}{T_2}$$

   C. *Gay-Lussac's law*

   $$P = k \times T \qquad T = {}^\circ\text{K}$$
   $$\frac{P_1}{P_2} = \frac{T_1}{T_2}$$

   From above:

   $$\frac{P_1V_1}{T_1} = \frac{P_2V_2}{T_2}$$

   D. *Ideal Gas law*

   $$\frac{PV}{T} = n\frac{(1 \text{ atm})(22.412)}{273\text{K}}$$

   $$PV = nRT \qquad R = 0.08206 \qquad 1 \text{ atm}/{}^\circ\text{K} \qquad n = \text{g moles}$$

   E. *Henry's law*

   $$V = \alpha P \qquad \begin{array}{l} V = \text{volume of gas dissolved} \\ \alpha = \text{solubility coefficient} \\ P = \text{partial pressure} \end{array}$$

   The solubility of a gas or vapor in a liquid (α) decreases as the temperature increases

F. Law of partial pressure (Dalton's law): each gas in a mixture exerts the same pressure as it would exert if it alone occupied the same volume at the same temperature; since pressure measurements cannot distinguish different molecules in a mixed sample, the contribution to total pressure made by a given constituent is in proportion to the number of molecules of that constituent

G. Graham's law: the velocity or rate of diffusion is inversely proportional to the square root of the density

II. Terms

A. Vapor pressure

   1. Tendency for a liquid to evaporate

   2. When a liquid and its vapor are in equilibrium, the partial pressure that the vapor exerts

B. Heat of vaporization: the amount of heat required for a liquid to evaporate

C. Volumes of a vapor

$$\frac{\text{Vapor pressure}}{\text{Total pressure}} \times 100 = \text{Vol } \%$$

D. Boiling point of a liquid: that temperature at which its vapor pressure is equal to the prevailing atmospheric pressure; generally stated for 760 mm Hg

E. Critical temperature: when a liquid is confined in a strong container, the temperature at which the contents of the container consists of vapor only

F. Critical pressure: when a liquid is confined in a strong container, the pressure that exists when the container has reached its critical temperature; liquid volumes may be converted to weight by the formula: volume (ml) × density (g/ml) = grams of liquid

G. Latent heat of vaporization: the amount of heat necessary to evaporate a quantity of liquid to its vapor state without any changes in temperature; expressed in calories per gram of liquid; this heat is stored in the vapor

III. Specific partition coefficients; the solubility coefficient may be expressed as follows:

A. Bunsen's absorption coefficient: amount of gas (volume) at standard temperature and pressure that dissolves in one volume of liquid when the partial pressure of the gas above the liquid is 1 atm

B. Ostwald's solubility coefficient: the volume of gas absorbed by a unit volume of liquid when the partial pressure of the gas is 1 atm, the volume of gas being expressed at the temperature of the experiment

C. The partition coefficient

1. May be expressed as the ratio of concentration of a substance in the gas phase and in the liquid phase (e.g., milligrams per milliliter)

2. Partition coefficients are also used to relate the ratios of concentrations in any two phases that are in equilibrium

a. Liquid-liquid (oil-water)

b. Liquid-solid

c. Gas-solid

IV. Useful tables (Tables 1 through 3)

V. Conversion equations for weight in kilograms to body surface area (m^2)

A. *Dogs*

$$\text{Approximate body surface area (BSA; } m^2) = \frac{10.1 \times (\text{Body weight in grams})^{2/3}}{10000}$$

B. *Cats*

$$\text{Approximate BSA } (m^2) = \frac{10.0 \times (\text{Body weight in grams})^{2/3}}{10000}$$

C. *Horses*

$$\text{Approximate BSA } (m^2) = \frac{10.5 \times (\text{Body weight in grams})^{2/3}}{10000}$$

TABLE **1**
STANDARD VALUES AND EQUIVALENTS*

METRIC WEIGHTS		
1 gram (g)	=	weight of 1 ml water at 4° C
1000 g	=	1 kilogram (kg)
0.1 g	=	1 decigram (dg)
0.01 g	=	1 centigram (cg)
0.001 g	=	1 milligram (mg)
0.001 mg	=	1 microgram (µg)
28.4 g	=	1 ounce (oz)
453.6 g	=	1 pound (lb)
16 oz	=	1 lb

METRIC VOLUME		
1 liter (L)	=	1 cubic decimeter or 1000 cubic centimeters (cc) or 1000 milliliter (ml)
0.1 liter	=	1 deciliter (dl)
0.001 liter	=	1 milliliter (ml)

METRIC LENGTH		
1 meter (m)	=	100 centimeter (cm)
1 cm	=	10 millimeter (mm)
2.54 cm	=	1 inch (in)
30.48 cm	=	1 foot (ft)
0.91 m	=	1 yard (yd)

CONCENTRATION		
1%	=	1 g/100 ml (10 mg/ml)

*International System (SI) units

TABLE 2
CONVERSION FACTORS

SI UNIT	OLD UNIT	CONVERSION FACTORS	
		TO SI (EXACT)	SI TO OLD (APPROXIMATE)
kPa	mm Hg	0.133	7.5
kPa	1 standard atmosphere (approximately 1 Bar)	101.3	0.01
kPa	cmH_2O	0.0981	10
kPa	Lb/sq inch	6.89	0.145

MEASUREMENT	SI UNIT	OLD UNIT	CONVERSION FACTORS	
			TO SI (EXACT)	SI TO OLD (APPROXIMATE)
Blood				
Acid-base				
P_{CO_2}	kPa	mm Hg	0.133	7.5
P_{O_2}	kPa	mm Hg	0.133	7.5
Base excess	mmol/L	mEq/L	Numerically equivalent	
Plasma				
Sodium	mmol/L	mEq/L	Numerically equivalent	
Potassium	mmol/L	mEq/L	Numerically equivalent	
Magnesium	mmol/L	mEq/L	0.5	2.0
Chloride	mmol/L	mEq/L	Numerically equivalent	
Phosphate (inorganic)	mmol/L	mEq/L	0.323	3.0
Creatinine	μmol/L	mg/100 ml	88.4	0.01
Urea	mmol/L	mg/100 ml	0.166	6.0
Serum				
Calcium	mmol/L	mg/100 ml	0.25	4.0
Bilirubin	μmol/L	mg/100 ml	17.1	0.06
Total protein	g/L	g/100 ml	10.0	0.1
Albumin	g/L	g/100 ml	10.0	0.1
Globulin	g/L	g/100 ml	10.0	0.1

TABLE 3

ALVEOLAR AND ARTERIAL GAS PRESSURES IN HEALTHY SUBJECTS AT ALTITUDE

| ALTITUDE (FEET) | ATMOSPHERIC PRESSURE (mm Hg) | PIO_2 (mm Hg) | SEA LEVEL FIO_2 | ALVEOLAR GAS TENSIONS (mm Hg) | | | | ARTERIAL GAS TENSIONS (mm Hg) | | | INSPIRED FIO_2 NEEDED TO YIELD SEA LEVEL PIO_2 |
				H_2O	CO_2	N_2	O_2	CO_2	O_2	SPO_2	
Sea level	760	149	20.9	47	37	574	102	40	95	97	20.9
6000	609	118	16.6	47	36	452	74	—	—	—	26.5
8000	565	108	15.1	47	37	416	65	38	56	89	28.8
10,000	523	100	14.0	47	36	379	61	—	—	—	31.3

PIO_2, Inspired oxygen tension; FIO_2, fraction of inspired oxygen concentration.

Appendix III

Drug Schedules

Controlled substances are obtained by prescription and must be used for legitimate medical purposes. The prescriber must have authorization from appropriate legal authorities (usually the attorney general), the Controlled Substances Act (CSA), to handle controlled substances. The CSA is the legal foundation of the government's fight against the abuse of drugs and other substances. All individuals and firms that are registered are required to maintain complete and accurate inventories and records of all transactions involving controlled substances, as well as security for the storage of controlled substances.

The CSA places all substances that are regulated under existing federal law into one of five schedules based upon the substance's medicinal value, harmfulness, and potential for abuse or addiction. The CSA list of controlled substance schedules describes the basic or parent chemical and does not describe the salts, isomers and salts of isomers, esters, ethers, and derivatives that might be controlled substances.

SCHEDULE I

The drug or other substance has a high potential for abuse
The drug or other substance has no currently accepted medical use in treatment in the United States
There is a lack of accepted safety for use of the drug or other substance under medical supervision

SCHEDULE II

The drug or other substance has a high potential for abuse
The drug or other substance has a currently accepted medical use in treatment in the United States or a currently accepted medical use with severe restrictions

Abuse of the drug or other substances may lead to severe psychological or physical dependence

SCHEDULE III

The drug or other substance has a potential for abuse less than the drugs or other substances in Schedules I and II

The drug or other substance has a currently accepted medical use in treatment in the United States

Abuse of the drug or other substance may lead to moderate or low physical dependence or high psychological dependence

SCHEDULE IV

The drug or other substance has a low potential for abuse relative to the drugs or other substances in Schedule III

The drug or other substance has a currently accepted medical use in treatment in the United States

Abuse of the drug or other substance may lead to limited physical dependence or psychological dependence relative to the drugs or other substances in Schedule III

SCHEDULE V

A. The drug or other substance has a low potential for abuse relative to the drugs or other substances in Schedule IV

B. The drug or other substance has a currently accepted medical use in treatment in the United States

C. Abuse of the drug or other substance may lead to limited physical dependence or psychological dependence relative to the drugs or other substances in Schedule IV

REFILLS (SCHEDULES III AND IV)

A prescription for a controlled substance listed in schedule III or IV may not be filled or refilled more than 6 months after the original date of issue of the prescription. They may not be refilled more than five times. Each refill must be entered on the back of the original prescription or other appropriate document (medication record).

When retrieving the prescription number, the following information should be available: the name and dosage form of the controlled substance, the date filled or refilled, the quantity dispensed, initials of the registered pharmacist for each refill, and the total number of refills for that prescription to date.

As an alternative to the procedures, an automated data processing system may be used for the storage and retrieval of refill information for prescription orders for controlled substances in Schedule III and IV.

ORAL REFILLS (SCHEDULES III AND IV)

The prescribing practitioner may authorize additional refills of Schedule III or IV controlled substances on the original prescription through an oral refill authorization transmitted to the pharmacist. The total number of refills (quantity) allowed, including the amount of the original, may not exceed five refills or 6 months from the original date.

A. A new and separate prescription must be issued for any more than five refills or after 6 months from the date of issue of the original prescription
B. The pharmacist obtaining the oral authorization records on the reverse of the original prescription the date, quantity of refill, and number of additional refills authorized and initials the prescription showing who received the authorization from the prescribing practitioner who issued the original prescription
C. The quantity of each refill must be less than or equal to the original quantity authorized

PARTIAL FILLING OF PRESCRIPTIONS (CLASSES III, IV, AND V)

Partial prescriptions must be recorded in the same manner as refills.

The total quantity of partials may not exceed the total quantity prescribed.

Schedule III, IV, and V drugs may not be dispensed more than 6 months past the original date of the prescription.

LABELING

A controlled substance in Schedule II must be labeled with the pharmacy's name and address, serial number and date of filling, the patient's and physician's names, directions for use, and any cautionary statements.

DISPOSAL

Any person in possession of any controlled substance and desiring or required to dispose of such substance may request from the Special Agent in Charge of the Administration in the area in which the person is located for authority and instructions to dispose of such substance.

A. If the person is a registrant, list the controlled substances on DEA form 41 (Registrants Inventory of Drugs Surrendered) and submit three copies to the Special Agent in Charge of Administration

B. If the person is not a registrant, submit a letter that includes the name and address of the person, the name and quantity of each controlled substance to be disposed of, how the applicant obtained the substance, the name, address, and registration number to the Special Agent in Charge of Administration

If you need to transfer Schedule II substances, the receiving registrant must issue form DEA 222 (Official Order Forms–Schedules I & II) to the registrant transferring the drugs. The transfer of Schedule III-V controlled substances must be documented in writing to show the drug name, dosage form, strength, quantity, and date transferred.

Reference:
http://www.dea.gov
http://www.deadiversion.usdoj.gov

TABLE 1
DRUG SCHEDULES

SCHEDULED DRUGS	LABELING SYMBOLS	DESCRIPTIONS	EXAMPLES
Schedule I	CI or C-I	No accepted medical use in the United States High potential for abuse A lack of accepted safety for use	Heroin, dihydromorphine, etorphine (except hydrochloride salt)
Schedule II	CII or C-II	Accepted medical uses in the United States (may include severe restrictions) High potential for abuse, which may lead to severe psychological or physical dependence	Morphine, meperidine, methadone, oxymorphone, hydromorphone, etorphine hydrochloride, fentanyl, pentobarbital
Schedule III	CIII or C-III	Accepted medical uses in the United States Lesser degree of abuse potential than Schedule I and II Abuse may lead to moderate or low physical dependence or high psychological dependence	Thiopental, tiletamine and zolazepam, ketamine, buprenorphine, anabolic steroids
Schedule IV	CIV or C-IV	Accepted medical uses in the United States Low potential for abuse of Schedule III Abuse may lead to limited physical or psychological dependence	Chloral hydrate, diazepam, midazolam, pentazocine, phenobarbital, butorphanol
Schedule V	CV or C-V	Accepted medical uses in the United States Low potential for abuse of Schedule IV Abuse leads to limited physical or psychological dependence	

The salts, isomers and salts of isomers, esters, ethers, and derivatives of these substances may also be controlled substances.

Guiding Principles for Research Involving Animals and Human Beings

RECOMMENDATIONS FROM THE DECLARATION OF HELSINKI (1989)

I. Basic Principles
   A. Clinical research must conform to the moral and scientific principles that justify medical research and should be based on laboratory and animal experiments or other scientifically established facts.
   B. Clinical research should be conducted only by scientifically qualified persons and under the supervision of a qualified medical person.
   C. Clinical research cannot legitimately be carried out unless the importance of the objective is in proportion to the inherent risk to the subject.
   D. Every clinical research project should be preceded by careful assessment of inherent risks in comparison to foreseeable benefits to the subject or to others.
   E. Special caution should be exercised by the doctor in performing clinical research in which the personality of the subject is liable to be altered by drugs or experimental procedure.

II. Clinical Research Combined with Professional Care
   A. In the treatment of the sick person, the doctor must be free to use a new therapeutic measure, if in his judgment it offers hope of saving life, reestablishing health, or alleviating suffering. If at all possible, consistent with patient psychology, the doctor should obtain the patient's freely given consent after the patient has been given a full explanation. In case of legal incapacity, consent should also be procured from the legal guardian; in case of physical

incacity the permission of the legal guardian replaces that of the patient.

B. The doctor can combine clinical research with professional care, the objective being the acquisition of new medical knowledge, only to the extent that clinical research is justified by its therapeutic value for the patient.

III. Nontherapeutic Clinical Research

A. In the purely scientific application of clinical research carried out on a human being, it is the duty of the doctor to remain the protector of the life and health of that person on whom clinical research is being carried out.

B. The nature, the purpose, and the risk of clinical research must be explained to the subject by the doctor.

C. Clinical research on a human being cannot be undertaken without his free consent after he has been informed; if he is legally incompetent, the consent of the legal guardian should be procured.

D. The subject of clinical research should be in such a mental, physical, and legal state as to be able to exercise fully his power of choice.

E. Consent should, as a rule, be obtained in writing. However, the responsibility for clinical research always remains with the research worker; it never falls on the subject even after consent is obtained.

F. The investigator must respect the right of each individual to safeguard his personal integrity, especially if the subject is in a dependent relationship to the investigator.

G. At any time during the course of clinical research the subject or his guardian should be free to withdraw permission for research to be continued. The investigator or the investigating team should discontinue the research if in his or their judgment, it may, if continued, be harmful to the individual.

Reference: http://history.nih.gov/laws/pdf/helsinki.pdf

GUIDING PRINCIPLES IN THE CARE AND USE OF ANIMALS

Approved by the Council of The American Physiological Society*

Animal experiments are to be undertaken only with the purpose of advancing knowledge. Consideration should be given to the appropriateness of experimental procedures, species of animals used, and number of animals required.

Only animals that are lawfully acquired shall be used in laboratory research, and their retention and use shall be in every case in compliance with federal, state, and local laws and regulations, and in accordance with the Institution for Laboratory Animal Research (ILAR) *Guide for the Care and Use of Laboratory Animals.*[†]

Animals used in research and education must receive every consideration for their comfort; they must be properly housed, fed, and their surroundings kept in a sanitary condition.

The use of animals must be in accordance with the ILAR *Guide for the Care and Use of Laboratory Animals.* Appropriate anesthetics must be used to eliminate sensibility to pain during all surgical procedures. Drugs that produce muscle paralysis are not anesthetics and they must not be used alone for surgical restraint, but may be used in conjunction with drugs known to produce adequate anesthesia. The care and use of animals shall be such as to minimize discomfort and pain. All measures to minimize pain and distress that would not compromise experimental results may be employed.

If the study requires the death of an animal, the most humane euthanasia method consistent with the study must be used.

When animals are used by students for their education or the advancements of science, such work shall be under the direct supervision of an experienced teacher or investigator.

Reference: http://www.the-aps.org/pa/humane/pa_aps_guiding.htm

---

* The Guiding Principles for the Care and Use of Animals are based on principles formulated by Walter B. Cannon in 1909. The APS Council first adopted them in 1953. Latest revision approved July 2000.
[†] Institute for Laboratory Animal Research (ILAR). *Guide for the Care and Use of Laboratory Animals.* Washington, D.C.: National Academy Press, 1996.

Index

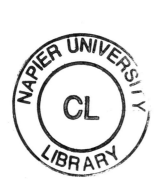